I am Kei

GW00362209

for
John V
with love
& respect
Keith

I Cured Cancer

at home

Puppy Pincher Press

All rights reserved

No part of this publication may be reproduced, stored in a retrieval system, or transmitted, in any form, or by means, electronic, photocopying, recording or otherwise, without prior permission of the copyright owner. All readers are however encouraged to use the information within to further the evolution of humanity and to help others to learn and to heal.

This is not medical advice. It is my story, it is comprehensive, detailed and impressive. It is based on my research and tells of my journey. It is a powerful story. I cannot and do not seek or intend to advise anyone on how to treat cancer. I do however advise that scientists and medical professionals take note of this research project for the benefit of humanity and I willing offer my services in that regard.

Copyright © 2018 Keith Mann

Keith Mann has asserted his right to be identified as the author of this work in accordance with the Copyright, Designs and Patents Act, 1988.

Keith Mann, ALF, nH, Rsr, IO, Vgn

PO Box 2174, Seaford BN25 94N

puppypincher@yahoo.co.uk

www.iamkeithmann.com

Published by Puppy Pincher Press

Only one greater treasure exists than the accumulated wealth of human knowledge that is preserved in books and that is love.

Chapters

I am Keith Mann I Cured Cancer

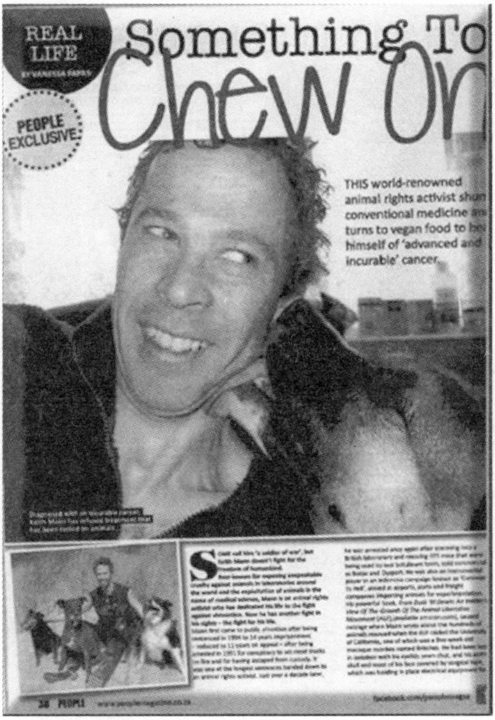
REAL LIFE

PEOPLE EXCLUSIVE

Something To Chew On

THIS world-renowned animal rights activist shu conventional medicine an turns to vegan food to he himself of 'advanced and incurable' cancer.

They'll throw tantrums
They'll throw fits
They'll get their knickers in a twist
But whatever they claim
Whatever they do
The story I share is for me and you

To share the truth is all that's meant
And the bottom line is ***informed consent***

I am Keith Mann

Introducing me

From the beginning of my cancer diagnosis in the summer of 2013 I made a conscious decision to write a book on the journey my experience was destined to take me. I felt a unique opportunity opening up and my goal was a cure for cancer. With such an ambition and no rules to deter me I felt I had a good chance. As we will see as I tell this story, when it comes to chronic degenerative disease the restoration of health is seldom the goal of our institutionalised medical researchers yet their limitations are boundless. I achieved my goal and became the very proud owner of a cancer cure and my options are now boundless. Taking my example to a logical conclusion millions of lives could be saved in no time at all from diseases our current medical system has enabled to be the plagues of the day. Profitable plagues.

I expected my therapy to work in around two years and the book begun to take shape the following spring as a kind of diary. It is now January 1 2017 and I am starting all over again, since my healing hypothesis (known to some as a "conspiracy theory") took on a life of its own and my story went widely off track on a journey of discovery I am bursting to share. I see this journey now as being absolutely on the right track. Same direction just a different route with some quite interesting views, I think you will agree. We expect that plans don't always come to pass and mine most certainly didn't, but it turned out even better than my wildest dream. And I did genuinely have a dream, one I have actively pursued for many years, in this I see a clear vision of a world that's a nice place for all earthlings to enjoy, as it once was.

And it will be again.

I have no complaints just a lot of observations. I was brought up in the northern mill town of Rochdale - **my** playground for 16 years. I left school in 1982 and in broadening my horizons I went to play with the animal rights movement, where my mischief would have purpose. I have dreamt up and employed all means at my disposal in the intervening years to stem the epidemic of human-on-animal violence. Vivisection [1] is an obscenity beyond reasoning in the 21st century and has been central to my actions. That evil word alone motivated me to push the boundaries

[1] Live experiments on other beings

and sod the consequences. Little else really mattered to me as I grew up but making it stop. I didn't want the costly car and alloy wheels, the nine to five and the other modern human desires, but I knew what I did want and I will always hold this desire central to my actions. Fortuitously I can now show and tell precisely how this may come to pass.

I try not to see the horrors in those live animal experiments as that would make my dream more like a nightmare. I have often considered how to most effectively turn my dream into reality. I know it must happen for the human creature/creation to survive and to thrive here, but how can it while so many benefit financially and are able to persuade so many more to think there is something in it for them too? They claim a "necessary evil" that is "rigorously enforced". In the UK we are told we have "the strictest regulations in the world", that our standards are "second to none" each experiment monitored closely by a team of inspectors. I imagine government gofers turning up with their clipboards must give those lab rats goosebumps with excitement.

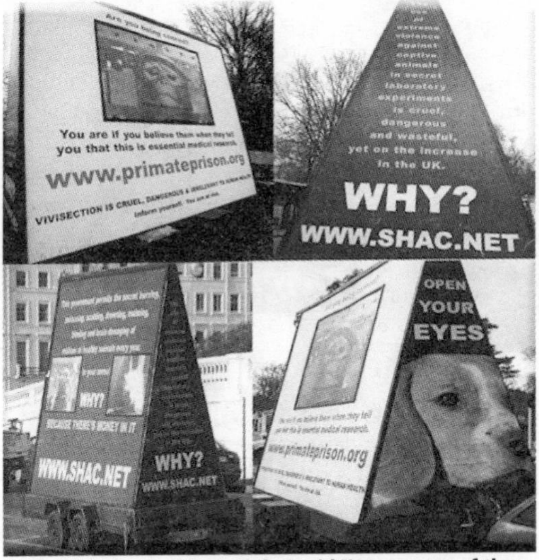
You are if you believe them when they tell you that this is essential medical research.
www.primateprison.org
VIVISECTION IS CRUEL, DANGEROUS &
extreme violence against captive animals in secret laboratory experiments is cruel, dangerous and wasteful, yet on the increase in the UK.
WHY?
WWW.SHAC.NET
WHY?
WWW.SHAC.NET
WHY?
WWW.SHAC.NET
OPEN YOUR EYES
www.primateprison.org

They said you must get a job. I said I've got one of these what do you do?

No one said it was going to be easy and maybe my dream will remain a dream in my lifetime but I don't think so. The story that has unfolded has, I think, made this task a great deal easier. I am living proof that there is another way to heal the human body that does not require an unbearable amount of suffering, vast research machinery and devastating poisons. And it is quite ingenious, by the way. I must make it clear I'm not the first to do this and there are many people healing naturally. But this is my story and as you will see I found myself at the messy end of the cancer process and we have devised a novel protocol to overcome it and if I can do it anyone can. Because someone says you have something incurable doesn't make it so, theirs is an opinion based on what they have been told by someone else. It's you who decides if you live.

Today's date is entirely in keeping with the synchronicity of events that have directed my journey to this point. We hear this thing about synchronicity a lot and I'm full of it. I believe there is something happening in our world enabling us to more readily sync and flow when we do the right thing. Humanity is moving into a new place in space, quite literally. It's a higher plane for body, mind and spirit. When our minds catch up we will be a very special being indeed. Today is the beginning of something amazing and I have a story to tell that is every bit amazing.

This is my second book, my first was a labour of love, 15 years from concept to creation spanning two prison sentences and I'm proud of that too. I crammed this one into about a year.

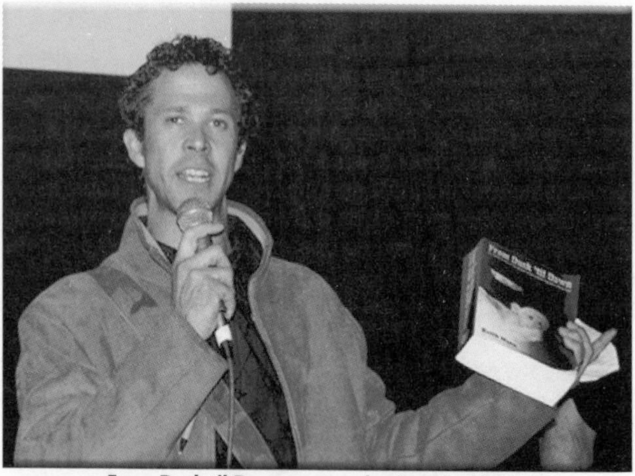

From Dusk til Dawn, on monkey's and a Mann.

From Dusk til Dawn is a big book weighing in at 600 pages and tells a big story of the growth of the animal liberation movement and my journey at the cutting edge, subtitled as a story the government does not want told. This will not be so big in volume but the content is colossal. This is **the** story they don't want told. It tells of a cure for cancer which costs nothing compared to the £rillion$ collected by drug companies and cancer fundraisers, which has rebuilt not trashed my immune system and by which animal experiments are obsolete. And it needs a big word. But this story is more than just that and I suspect you will be as intrigued as I was about how this all unfolded.

I say we can pull out of Big Pharma's game of hide and seek, where the real cures are hidden and fake ones sought, and we will be just fine. We alone, from home, stopped in its tracks and reversed an ingrained "incurable", recurrent stage 4 non--Hodgkin's lymphoma. This is a notoriously deep-rooted lymphatic/immune system/blood cancer that had returned angrier than ever following failed treatment. This is a disease that has always swept aside the best of the orthodox arsenal of cancer treatments, but it has been eradicated from my body through an extended, organised healing process. This experience I now see clearly as something that has been laid out for me from a very early age and I am delighted to have the opportunity to share it. I have been a vocal opponent of the scientific fraud of vivisection for many years and so my support network was ready made and I was good to go with my plan of action when I announced it. We found a way to heal without gruelling stem cell transplants, re-engineered species, gene therapy, devastating poisons, and there are no baby rats and mice needed. Just natural simplicity, sound logic and sensible science. As important, I have the willingness to invite the wrath of the devil and his gate keepers for telling the world all about our discovery of the Holy Grail of medical research. There is no coincidence in all of this and for all I am worth I shall use the second chance I have been given to be of service to the greater good by telling my story to all who are listening.

I had two goals when embarking on this very public challenge. One was self-preservation. That was my priority. The other was to get this information out to as many people as possible. That is my priority. Well folks, join me as I take you on a roller coaster ride to somewhere very, very special, to a place more magical than Narnia and more valuable than Christmas (and to some places a little bit creepy).

Funny enough they told me I'd always have a criminal record and that it would affect me for the rest of my life and sure enough they have never let me forget it. Well now it's my turn! I'm proud of all my past efforts and achievements and it just got better! I doubt there's much more I could have achieved even without a criminal record on my CV so I'll just have to muddle on through as a cancer curing criminal. They also instil the notion that you can't beat the system; everyone repeats it over and over so we never forget to obey, but I beat the system. Mine is a feat which all the experts and their loyal followers assured me with all certainty and some anger could not possibly be done.

Oh, you experts you!

I'm so proud I cannot begin to tell you. But I will enjoy trying. I am pretty chuffed with myself and am in absolute awe of my dear wife Alice for making my dreams come true. This project was always going to have her at the centre. I am also in deep debt to the many friends of old and new who have stood by us on this journey, and to my family, especially my mum, now 88, who hasn't left my side since the day I was born. Dawn Parkes has been our rock. Kerry Duggan also stepped forward as soon as she heard I had cancer and a plan, so did Maria & John Daly and Virginia Alexander, Margaret Whymark, Linda Furness, Terry Stringer, Jon Grimble, Marilyn Fahy, Katherine, Charlie, Hannah and Jess and they stayed loyal. We lost Terry along the way. His quack GP told him he didn't have cancer when he did, he died soon after. Oh, and Marilyn. She told her quack GP repeatedly that she had cancer, he told her she didn't. Sadly, she was right. She was preparing to do the Gerson Therapy and B17 but she never stood a chance. It was all over her before they could say "must do chemo". Neither made it to the end of my journey but they would both be very proud of what we have done. There are many more, without who we would have struggled. Too many to name, every one a treasure; you know who you are and you should be proud of your canine loyalty. I am. For the many terrible experiments human beings inflict on dogs, unconditional love is what they are trying to teach us to make us whole, and from that we will achieve great things. True friends made a success of my pre-prison exploits; they guided me through two prison sentences and made life as a fugitive easy. And were it not for that loyalty, I wouldn't be here now with a pretty amazing story to share that goes way beyond 'just' curing cancer, if you can believe that!

Believe it or not, this is a fairy tale with a happy ending. And I'm a fairy.

It was no coincidence that just at the point when I was diagnosed with cancer I was freshly informed on the wide potential of natural cancer therapies, about which many readers will be surprised to hear there is a great deal of invaluable information. There isn't just one way to cure cancer there are many. My laptop and book shelves were littered with material and I was excited to be sharing it, hoping I could help others. Little did I know I had a bigger opportunity than simply sharing what other people have to say about these things. I'm grateful to all the authors I reference; I have taken the liberty of incorporating only a snap shot of their work into my story. Their work guided my research and fed my desire (and accompanied my enemas) and they leave a valuable legacy. In testimonials, survivors often say they'll be happy if their success story helps save just one other person. Not me, I want them all but I remain perfectly content with me.

So before I get to the bit we are here for, the answer to cancer, I really must preamble and touch on some other touchy subjects and give you a feel for who I am and how I got to this place. The stuff we don't want to hear represents the problem but we have to work through the problem in order to get to the solution otherwise we will remain stuck with the problem. I don't belittle the subject, but cancer is not as complicated as they make it out to be. Simply, we have cause and effect and we are seeking to affect the cause. Problem - reaction - solution.

Curing cancer I suggest is in principle very straightforward, although my journey was anything but straightforward, until we found the correct tools from which point on it really has been a breeze to cure cancer. I offer myself as a guide to ease this journey further with a list of the tools you can use to create your new you. Finding the courage to walk away from old habits, the peer pressure, the terror threats and the fear mongering of the ortho-docs and to take control of our own life is the bigger challenge. I hear that I am something of an exception in this regard and that most people simply want someone else to tell them what to do. There is some truth in this and it has pained me a little. It poses the question: if true, what is the point of this book? Does anyone else care whether cancer can be cured at home using organic nutrition, energy medicine and an open mind? There is no doubt that not everyone is ready for this kind of extra terrestrial information, but for those who are, here it is. And much more.

Part of the problem - and it is the big one at this stage in our evolution - is the fact that the majority of us are still under the spell of the witch doctors, spin doctors and parasites, and there is a very real tendency by default or design for humans to try and keep each other spellbound. There are some who are desperate to stop the evolution of our species for their own ends, such as the managers of the mainstream media (MSM) and those who advertise their product through it. And those often referred to as the useful idiots who don't just believe what they are told but demand the rest of us believe it too. I have always felt like something of a loose thinker with a flexible mind and I don't get my knickers in a twist about what anyone else believes. I am not a fan of political correctness, censorship or fascism, which is all about control.

I feel my hackles go up when I hear lies told to excuse or create suffering and it only takes one attempt at this deception for me to become irritable and alert. I am a suspicious character. The state machine is based on lies and our reality is formed on lies. It is normal for serial liars, the really evil ones who run the show, to punish the victims. I compare the dead football fans at Hillsborough, the protestors of Bloody Sunday, to the people of foreign lands and to the parents of the child victims of the dodgy vaccines. We accept the word of Superintendent This or That, Lord Posh, Sir Stuck-Up and all manner of establishment scientists and affiliated experts and spooks as they defend with proud arrogance the dark and destructive lies they tell daily because they are officials with a suit, a tie and a platform. Even when the truth emerges from conspiracy theory into conspiracy and from the independent media into the public domain, we are outraged for a while. But soon we forget. Our attention diverted by the promise of inquiry, of justice just around the corner, or by another outrage, a little bit more shocking than the last, one that can be fuelled far into the future and stoked as required to oppress some more.

Just look at us!
Everything is backwards
Everything is upside down
Doctors destroy health
Lawyers destroy justice
Universities destroy knowledge
Governments destroy freedom
The major media destroy information
and
Religions destroy spirituality

But there is never justice and these wounds are buried to fester. The human being is a wounded animal and I think it will finally rise up and bite back when it realises what is being done to the children. Since I was once one and I have healed my wound, I am going to begin with me as an example.

For many years I have placed myself at the forefront of the animal rights movement, working diligently all hours, at my expense, to impact animal laboratories and animal supply firms and to expose the truth of animal abuse. I was a hunt saboteur, at great risk to my health, an Animal Liberation Front (ALF) spokesman and coordinator, at great risk to my liberty. I am prone to pushing my luck and the boundaries in the hope of a breakthrough, of something big. Just because. I was happy as a pig in the compost heap and cherish every moment, as hair raising and challenging as some of them were and even when 'big' meant big prison sentence. In this capacity I have become increasingly disillusioned with the system and driven to spend more of my time outside of the box. This means thinking different to the general norm, where thinking is generally guided by what comes out of the box at the centre of our world, in our living room. Interestingly, introducing natural cancer therapies into my CV, while less mainstream and thrilling than animal activism, is by far the most extreme in the eyes of most, even some animal rights extremists go into meltdown! I guess I have taken extremism to the extreme and they will probably have to think of some new labels just for me! I freely admit I got a thrill from my covert operations, but I'd swap it all for this.

Not that I have to swap it, I am rewarded by getting to add to it!

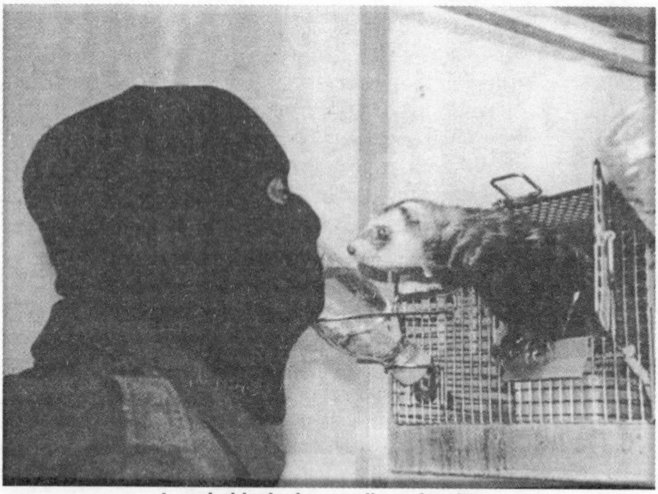

Love holds the key to all our freedom.

It dawned on me very soon after leaving school that it was a lie that we are a nation of animal lovers and wiped out any hope that the overly touted claims of *the best animal protection laws in the world* had any real meaning. Why else would there be a need for me and so many people like me to take the law into our own hands and force all these horror stories into the news? I never bought into that never-ending narrative about the need to torture and kill ever greater numbers of animals in secret laboratory experiments in order to discover hidden cures for human ills and guess what? I was right.

Then came the police, all angry and bothered, deeply loyal to the status quo. We are told they are here to keep us safe but they chase around after campaigners and cannabis smokers like their lives depend upon it. They have seldom left me feeling safe and they protect perverts. Right and wrong is part of the picture but they are used primarily to keep safe those with the power and money and to divert attention from their criminal overlords. And then there were the prison stays, first an 11-year sentence through the 1990's and another 18 months through 2005.

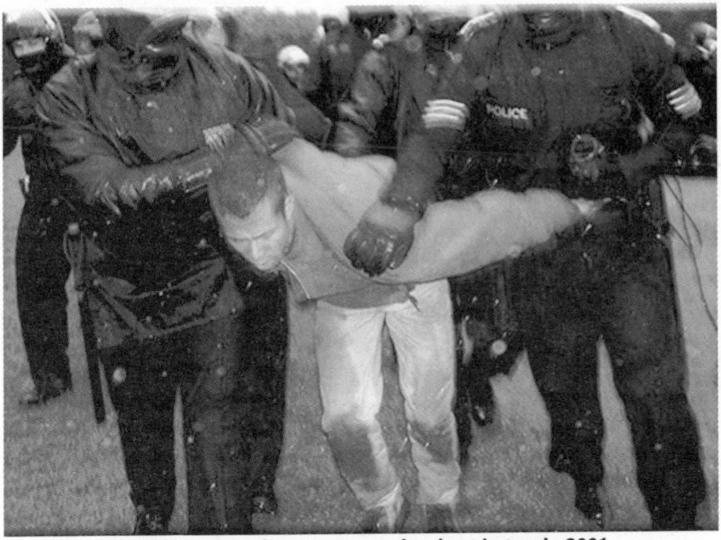

In between my prison sentences they kept in touch. 2001.

Prison is not meant to be fun of course but nor is it meant to be cruel yet it is and prison does not make a bad man good. I spent a considerable amount of time in a great many prisons and consider myself something of an expert in prison life and to me it is quite clear they are not rehabilitating people but churning them out angry and more disillusioned than ever. And usually with less than they went in with! Justice is for a large part not being served and too many inmates are wrongfully convicted or have mental health issues and should not be there in the first place. And there's a striking absence of the anti-social bankers and the perverted politicians who do the most harm to society.

I knew the rules and earned my jail time but these people who make all the rules don't keep their end of the deal, so they have no authority. I duly returned to the streets in 1999 after seven years, unrepentant and unpersuaded by their half-hearted ill-conceived instructions in how I should stick to the rules simply because the rulers know best. But since the rules are written by the rulers and since my teachers were ruled by the rulers and were not prepared to evolve their thinking to consider that conflict of interest, we would remain conflicted. I carried on as normal driving toward my dream and busied myself on projects of a borderline legality, some were even legal, but I didn't have a hope of dodging all the traps whatever I did.

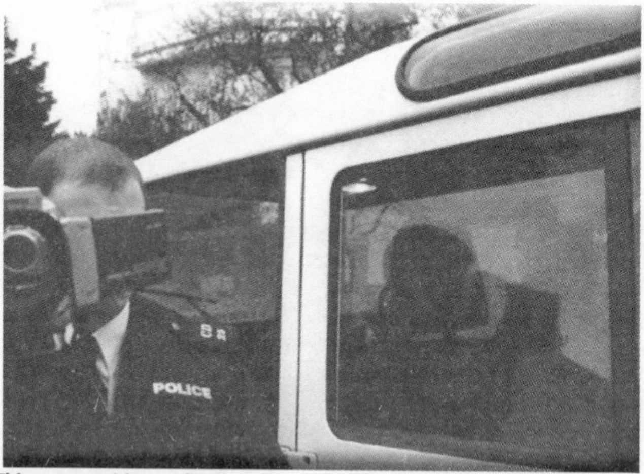

This was outside our flat in Brighton early one Saturday morning in 1999. I had been out of prison a few months. Land Rover full of them, lurking, following us around, looking for trouble. You don't need it!

We swamped many of the ne'er-do-well lab animal suppliers with our energy and caused their extinction, including the notorious Shamrock monkey farm near home in Sussex. Today protesting is more a criminal offence and so the protestors need to adapt and to encourage each other to think of new ideas, not park up, hark back and turn on each other. The point of a movement is to take humanity forward, to where the good ole days really are.

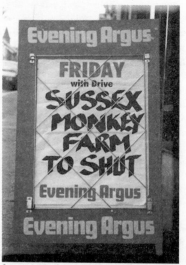

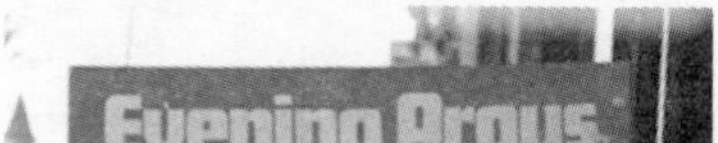

A few months later. 2000. This was why they were crawling all over us. We had plans for change and they wanted things to stay the same.

And in due course I would be back in prison.

Leading a raiding party into Wickham Laboratories in Hampshire in 2003 we cleared offices of files and cages of mice and exposed the lie that cosmetic experiments had been banned in the UK. This claim was made in 1998 by the Labour government of the day, politicians: professional liars. The same people who killed Barry Horne in prison for shaming them on their broken promises over the vivisection programme. They lied. The same people were spreading conspiracy theories about Iraqi vaccines of mass destruction, or whatever.

Extensively detailed in our haul of recovered documents were thousands of experiments on mice and rabbits to test the toxicity of botulinum toxin batches. Botox is used an awful lot for cosmetic purposes and each batch gets tested on animals. Tens of thousands of animals every year die just in this one creepy location alone subjected to the vile LD50 death test in which subjects are injected, in this case mice into their stomach with the poison and are casually observed until half are dead. I say experiments, and this is how they are often described, but the truth is that the majority of lab animals die in these tick box toxicity tests. Vivisection is mostly about monitoring how much poison an animal can take, for a data package to be generated and that poison be made available to the public. Safety tested on animals! It's the animal's eyes they target in some tests, raw skin irritation in others (sand paper/bleach kind of thing), acute oral poisoning... foot pads injected... The list goes on and on and at the end of it one might hope at the very least some level of safety or benefit has been established, but as we will see nothing could be further from the truth.

Humane slaughter and free range are not what they sound either, not even close. Like giving lab rats the key to the lock and claiming they are free to leave – it's more deception. I would energise my soul creeping around these camps they call free range farms taking animals, documents, footage, liberties... Firmly of the view that most people would be truly sickened by the depth of this cruel deception. I could go on for pages but I already did that in From Dusk til Dawn. These places were my introduction to the real world once I left the indoctrination of state-run school and it grabbed my attention. In a nutshell after years of being attacked, harassed, imprisoned and misinformed about almost everything, and observing the utter failure of the many wars those in power fight on poverty, drugs, crime, terror and so on, it struck me that on the balance of probability the war on cancer would be a failure too, in spite of the claims to the contrary.

But then some of us, the cancer curing "conspiracy theorists" as we are labelled as a deterrent to others, we suspect this is exactly as it's meant to be. We think that the greatest profit is not in a cure, but in a chronic disease that can be maintained long term with high profit drugs. We think that some people would do anything to maintain high sale of their product and we think they will do anything to keep anything alternative they couldn't own or control out of public view. We think they will then happily continue to sell not one product per customer but multiple, which is how to do good business under the current model.

A cure is not the goal. Profit is the goal. A cure would be an accident. The continuous cycle of animal testing/drug testing has much more to do with generating income, employment and maintaining the status quo. Don't the vast, unimaginable profits of the drug cartels hint at this? Why on earth would today's rich and well connected men want cures for the vast array of human ills and an end to all those treatments that keep them rich and powerful? Why! A cure for cancer based on anything but synthetic drugs would bring down an industry built on synthetic drugs and there would be a lot of high earners on a minimum wage stacking shelves, or growing organic vegetables, perhaps?

I choose not to trust these businessmen based on an appalling track record of deception, crime and cover up and my own personal experience. And the drugs don't heal. In fact the drugs often make things worse. Chemo is not sold as a cure nor does it serve as one. It is a treatment. We could use literally anything to treat cancer, such as paint stripper, melted chocolate or mustard but in order to eliminate disease permanently, and to heal so it doesn't come back, a different approach is needed. Besides which a cure in medical terms is rather evasive, both in terms of definition and practicality.

A cure is the end of a medical condition; the end of a person's sufferings; it is to be healed. When we are cured the disease has gone away, otherwise we are in drug-induced preclinical disease state, awaiting its return.

What the medical profession refers to is not a cure it's false hope. As a clear sign of things to come, even the simple word cure and all its implied beauty has been corrupted not to heal the hopeless but to create an illusion. If a cancer doctor says the word cure they are alluding to five or maybe even just three years of your life where you are symptom-free following chemical 'treatment'. It's an arbitrary, random cut off point one might consider, especially when it is so common for 'survivors' of the chemo, the cured, to have the primary or a secondary cancer emerge in the months and years after this calendar cut off point says you are cured. Cancer didn't go to medical school and doesn't follow these rules of science. So we have a community of the 'cured' who are dying of cancer! Going through it once is enough for anyone and it is more aggressive and ingrained when it shows up again. Good from a business perspective though. Returning customers are the capitalist's wet dream. Some think this is just an unfortunate side effect of a desperate frantic push to find a cure for a complicated disease, but I have a different perspective. I took the red pill, which has no side effects. Except for some repetitive, monotone name calling.

When I first began to share widely the information I was finding on holistic cancer treatments, which were evidentially effective in restoring health in adherents, I had this fluffy naïve notion that my immediate audience in particular, the activists fighting for change, would be all over this stuff like a fast growing cancer. Oh Keith!

Here's what I was thinking. Few people I knew especially in the animal rights (AR) community were investing any time or energy in researching this field of knowledge and even less sharing it. Yet here is information which could bring an end to vivisection and clean up farming and heal disease on a scale never before witnessed. Oh my god - imagine that! Many of the people I grew up with invest a lot of energy in saving a single life and we gather in groups to protest, but in line with the wider society most believe that cancer remains largely incurable and requires heavy industry investment – someone else - to combat it (albeit excluding the use of animals). The general consensus is that cancer is not curable - animals in the mix or not - and if a cure was found "it would be on the news". That one simple naïve belief stands in the way of all further investigation of a vast field of intrigue and of us moving forward as a species. And such is the power of this advertising, which can be confused with education that it causes some people to protest angrily that anything that isn't on the news couldn't possibly be true!

I have been drawn to be a little more discerning and wander the fields as far as they may go. In doing this, while I am immovable in my love and respect of the animal kingdom and share this story with their wellbeing in mind, I have adapted my interpretation of the struggle for animal liberation being the greatest struggle we face. The greatest struggle we face is for the human mind and that goes way beyond simply recognising the beauty of the animals as living beings, as we must. Kindness of heart does not come from kindness for animals, a kind heart just is.

My evolving understanding of the bigger picture was helped in no small part when my soul mate, Alice, had her health collapse in 2007. She was 19 at the time, 22 years younger than me and her life had never really got going. On the face of it this was not something to get too excited about especially for someone so young. Well that's not strictly true. What was expected of her by others didn't come to pass, but we have spent the intervening years together entwined in a magical mystery tour from which we cured cancer together and this is only the beginning for us. And does it get much better than that?

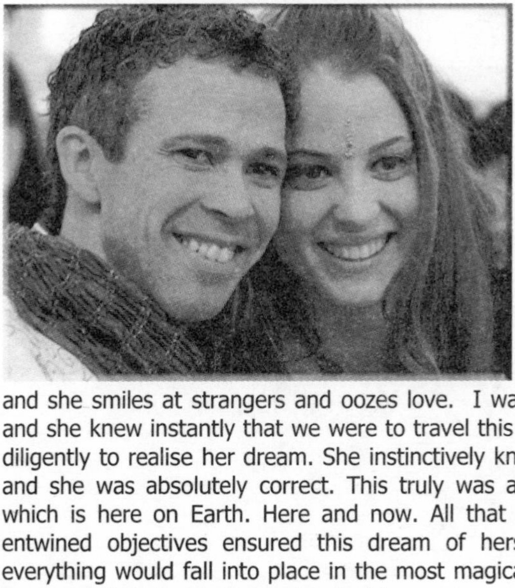

2010 we married.

I was a friend of Alice's parents for some years before Alice and I realised what was meant to be and we bonded and blended into our one. Alice is my counter balance, she's an angel; way ahead of her age, smart, loyal and she smiles at strangers and oozes love. I was her first crush a long time ago and she knew instantly that we were to travel this life journey together and worked diligently to realise her dream. She instinctively knew what was best for both of us and she was absolutely correct. This truly was and is a match made in heaven, which is here on Earth. Here and now. All that and her natural beauty and our entwined objectives ensured this dream of hers would become mine too and everything would fall into place in the most magical way imaginable, in spite of the immense obstacles we were faced with.

Alice's health was unbalanced for many years, in spite of the fact she was vegan from birth. Some will say *because* she was vegan from birth. There is some truth in both statements, but for her early years she was healthy until events conspired. Junk food vegans risk illness as do junkies generally and she was the queen of crap who could happily gobble her way through two packets of crumpets dripping in margarine and yeast extract, a plate of fat fried potatoes buried in salt and enough HP sauce to paint a wall. That would be breakfast. She chomped through packets of veggie burgers, pies and sausages and ice cream, hash browns and cheese and all the other fake food we crave so much like she was in some sort of competition. This mountain of waste would gradually help break down her system in a kind of high speed version of what we are all going through. She had been born 2 months premature, weak and jaundice which didn't help matters and with other more structural issues which it would take literally 26 years for the experts to discover. In the meantime these mechanical misalignments would join forces with the weak immune system, the junk food, toxic vaccines and mercury and together create all manner of crippling disturbances. This mess of stuff we take for granted in our everyday lives is not nurturing our future.

Our journey together was just beginning in 2006. Alice had recently left home to start university at Bristol. She is much smarter than university and has so much more to offer than simply being sucked into the system and spat out programmed to think and behave the way the system says, but this, as it so often is, was a case of being persuaded to follow the herd. Nevertheless she set about with admirable enthusiasm the role of soon to be *educated* student in a whole heap of debt. Except this was not the direction the universe wanted Alice to go in and the divine plan of that entity matters more to the universe than what we might like to think.

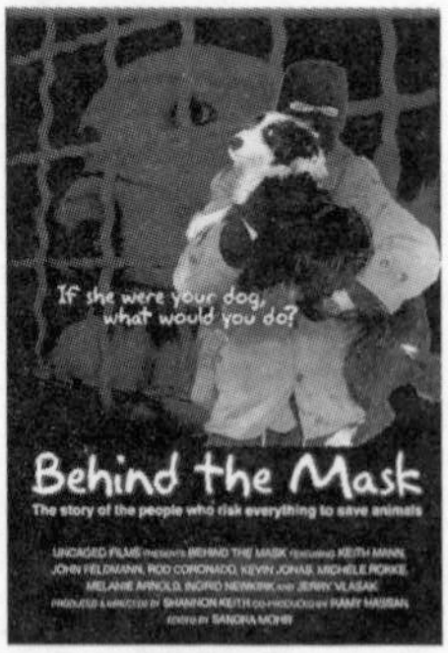

Soon after settling in to student life the periodic bouts of abdominal pain, nose bleeds, diarrhoea, vomiting, passing out and exhaustion begun to manifest ever more frequently to the point where more time was being spent in hospitals than classrooms, which she was increasingly struggling to get to.

I was busy as a bee at this point on tour promoting my first book and the film Behind the Mask,[2] and their honest unmasking of the Animal Liberation Front and its cause. This cause was the centre of my day every day. Not just active in ALF operations, (which would be mostly in the night) I had also morphed into a public spokesman and ultimately a long serving prisoner. Fourteen years was my original sentence, handed down to me by a freak in a frock in the Old Bailey in 1994 but later reduced on appeal to 11 years. Being happy at that point in my life with 11 years, rather than 14, reminds me it is always possible to adapt to life's challenges. You learn patience in prison, where nothing happens,

2 https://www.youtube.com/watch?v=FfKXq9BL29o

slowly and about who you are and who your friends are. It was an interesting experience and some kind of primer for my future.

Big Chief Running Mann.

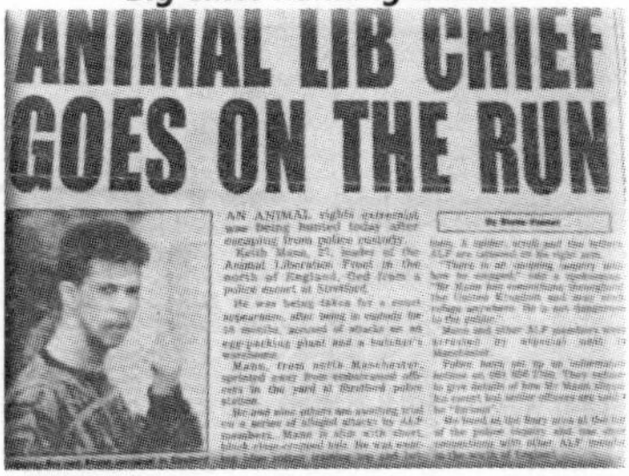
ANIMAL LIB CHIEF GOES ON THE RUN

In 1993 after the best part of two years held in prison awaiting trial I executed a long-established plan to escape. Always good for morale! I pledged I would get out if they ever locked me up and had a rendezvous arranged with a friend who was herself a fugitive and duly anticipated my eventual arrival. That plan was now the centre of my day and I worked at it industriously from my cage. It took me 20 months and by the time I pulled it off I figured I'd earned it and we did rendezvous as arranged 2 years earlier. The rather obsessive trial judge and a few over enthusiastic detectives with reputations in the mangler were furious I'd gone AWOL, but sometimes you just have to think about you!

I was free and freedom should always win over what someone else thinks. What I have now is a similar kind of freedom. Forbidden freedom! It's a spine tingly kind of free. Content and excited. It sounds cliché but you only really understand what freedom is when you lose it. You hear it a lot and I agree, health is only appreciated once it's gone and that's a shame because so few of us are lucky enough to recover it and fully appreciate what that feels like. It's good!

I had no idea where my schoolboy discovery of animal exploitation would lead but once I was alerted to the extent of it I just wanted to save some animals from their hell. It's not just lambs - they kill them all at a few months old! I became absorbed in my goal. Speaking publicly about the ALF and our 'game plan' during the day, while enacting that plan at night was always going to get me into trouble, and I knew it, but I'm living my dream. Although I had a hope I was invincible, I knew deep down me and my balaclava had a sell-by date, because none of us are elusive enough or youthful for long enough to get away with it forever, so I made the most of every opportunity. Anyway, clearly this was all meant to be and aside being something I'm proud to be a part of it has given me a great foundation. I like to challenge myself physically and intellectually, I'm not afraid to debate the issues in public and I don't mind being wrong. I am keen to do what I do to the best of my ability and nothing matters more to me at this time than creating a new reality and changing the direction of our world from violent, cruel and greedy to loving and compassionate. It will be so beautiful and so simple when we finally realise what it is that we need to correct.

And maybe, just maybe, I got it wrong about not being invincible! I jest of course. I'm working on longevity and I have certainly extended my lease, but we have a lot of work to do to make our home a safe place for all to grow old in good health. Thank you for allowing me to share my story. I hope it may be of assistance.

If you keep your wits about you you'll hear quacks quack

Quack: an ignorant, misinformed, or dishonest practitioner of medicine

Mann banned from New Zealand

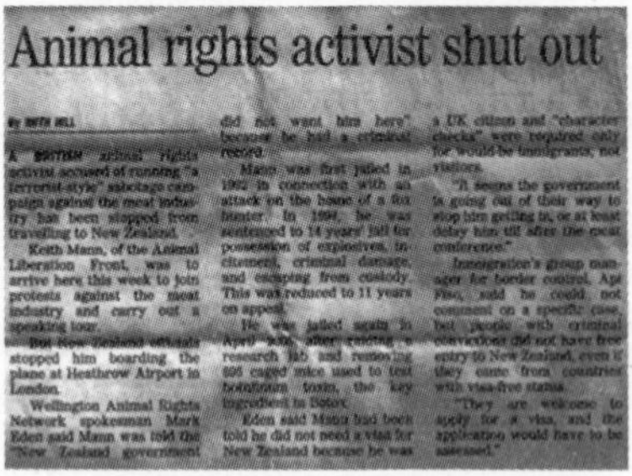

Alice had been accompanying me on the tour across Europe through 2007/08, I'd been to South Africa, barred from entering New Zealand and Australia and Canada. We were living our dream, but this health thing of hers was increasingly getting in the way and was set to ultimately ground both of us and make sure that balaclava of mine stayed neatly folded in the drawer. By the spring of 2008 during the Scottish leg of the tour this thing had hit her so hard she was floored with a heap of symptoms and couldn't get out of bed. Alice was in a mess and was terrified. We cancelled all plans and managed a difficult journey from Scotland to my mum's house three hours south where we settled for a while until things eased. Well, that was the plan but plans just now weren't working out too well and this temporary stop-gap until things improved never quite ended. It's almost exactly 11 years since that trip to Scotland and we have not even come close to getting back to our plan of the day.

It was a fantastic experience but we've moved on. We were actually eased quite forcefully in another direction and now have some bigger plans. You have in your hand my plan B, which is really the beginning of more of the same but with a highly developed theme. We've been recycled!

Over the next few years we were in and out of more hospitals and surgeries than I care to remind myself but we couldn't get sense from anyone. And as Ali's health deteriorated under the 'care' of the experts it got to the point where I could barely leave her side. Just getting to appointments was a real struggle physically and emotionally. Then they'd do the same tests over and over and conclude on finding the same nothing that there was nothing to find. It's not all of them but there is this odd thought pattern many share. They'd give her drugs for pain and anti-sickness and send her home with an appointment in 6 weeks. Then comes an appointment date for test results 6 weeks later to find they want to repeat the same test in 6 weeks and on it goes. It adds up to a lot of miserable weeks going nowhere.

One doctor discharged her from hospital with 5 bottles of morphine because he didn't know what else to do! First do no harm? Morphine was not good. All of the drugs she was prescribed during this period were junk and the side effects everyone talks about are direct effects. A cure would be a side effect. Almost everyone suffers *side effects* and the more you take the more of these effects you will suffer. Few are actually cured by these drugs and the more of them you take the less likely you will be. You see what I see? Drugs destroy health.

It first took a feat of endurance to actually get Alice into a hospital so they would carry out their stupid tests and figure out nothing but once discharged we were back in no man's land again. The tests were invasive, repetitive and futile. With localised abdominal pains seeming to provide a clue, tubes and cameras were with painful regularity shoved in any which way, images and samples taken and tested but everything was found to be normal. Or rather they couldn't find what **they** were looking for. It isn't so comforting after a while when the doctor can find nothing wrong with you, but adds insult to injury when you are suffering in so many ways to have all the experts and their fancy equipment bring up no answers, implying there is nothing wrong. Then there were X-rays and more drugs for pain and to prevent clotting and to ameliorate the sickness caused by all the drugs, and just to "try" because they don't know what else to do! But since the drugs don't work the same tests produced the same negative results and no one could give a label to this variety of debilitating symptoms other than some half-cocked speculative diagnosis, the cycle was destined to continue ad infinitum.

We went through many different departments specialising in this or that and learnt quickly of their limitations. Doctors were making this patient sicker because they didn't know what else to do and it wasn't just the drugs and ill heath making life miserable, there was also the odd innuendo (with legs) that this was all perhaps imaginary or "growing pains", psychological or stress related and something she would get over. Some would tell her to "exercise more" encouraging her to "work through it". This is awful advice for such patients and always made matters worse for Alice and we would later understand why. One particular quack had her down to her underwear and then quizzed her about possible sexual abuse as a child. I mean, seriously! We often hear medical people described as experts and we are expected to worship the ground they walk on but some of these people are as messed up as the rest of us. Here we have a very sharp teenager who has just left home to jet off with the man of her dreams and follow her passion and some over inflated half wit incapable of doing his job properly, or at all, is concluding she is screwing it all up by allowing her mind to cause her to think she is so seriously ill she can barely function. For a community driven by science this is a rather peculiar conclusion to draw but it is not at all rare among this class of professionals and it only takes one bozo such as this to mess up someone's life.

We had come to expect nothing in the way of answers from the ortho-docs by this point, but a quack-led accusation that the patient is at fault often carries great weight, because it comes from an 'expert' and to a believer this is like the word of a god. In this case some of those closest to Alice saw it as their way out and abandoned her in the midst of her worst nightmare. Alice had suffered more than many young adults by this stage in her life but this was the sucker punch that sunk her into a deep depression that it would take two years to come out of. But come out she has, as a shining example.

This simple but powerful belief in the word of an expert or an official absolves adherents of all personal responsibility and is critical in our discussion. This was unfathomable for us at the time and marked the end of innocence and of a fairytale upbringing for Alice. The end of her dream of happy families was perfectly in keeping with the moment. We joke about how we seemed to have fallen into a swamp at this time in our lives and how as we struggled to get out felt we were being trampled on. We laugh now, a lasting laugh.

As painful as all this was we were lucky with our experience. As we would later discover this deflecting of attention is not uncommon in orthodox medicine and has had grave, irreversible consequences for countless patients.

I had for some time been raising other issues for inquiry, inviting consideration when formulating strategies for changing the world for the better. There are the animals of course and every one is equal and they are part of something bigger and it all joins up. Such as cancer causing animal DNA vaccines, suppressed cancer therapies, shady governments, control and depopulation agendas, hidden human history... You get the picture! And that which holds together, the ultimate weapon of mass distraction: TV programming and what they call 'the news' controlled by a small number of perverted murderous lying monsters who lack all empathy and seek only to service their agenda for consolidating control of everything. We hear lies and see cover-ups everywhere we look yet still we cling to a belief that some of it must be the truth because we are told it is, while rampantly assassinating the character of anyone who says it isn't! For my efforts I was under a barrage of name calling as Alice took hers.

These are big issues that matter yet most of us are completely clueless and are often wilfully so, hence the focus on the messenger rather than the message. I don't wish to take that away from anyone but I don't think stifling initiative helps us grow so I'm standing my ground. Equally unsustainable, and arrogant, is claiming that science is settled and that we have nothing more to learn so nothing more to discuss. Stagnant science serves egos and commercial agendas in the here and now but what of the next generation and the one after, what will become of their innate human desire to invent, explore and discover new ideas and to think bold? I can see from the food I grow that a healthy plant produces its best fruit when it has access to the widest variety of nutrients, yet we teach and feed our children junk. Who will take the human race to another level if the experts and gatekeepers of today are telling our kids that we, in 2017, are the best the universe has produced, that the cure for cancer is a few more vile animal experiments away and all disease is preventable with crude preventative injections. At the present time in order to maintain the order, the take home message is that anyone who dares to question the supreme knowledge of the TV newscaster and their 'inside sources' will be isolated from the herd and banished to the land of crackpot conspiracy theorists.

The thought controllers among us filter errant thoughts into their overcrowded conspiracy theory prison and shut them away, ill prepared and uninterested to know that ancient and futuristic solutions to all our woes are being buried away by people who are interested. We are a steadily deteriorating species on a ravaged planet and it doesn't look to me like an accident or a coincidence but whatever it is it's clear we need to change the way we think, because it's of our doing collectively. That's how we do everything, by thinking it through first. From early in the morning to the beginning of time we shape our reality with our minds. Think about it, do it. At least that's how it works for me.

The trendy thought stopping classics "it's just a conspiracy theory" and "it's quackery" weren't just passing commentary on one or two subjects, such as moon landings and cancer cures with carrots, oh no! These simple retorts have stood the test of time and have been used to brush off a storm of information. The kind of stuff that comes like a package deal once you sign away your pre-conceptions and everyone tries to stop listening anyway! We question none of it or see all of it. This gives us some idea why so many of us are in the dark about so many important subjects, such as curing cancer, and why we become slaves to the agenda of others. This simple word association shuts down critical thinking, as it is designed to do. No one wants to be thought of as stupid or uneducated so we stick with the majority who only believe in orthodox science, scientists and whatever is on the news. I discovered very quickly when hearing repetition of "the best scientific research in the world" says it's impossible to heal naturally or "you're just into conspiracy theories" or when someone recites "double blind randomised placebo trials" like it's one of the Ten Commandments, that my time was being wasted.

This is a form of chronic cognitive dissonance, an acquired psychological condition which requires patience and understanding. There is no quick fix and in serious cases the damage may be irreparable in this lifetime. Fear lies at the root and questioning the gospel of official authorities in the presence of a sufferer can cause flare-ups of anger, aggression and resentment. A common physical symptom is expressed through them trying to inflict their disinterest onto those of us who clearly are interested.

Those most often using 'conspiracy theory' as a retort are the most averse to asking questions so are by definition prone to believe conspiracy theories, albeit popular ones! And those who allude to others practicing quackery are the very people most often peddling medical products and practices that will more likely than not do harm. This is what judge-mentalists typically do – they reflect themselves onto others.

The term conspiracy theory was first introduced into the popular culture by the CIA in 1967 following a stirring of consciousness after the president was gunned down in public and the Warren Commission covered up the truth. Too many people saw through the lies and figured the murder of Kennedy was not the creation of a crack shot crackpot. If this awakening wasn't quelled and the real plot was unravelled some key people and institutions would have been implicated and the world would probably be a very different place today. But we weren't yet ready to face down our demons and by the end of 1967 we were instead being trained by those demons to brand as a conspiracy theorist or nut job anyone among us who questions anything those demons say.

Tragically, Lee Harvey Oswald is still blamed for killing the president. No evidence of this has ever been presented to a jury, but a few official experts are all it takes to spread an untruth that will sweep like a viral infection through humanity and persist a great deal longer! No matter what the evidence says. Dead suspects and trial by

TV is a pattern often repeated in the years since 1967 while the bold are branded as loopy for expressing any hint of doubt about this Orwellian style of justice.

Significant effort is made to keep people in line regarding orthodox medicine, where the white coats and their gadgets are seen as holding all the answers, and the queue to the pharmacy grows longer. The high and mighty who claim health expertise can actually cure remarkably little yet we generally believe the opposite. For the grotesque sums of money spent and the equally grotesque 'scientific research' inflicted on vast numbers of living beings going way back through modern human history, the truth is a travesty. Yet still we usher each other along to the slaughterhouse, with a great deal more enthusiasm than the sheep ever would, for the high priests of medicine to do with our bodies what they will, seldom thinking to ask to what end.

I have been treated to a feast of fury since I opened my mind and connected my mouth to what I saw, and have become a regular enemy of someone else's state of mind. And with honours! It's not what you expect in response to your curiosity but I understand; it's nothing personal. And so what if I am a nut job and what I say is therefore crazy and can be ignored. Then everyone is happy! I've had comrades in arms up in arms for raising intellectual dialogue and have been blacklisted and even banned from Animal Rights forums by self styled 'anti fascist' fascists under a barrage of branding for asking simple questions. They do say a little bit of knowledge is a dangerous thing! This is a devolutionary process through which survival of the thickest would ultimately rule the roost if followed to its ultimate conclusion.

The entertainment value in this is priceless and I am honoured to remain an irritation for thought police and variant lost souls among us. Even in light of establishing my natural cancer cure conspiracy theory as a walking-talking forthright fact, I am according to citizen stupid still "just into conspiracy theories" and must be segregated. And good luck with that.

What is a conspiracy theorist anyway? Someone who asks questions about topics involving more than two people? Like a private investigator or a detective perhaps? I guess someone who doesn't ask questions or believes the first thing they are told is an idiot? Is a highly qualified medical researcher who hypothesises with a colleague about a method of curing cancer using a rainforest plant a conspiracy theorist? What about a newscaster who has done no research of his own banging on about weapons of mass destruction? Or Cancer Research UK supporters telling everyone about chemical cancer cures coming soon? When does that prediction of a future miracle become hocus pocus and worthy of a few scathing words or campaign ideas from the sceptics? Is anyone allowed to think for themselves? It is very confusing, unless you think for yourself and then it's just fun.

For years I've had this curious jumble of anger coming at me from all over the place and it's all terribly disjointed. The mainstream media have all the resources and plenty of practice but they can't really get a handle on anything either so they invent a monster, but not any old monster...

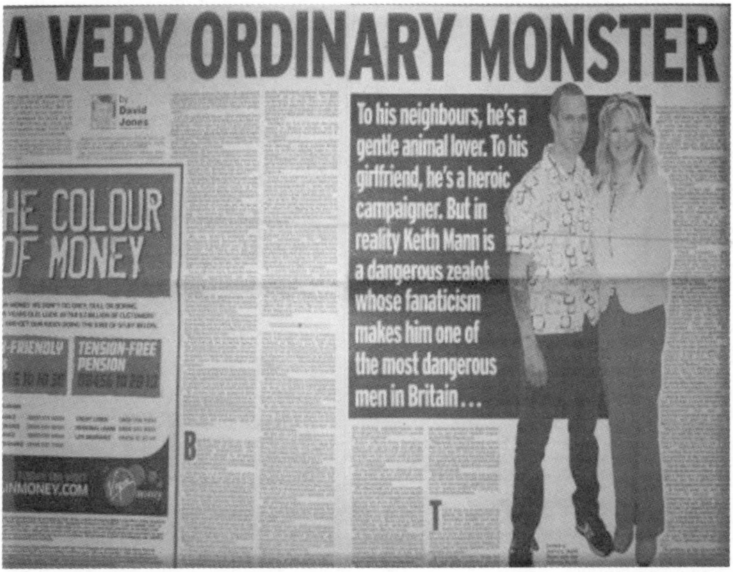

A VERY ORDINARY MONSTER

By David Jones

To his neighbours, he's a gentle animal lover. To his girlfriend, he's a heroic campaigner. But in reality Keith Mann is a dangerous zealot whose fanaticism makes him one of the most dangerous men in Britain...

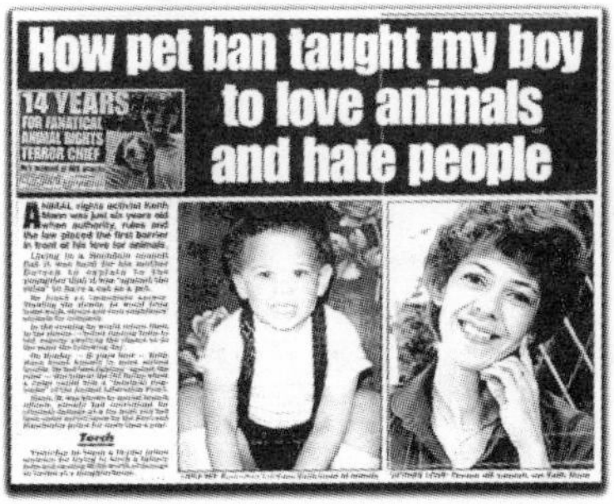

How pet ban taught my boy to love animals and hate people

14 YEARS FOR FANATICAL ANIMAL RIGHTS TERROR CHIEF

ANIMAL rights activist Keith Mann was just six years old when authority, rules and the law placed the first barrier in front of his love for animals.

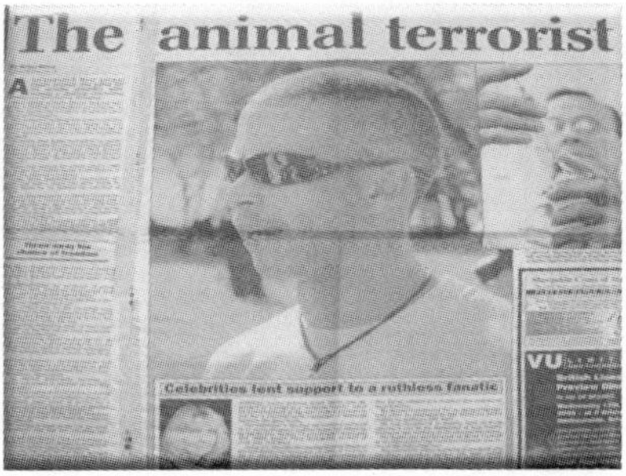

The animal terrorist

Celebrities lent support to a ruthless fanatic

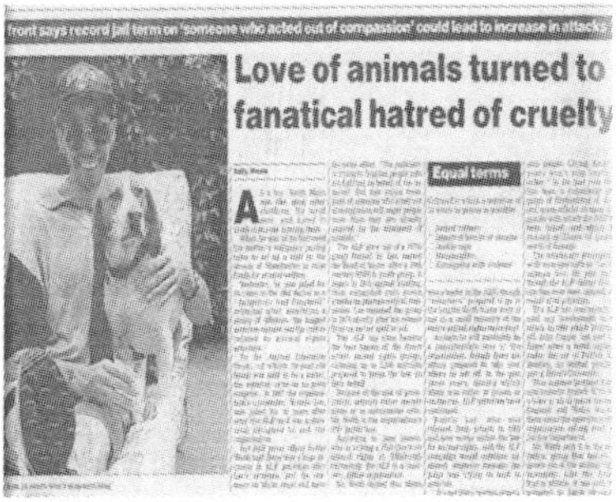

front says record jail term on 'someone who acted out of compassion' could lead to increase in attacks

Love of animals turned to fanatical hatred of cruelty

Equal terms

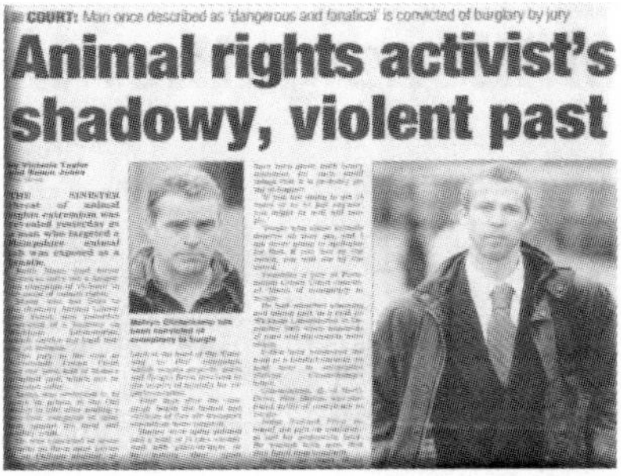

COURT: Man once described as 'dangerous and fanatical' is convicted of burglary by jury

Animal rights activist's shadowy, violent past

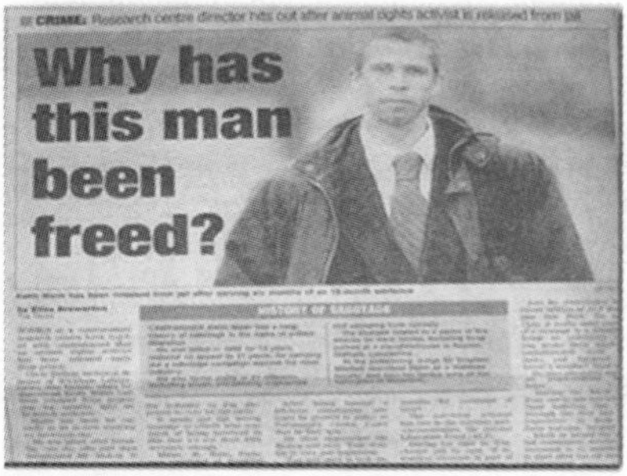

CRIME: Research centre director hits out after animal rights activist is released from jail

Why has this man been freed?

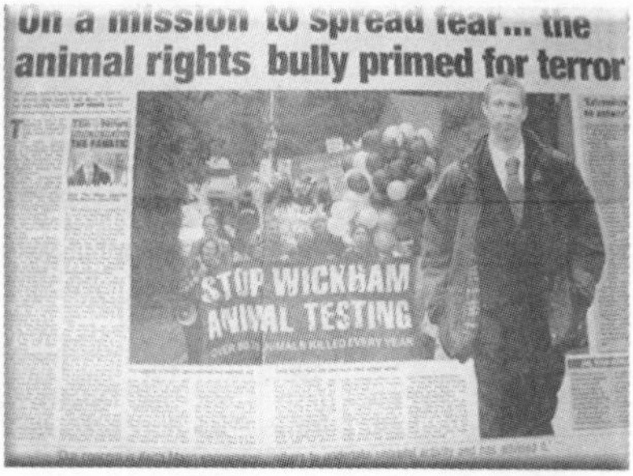

On a mission to spread fear... the animal rights bully primed for terror

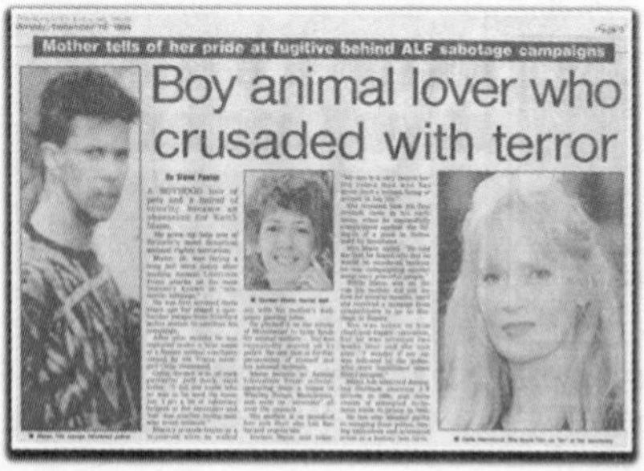

Mother tells of her pride at fugitive behind ALF sabotage campaigns

Boy animal lover who crusaded with terror

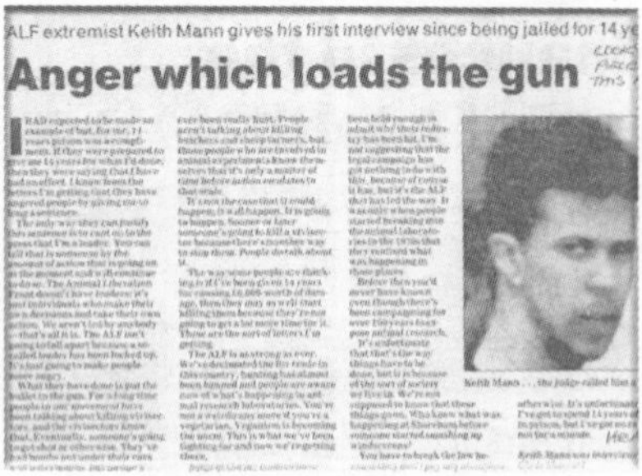

ALF extremist Keith Mann gives his first interview since being jailed for 14 y

Anger which loads the gun

I turned out OK though, eh? See a pattern? Just say things! Anything! Guns, terror hate, fear, bullying, anger... The opposite of me! Throw stuff, repeat it and something will stick or at least it will create a diversion or division. It's like advertising; some of us get confused between advertising and education, information and indoctrination so they play on it to keep us all orderly.

Next over the hill came the university medical students, some proudly from Oxford, calling me a "nut job" with no "formal education" and accusing me of spreading "pseudo scientific claptrap", snake oil therapies and quackery. They protest that I am "harming medical science" by rejecting vivisection. And to complete the circle of crazy talk around my wagon came some 'activists' (comrades?) who could be found protesting *outside* the Oxford labs, now calling me a conspiracy theorist who is informally charged with "discrediting the movement" and "harming the cause" for drawing attention to the bigger picture you have in your hand. I was starting fires all over the place and I wasn't even getting out that much!

On some level the two opposing sides on this for/against lab-animal battlefield are united in killing any notion of exploring other ways. Seemingly settled into their ways the representatives lead their sides nowhere in particular while attending to any initiative seen to be breaking ranks.

Assassinating a character is what an ego does when cornered, desperate to guide the discussion away from the trauma inflicted by a truth. We can learn from them. I found this on one so called animal rights activist's website:

In the 1990s our movement had a variety of articulate, savvy spokespeople, and the release of Angels of Mercy? quickly made Keith Mann foremost among them. His voice-overs from a prison phone are heard over shocking footage of animal abuse, and interviews with his family and supporters act to assure the audience that he is a rational, and passionate activist to working to stop what can only be described as horrific cruelty. When Keith was later released from prison he was highly sought after as a speaker and a source for reporters. I always felt reassured when I saw his face in the news since I knew it meant that at least one positive quote would make it's way to the public.

Sadly, in the last few years Keith has become a devotee of British new-age guru David Icke, a man who believes that a race of reptilian shape-shifters secretly controls the world, that cancer is a fungus, that some humans are actually half-dead, inter-dimensional beings, and a host of other pseudo-scientific nonsense. After being literally laughed off of television in 1991 when he wrongly predicted the end of the world, he has resurfaced in recent years as a lecturer and author with a depressing number of followers.

Since his conversion to odd-ball conspiracy theorist Keith Mann has lost much of his credibility both inside and outside the movement. Most recently he has become a holocaust denier, thereby severing his ties with many of us who still held some hope that he would come to his senses. It's a shame, because as I watch Angels of Mercy? I am reminded of the rare power he once had to make everyday people understand direct action and animal liberation, a power whose benefit is now lost to the animal nations. It is my hope that by posting this video others will consider how desperately the animals need trustworthy advocates, and how easy it is to damage that trust.

Who needs enemies! I can be persuaded to change my mind but this isn't meant to be constructive, more the opposite. Toxic tabloid projects such as this are a perfect example of why the animal rights movement needs a detox of its own, and why we encourage people to try and get a grasp of a subject before claiming knowledge! These people can be found in all social groups, some are placed here to do just this, others have their own agendas but the MO is the same: mix things up with a little bit of the truth, make things up and go for the messenger.

I don't think anyone who posts around things like this would know where to start looking for the truth on anything they ridicule so irresponsibly.

I work purposefully to create a society based on compassion where all are respected as unique individuals, where discrimination is an unknown and where we live and let live. These kind of campaigners take us backwards to a backward time. I say we need to further develop our social conscience, not close it down; we need to stop vaccinating animals and babies with cancer causing pseudoscientific potions; stop assuming we know it all; stop attacking the 'other' humans for their personal characteristics; the food, the cancer tumours and the truth and try a different way.

When we work together not against each other we grow. Dr Max Gerson observed this 60 years ago when healing cancer...

> ***It is important to recognise that, in our body, all the inner-most metabolic processes work together, are dependent upon one another, and will be deranged with each other in disease.***

Dependent upon or deranged, it's a choice.

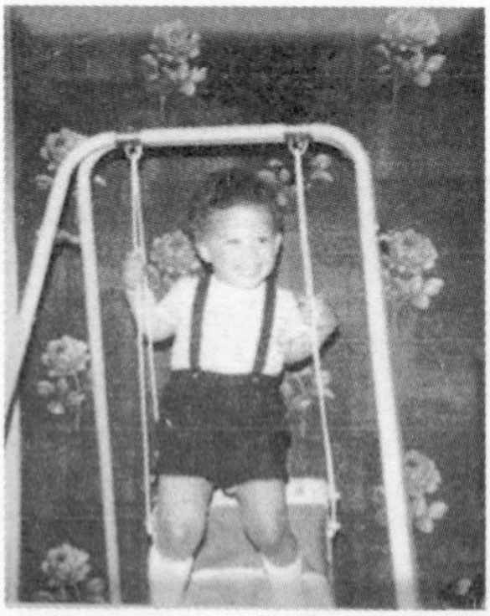

When I was at school one group of boys would pick on me and call me names because I was a little different to them. I remember clearly 1976 when a long hot summer was raging and this little brown boy was climbing trees and soaking up that sun while some of the little white boys burnt. Being called "Monkey Mann" and 'a nigger in a tree' and all the other silly names they could think up was a deeply painful experience for me at the time but I can see how it helped. And Monkey Mann was incredibly predictive as you will see! I find bullying repulsive and this pre-teen taster of ignorance and envy gave me an added sense of urgency for the underdog. I soon figured out how to deal with the small-of-mind and by the time I had left school I'd stopped eating animals and became a hunt saboteur and faced the brave men hunting the animals and singling me out - partly for being annoying but also - because of the colour of my skin, I had developed my immunity. Ignorance is like water off this ducks back and it fuels my determination to be me.

Quack, quack.

Now I use the ignorant to advertise my cause.

Incredible as it seems to me, 40 years of human evolution later and it's still perfectly normal for the same like-mind to single out others for ridicule. In my case it would now appear to be for having mental health issues. I think! Eek! What do I do, change my mind? Stop thinking for myself? Curious, to me, in looking for a pattern in what these people say in their attacks, even if their true agenda is unclear, I've noticed it's the same very narrow demographic using the same limited library of labels. This is quite interesting. Were we to stereotype and pin up their mug shots on a 'suspect board' alongside their poor communications and evident disapproval of the other, we might expect to see a Union Jack or two floating about, if you know what I mean! But we don't because they present themselves vocally at least as anti-fascist while actively trying to control the thoughts and actions of others. Bit bonkers!

Perhaps I'm mentally deranged because of the same like-mind that bullied me when I was 10 years old when boys will be boys and ignorance can be excused? Perhaps the efforts of the not so grown-ups to undermine others' exposes a vulnerability of their own that makes them act like adolescents?

I think so.

The only real 'movement' there is is guided by a vast loose collective of human compassion united not at the hip or by a set of rules or commandments but by an instinctive intent to bring the animal kingdom into the circle of love. Love alone 'moves' us to that brave new world we are all looking for, guided by example. It's steady and reasonable and easy to understand; everyone is welcome and no one gets hurt.

I don't get into bickering with these people any longer. No point. Nevertheless I occasionally pleasure myself enquiring just what is really troubling them. I query what thoughts they recommend I amend in order to be welcomed back on the team, so I may again save some animals. Am I to revert to thinking of cancer as incurable? Should I join in with mocking David Icke for having courage? And embrace bigots as bringers of light? Could there be a retrial before a jury of the self-appointed thought police, with evidence of my blasphemy for me to defend? I need to know the rules! But there is only silence! I am here if needed, not in theory, but for real. For a cancer cure maybe? This story is for everyone, friend or foe let me know.

This kind of bullying is meant to change how we live our lives so we fit back in again to someone else's view of acceptable or appropriate. It creates division and implies superiority; it's based on fear, presents as envy, ignorance and a little bit self-righteous. Had I allowed myself to be pulled back into 'the box where all is known', and from where I have clamoured, I'd be dead now and they'd be looking for someone else to subdue. It's happening all around, this self-imposed ignorance of the possibility that we may be mistaken about what the truth really is. My interest, aside the unpalatable stifling of inquiry, wherever it may lead, is to ask in my best royal accent: *How does one propose to influence those with whom one disagrees, if one invests one's energy so heavily in excluding them from one's sphere of influence? Is one bonkers?* Lead by example, much as you might set a world record as something for others to aspire to. This little monkey kept climbing not listening to the attack dogs down below and is now sat at the top of that tree.

With me a target of lost souls, up stepped a former hunt supporter to publicly pledge her unconditional support. Not for them, for me! Claire is the daughter of my local huntsman who I'd pestered relentlessly through the 1980's. She had heard of my plight and wanted to help. Who wouldn't! Claire and I met 25 years earlier on the battlefront. She was one of 'them' for years but was now revealing how much her huntsman father, Alex, who had died of cancer recently had greatly admired me in spite of our vast differences. With all due respect for him as a fellow human being, I did everything in my power to mess up his days and stop him killing wild animals so I welcome the accolade. Claire is now one of us, she is a friend of mine and a hard working animal activist. Now that is upside down – 'hunt scum' helping me and the animals and the other lot, whatever they label themselves, are throwing tantrums and wanting me dead! In my lifelong search for irony you can only imagine how happy this made me!

The animal rights community is my immediate point of contact with the wider human family, but my observations are not isolated. This is a reflection of how the control system ties up the rest of society in the straightjacket of conformity and creates a stigma toward honest expression and independent discovery, helping to maintain the status quo where we all stay in our place. No one likes change but it is getting silly! Stockholm syndrome is another way to describe this kind of unhealthy emotional attachment human beings express toward their oppressors.

It also helps to highlight the resistance that certain animal advocates place on something so profoundly beneficial to all of us as a natural route to health (animals equally) and gives some sense of where the rest of society is on the issue of taking back personal control and taking health seriously. If our radical animal allies don't want to see how profound this opportunity is for shifting the paradigm from dead end cancer research to delivering natural health from the land, what lead do we set the wider society?

Seeing beyond societal norms and its lies has generally been frowned upon but times are changing fast. We have a stunning map from the ancient Maya of this time in the universal cycle and there are many others, some more 'local' observers such as George Orwell who could envision a future outcome. New thoughts are indeed peer reviewed and kept in check, as with medical treatments. Ask a doctor or best friend about coffee enemas or mega dose Intravenous vitamin C or anything else we use to assist natural healing and you'll see what I mean. If they become angry or defensive or give you that condescending look, or they mock, or their eyes roll, or all of the above, take note. Central to the illusion is that only those trained in a particular field can find the answers, when overwhelmingly those who have been trained have become so locked into their programming that they are unable or unwilling to look beyond it.

Think too much outside the box, like about natural medicine, and you risk demonisation and isolation by those living in the box. This is actually a good thing, it's like a pill that worked, it just takes a little while to figure out that living outside the box with that separation from the heavy weighted energy is liberating. And there are a lot of good people here now leading in a new cycle of time, thinking differently. Just thinking. Hence the Orwellian push to distort the message with claims of fake news from the professional purveyors of fake news and quackery from the quacks. If we allow this to continue they will simply call themselves the Ministry of Truth and do away with all pretence!

It seems clear to me that drug companies have a monopoly on illness and would logically, mechanically work to not only keep it but to build on it. This makes for either a conspiracy or a heap of coincidences. I can see the conspiracy but it doesn't matter how we view it, it's out of control and it doesn't serve the best interests of the average trusting individual or of the collective. It is clear also that the status quo does work really well for some people. People with a lot they'd like to keep. No broke, no fix, no matter how many claim injury. Big Pharma makes big bucks and not from cures but from treatments and better still from treatments that cause the need for more treatments. Introduce a cure into the market and it is game over.

The Big Pharma group of special interests brush off billion dollar fines and compensation settlements like flies. They factor the fines into expenses. What do they have to care about? The animal rights (AR) movement is the most vocal anti-pharma community in many parts of the world yet all too often those of us who protest vivisection end up knocking on those same industry doors when the illness sets in asking for the very drugs we don't want testing on animals while fighting against alternative ideas. What for industry needs to change? I pass no judgement by the way, been there myself, and these products would still be around in spite of the animal tests, and safer. My question is and was, to ask how will we ever bring change if we don't change our approach and open our minds to new solutions? We used to target a boycott of animal testing, but we don't really press the issue beyond specific products and cosmetics, so can't then expect others to bother. It was a rhetorical question and one I was asking myself as much as anyone else. I knew the answer then and of course I know the answer now. We do something different. Starting now by first thinking about it.

The animal tests aren't just a remnant of a dark age; they are more importantly an intrinsic cog in the wheel of fortune that churns out dangerous products often leading to the additional use of further dangerous products with the animals there as the scapegoats when it all goes terribly wrong or simply doesn't work. And each one of the many billions of animals they consume in this pretend search for cures is a valuable business commodity in itself. If we think those who profit heavily from this highly efficient and deeply embedded machinery are going to let any of it slip away to please us, we need to take a step back and think again.

I don't have all the answers because I have so many questions but I get more and more answers the more questions I ask. It's important to ask the right questions and to keep asking. I asked about cancer cures and got called some silly names by one group of people and was advised on my options by others. I naturally followed the advice of the bringers of light and what did I find? Everything!

The highest form of Human Excellence is to question oneself and others.
Socrates (469 – 399)

Outside the Box

Darkness cannot drive out darkness; only light can do that. Hate cannot drive out hate; only love can do that.
Martin Luther King Jr. (1929 – 1968)

Being trapped in no man's land through 2008-9, with nowhere of our own to settle, we were sofa surfing around the homes of friends trying to find a hospital to help Alice, but no matter how hard we pushed they had nothing to give. After six weeks of procedural recycling in one hospital, where they were unusually keen to help, we'd had enough. We would return her as an outpatient in exchange for pain relief prescriptions. With pain manageable out of hospital and with me providing all the food she ate anyway we were better off finding our own way in our environment to which we eventually settled. We had learnt lessons about a wide range of allergies which the hospitals little understood and would aggravate symptoms. The nursing staff were good here and in most places for the most part, with the odd sociopath or two thrown in, but they aren't the problem. They are forced to use mainly junk drugs and radiation and junk food all based on junk science with all its glaring politically imposed limitations.

With all my campaign projects, my big ideas and dreams suddenly halted and steadily drifting out of reach and little hope of a quick fix for Alice any time soon, our garden wasn't looking rosy. But we grow through our suffering. That seems to be the deal. Or one of them. So this was all a good thing. It's pretty cool if you think about it. Learn your lesson from your suffering and your suffering lessens. If we choose to ignore the lesson and carry on as normal we will suffer the consequences. Resistance breeds resistance. I resisted my latest confinement for long enough but eventually I learnt to accept it and settled in. I'm no expert in the workings of the universe but I have a good idea and I know how it works with me. This latest enforced restriction of mine was my gift once I figured that out.

This cancer experience for me has never meant any physical suffering, all mine has been mind inflicted. I'm learning to deal with the mind. We can observe how this invisible entity plays with us just by paying attention. Native Americans call it Wetiko. It's a parasite that feeds off our suffering and fears, our negative emotions. So it creates those heavy energies. Makes us 'think' about what was and what should be. I spend time observing the thinker and I notice a pattern of repetitive chatter that creates tension so I switch off the thinker and I do something constructive or nothing at all. I find solace in silence. And when you put your mind to work *for you* great things can happen.

The silver lining in all this was our forced confinement. I now had nothing else to do but to accept my reality, take a step back and occupy myself another way. So I read and researched and got taken on something of a trip. There's so much information out there but we don't make the time or dare to look at it and instead get most of what we hear from the same unreliable sources, so we easily become susceptible to manipulation. We are programmed to think a certain way. It's subtle but it's super effective at containing the herd. My days before Alice's medical meltdown consisted of one project after another, day and night: I had to save the animals yesterday. All of them! Suddenly I could barely leave the house, but I can read I had access to the internet and I'm curious and once you get interested there's no end. I only needed a glance through the fog of deception to find myself hooked.

I had cancelled all future public speaking dates from 2008 and such was the extent of my campaign work for the next 10 years. All but for one imaginative little project we engaged in from home in 2010 I was in early retirement! In this I agreed to stand as a candidate on behalf of the fledgling, now defunct, Animal Protection Party in the 2010 General Election, but I didn't actually stand so to speak, rather stayed at my desk. Politics as we know it does not float my boat and I'm not drawn to playing in a game whose rules are fixed but this was by our rules. And never say never, right? Rather than stand to try and grab a seat at the table we were going to target a career politician with an obnoxious agenda and take away his seat at the table by asking voters to tick any box for any candidate but his. Our job was simply to unseat Evan Harris, or Dr Death as he had become publicly known, by raising some big issues. I'm drawn to that.

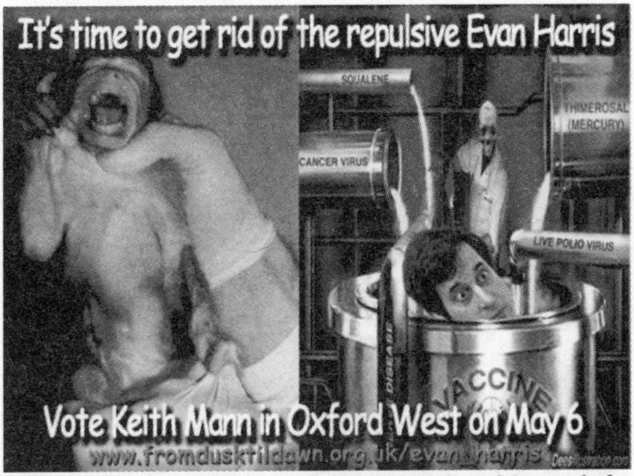
It's time to get rid of the repulsive Evan Harris
SQUALENE
THIMEROSAL
(MERCURY)
CANCER VIRUS
LIVE POLIO VIRUS
VACCINE
Vote Keith Mann in Oxford West on May 6
www.fromdusktildawn.org.uk/evan_harris

This was 2010, 3 years prior to my cancer diagnosis and 6 years before I would discover the cause and the cure of my cancer. As you will see as this story unfolds this banner is littered with hints of what was to come.

Harris was one of four MP's we stood candidates against, all vocal anti-animal politicians. But Harris stood out a mile. He called for forced vaccinations, he wanted to extend the abortion time limit to beyond 6 months, he was an aggressive secularist with little time for a Christian community, he was a fanatical promoter of animal experiments, he advocated the use of hybrid human/animal embryos for research and wanted to remove the human right to refuse the mass fluoridation of the water supply. It was Dr Death for a reason! He was a long-standing MP in the conservative, god fearing county of Oxford in what was seen as a safe seat. But we figured if we made public this heavy agenda (an opportunity in itself to open the debate) the people might not like it. So we made ourselves busy in the weeks leading to the election.

Well that turned out to be a really good idea.

The one time I was able to leave Alice alone for more than a couple of hours during these two years was for the general election count in Oxford in May 2010, and it was a curiously good night out. We had tried something new in Oxford and succeeded and had shown what could be done with a little imagination. Harris started the night with a safe 7,683 seat majority and he was the last person to expect to be unemployed by the morning. But following repeated recounting of a narrow margin, by 4.00am the Oxford West numbers were confirmed and we'd achieved our goal! Told we couldn't, did. No one really expected such a majority to be overturned and it was pretty impressive but Harris was not a happy bunny. In his loser's speech he bemoaned the 'dirty nature' of our campaign, which was in fact entirely honest and informative. It was the Daily Mail that had branded him Dr Death, we thought this perfectly suitable and attached it to our story of his hideous agenda and told as many people as possible. The Times described the outcome as "a terrible night for science". And the Independent recorded that

> *Science lost one of its strongest parliamentary supporters with the surprise defeat of Evan Harris. Professor David Nutt, who resigned as chairman of the Government's drugs advisory committee, said that it was a sad day for science and the Government.*

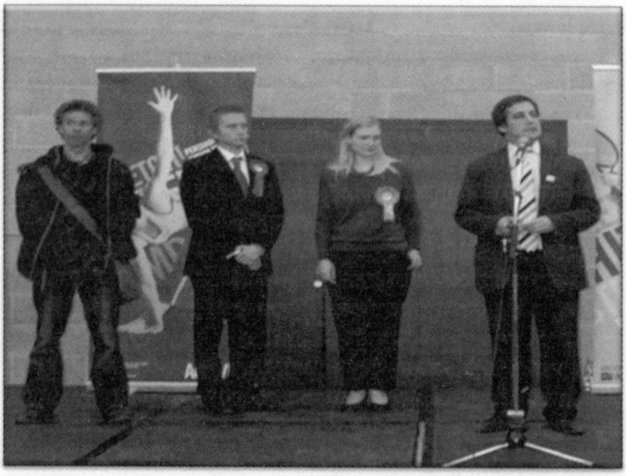

Ah, the science! We're coming back to that. The scientists were still not helping Alice recover her health, its experts couldn't even figure out what was wrong and getting rid of Harris was hardly going to topple the death cult feeding off the planet, but we'd poked them in the eye and broken our monotony. In reality, all this time we felt was wasted to ill health was actually the ground being prepared. As the days and the multitude of medical experts passed us by we weren't so much as wasting time as filtering out the waste. Had we stopped searching we would never have found what was waiting for us.

Patients who heal themselves write books and these stories hold patterns and clues. An early clue to the puzzle of Alice was laid out in a book called Tears Behind Closed Doors by Diana Holmes. In this she documents in detail her discovery of a simple and superior urine diagnostic test for deficient thyroid and adrenal function. A test which was, and is, being suppressed by the orthodox in favour of their outdated and dangerous gold standard blood tests. The book told of her struggle with the medical profession and her saviour, a maverick GP, who had been suspended by the General Medical Council, accused of the unapproved healing of these debilitating disorders. This story rang alarm bells and peaked our interest and it would turn out that Alice had the same debilitating set of symptoms being incorrectly diagnosed by the same inadequate experts, unable to admit they've got it wrong again.

The thyroid function test being used by the ortho-docs amounts to a blood test of thyroid stimulating hormones (TSH) and sometimes a more thorough doctor will measure T4 and T3 levels in the investigation. Diana Holmes revealed a critical flaw in the gold standard test which is notorious for returning the patient within the normal range irrespective of thyroid dysfunction, thereby putting an end to the matter for the medical profession. But the patient still ails, undiagnosed. Most doctors within the controls of the system, if they even considered investigating the patient's thyroid function further than the gold standard would be unable to do so because the computer would not permit. Dr Barry Peatfield ignored the rules in favour of the patient and became a quack.

In addition, some patients already diagnosed with thyroid dysfunction are being inadequately treated because the doctor of today relies more heavily on the blood tests than the patient symptoms and story. Therefore some patients can be diagnosed hypothyroid via the gold standard and are prescribed thyroxine (T4) medication. The doctor will adjust the dose according to the dodgy blood readings that will soon show normal range, yet symptoms persist so the patient needs more. And here begins the clash of civilisations. The computer says they are right; you are now healthy, go home. You only *think* you still have symptoms, perhaps they'll suggest because of the length of time you have been ill you will have forgotten what it feels like to be well. They say that! In addition to this problem some patients cannot convert T4 to the active thyroid hormone T3, T3 medication can be prescribed to bring balance but rarely is. GP's usually focus only on TSH levels but the patient is not going to improve symptomatically unless they have enough of the active thyroid hormone and they aren't going to get it within the rules of the system.

Further, there is a problem with diagnosing adrenal insufficiency. The gold standard for this is a test, of blood, of the hormone cortisol. But these blood tests are critically flawed too. Often a thyroid and adrenal issue combine, and if we consider nothing happens in isolation and that this happens all too often the likelihood should be taken into account. But alas, still emerging from our slumber, it's only once the adrenal glands (which sit on the kidneys) collapse causing a medical emergency that the medical experts sit up and listen and then prescribe the urgent intravenous cortisol infusion. It is like cancer, you don't wait for it to deteriorate before getting your act together.

We found this combined calamity is much more insipid and widespread than anyone will admit and is often disguised with other medical mishaps as a mystery syndrome. Patient groups such as Thyroid Patient Advocacy have sprung up seeking to raise awareness.[3]

This is another very big medical problem that has a very simple solution. At the moment in time when the blood is taken it is possible that the patient's typically low cortisol is elevated into normal range, especially factoring in the heightened state of anxiety the patient may be in while anticipating a needle in the arm. What if you are someone with veins they have to fish around to find and you know that's coming? Anyone taking the temporary rise in cortisol from low to just about normal into consideration? Not so you'd notice. And even then, what is normal? Not everyone fits into the normal box. Further, the orthodox typically only look for extreme adrenal failure, a medical emergency, and nothing in between. Like looking for stage 4 cancer and ignoring 1, 2 and 3.

Diana Holmes discovered that there was a more accurate test available which was in fact cheaper and which saved her. This lady was never into conspiracy theories but she asked questions and challenged the orthodox and by sharing what she found in fighting for her life, she now fits that label. And she is in turn back to full health. This is an interesting model and as we will discover it is often those branded a 'conspiracy theorist' that heal! No one else thinks it possible! In this case all it took was the application of a simple urine test which monitors thyroid output, free T4 and T3 over 24 hours, and is much more reliable than the orthodox approved snap-shot blood test. This is marked by the fact that those who take this test, who were previously found within the standard medical blood range reading to be normal, and by some convoluted logic therefore healthy, may now be found deficient in the thyroid hormones and in need of help. And who, upon restoring the hormone balance, recover full health. Additionally, adrenal function can be more accurately assessed by a 24-hour urine test and 24-hour saliva test. Yet this novel approach is frowned upon because there are rules that must be obeyed at all costs. Say you discover this and buy yourself a test kit, pay for private analysis and discover a thyroid/adrenal issue, as we did, then what do you do? Can't go to a system GP because they aren't allowed to believe in unapproved diagnostics, only in their blood test, and that says your thyroid and adrenals are healthy.

In 2001 the General Medical Council suspended Dr Barry Peatfield over the use of what they called "controversial treatments". This represented the unapproved use of those urine tests and the therapeutic use of approved medications in response to positive test results. These were patients with deficient thyroid function which may be labelled Chronic Fatigue Syndrome (CFS), fibromyalgia, Myalgic Encephalomyelitis (M.E.) or some such.

Peatfield had stepped into the pond after he'd watched a young patient of his die for the lack of official recognition of this test and from then on he adopted it into his practice. In doing so was able to identify thyroid dysfunction in otherwise hopeless

---

3 http://www.tpauk.com/main/

cases and heal them. But you can't get away with that for long! In doing so he'd broken the rules and was restoring health and such deviant acts of humanity bring down the wrath of the orthodox high priests in an ugly pattern repeated over and again in this controlled environment. Peatfield found himself in front of the panel of suits who insisted he must stop or be evicted from the club. So Peatfield walked away to become an outcast among his peers and a hero to humanity. Dr Barry Durrant-Peatfield tells it as it is in 'The Great Thyroid Scandal and How to Survive it' and for anyone still in no mans land with a vague diagnosis and thyroid and adrenal symptoms, I urge you get a copy.

We tracked down Peatfield who now operates privately but is unable to prescribe treatment for patients. He will, as he did for us, offer advice, interpret test results and suggest options. In reality you have no choice if you want your health back and that is your ailment. It had taken just half an hour for this kindly gentleman, who we called Dr Robin Hood, to do what the orthodox medical system had failed to do in 3 years, leaving us with our first real solution. Take the patients blood pressure while seated, stand the patient and test BP again. A drop in BP is suggestive, as seen in Alice, and adrenal insufficiency was indeed confirmed by lab tests.

Dr Peatfield is a gentle man who empathises with others. I was carrying Alice around on my back at this time, he realised she had other issues out of his field and he charged us next to nothing for his time. But lab tests come with an invoice and her medication had to be sourced from a Mexican pharmacy, too, can you believe it, because without an official diagnosis such treatments are forbidden under the control of crazies!

Within a matter of weeks of our self treatment of Alice's significant adrenal insufficiency some symptoms begun to improve and her health stabilised. Further tests confirmed this improvement. This was quite remarkable and for people we met along this journey this was all they needed to return to full health after years of struggling. But for Alice there were more layers to unravel. Peatfield, while he was a light year ahead of the crowd and had done much more healing than most, had himself parked up on these treatment options which are themselves dated and don't always suffice.

Keen to work on this chink in the armour we arranged to see a private doctor based on the over priced Harley Street in central London who had also stepped away from the restraints and went on to practice functional medicine. This is a fluid health discipline that incorporates new ways to measure and balance the functions of the whole body system so it may restore equilibrium and heal, in place of the drug-induced symptom suppression we are used to. This is the immediate future of healthcare once we retire the Pharma. Cancer, as a suitable example, is a whole body dysfunction and conventional medicine, using all the power tools it has focuses on a late stage side effect of this dysfunction and drills away at tumours. This tradition of disease management hints at why cancer still cannot be cured.

Dr Mantzourani was sharp, determined and clearly ahead of the game. She recommended a battery of stool, blood and urine tests little understood by regular doctors. We got more information from a single dollop of Alice's poo sent to the US for a Metametrix 2100 Gastrointestinal Function Profile at a cost of £400 than we had over 3 years of cameras, blood tests, x-rays, and scans and specialist consultations. And we discovered multiple serious health issues including mitochondrial dysfunction, invasive candidiasis, pancreatic insufficiency, impaired liver function, adrenal insufficiency, low oestradiol and progesterone, gut dysbiosis, a catalogue of IgE food allergies, including fruits such as bananas and nectarines and nutrient deficiencies (no doubt partly due to her digestive issues).

This was the kind of doctor that quickly knew how to find what she was looking for and seldom appeared stumped. An allergy to fruit was certainly a little odd, until more recent times when it has become quite common. I'll come back to why this might be. Another thing she couldn't make sense of very early on was the medical investigation of Alice thus far. Same tests recycled and a deteriorating patient. And, the very tests that would later help diagnose were never done! Alice had numerous neurological symptoms yet no one ran a brain scan. That day Alice was referred to a competent neurologist and within a few weeks of our first appointment with the doctor of functional medicine we discovered Alice had brain lesions. Brain damage! All clues building a puzzle.

This was all very curious. Mercury was another finding of tests carried out by Dr Mantzourani. We would later in our journey discover the exact storage location of this mercury inside Alice (using other advanced technology unknown to bog standard medicine) was in her brain. Just how do you get mercury into your brain? And brain damage? Are they linked? It's quite a common association it turns out, in young and old and has a devastating impact. Alice got off lightly because we found the metal poison and got rid of it, but how much information does a vast industry of medical experts miss? Alice was officially in a mess and to be fair her symptoms overlapped, as is most often the case, but all it took was one smart doctor assessing the whole patient and her blocked biochemical pathways using simple tests that the orthodox choose to ignore and it was actually very easy to take science and medicine to another level, where it works. The fact that her liver was struggling was of concern to the good doctor who linked this to the gut issues and went some way to explain the typically negative effects of the wide range of pharma drugs she had been fed by nearly every other doctor she had seen in the previous few years. Pharmaceuticals are liver toxic and every single one, and there were a lot, was prescribed to manage some symptom and maintain the need for the drugs, never to make her better.

We desperately wanted answers and were now collecting information quicker than we could process it.

Each test result confirming a deficiency or imbalance needed a remedy and working through each element naturally takes time. Healing is a process not a pill. With mercury a serious issue, the amalgam fillings needed replacing, one at a time, by a holistic dentist, privately. The ortho-docs are in such a state of denial about the danger of mercury they're even injecting it into day old babies, so they won't help! Same old, if we see a problem we need to fix it. Money was an obstacle to quickly healing Alice and at £300 for the doctor consultations alone we soon cut back on them and gathered together what we had learnt so we could manage things ourselves. This was money spent the best way possible and had included a crash course in the science of functional medicine which is priceless and gave us a much clearer picture. Alice was prescribed merc-sol by a homeopath for six months at the end of which she was clear of mercury contamination.

We sourced stacks of supplements as the good doctor advised and made radical dietary manoeuvres. Over the next few months Alice consumed copious quantities of supplements and bio-identical hormones from Germany, all of which were quite harmless and which accelerated this lengthy healing process, more a scientific work of art, which at first involved stopping the rot and then detoxing and more tests and more tweaking. This discovery of a new approach to health came to us with good timing as other events were converging that would ensure we didn't come close to completing this process as prescribed for Alice, who would just have to hang in there half fixed that little bit longer.

We had made significant inroads and she was at least stable but still there was a peculiarity about the pattern of symptoms Alice presented that even had the new wave of doctors we were encountering utterly baffled. The cause of physical disability would remain undetected for some time to come and confine her to a wheelchair from 2009 to the present. But the mercury was gone, allergens were removed and managed, thyroid and adrenals working correctly, liver better... Her mitochondria, gut dysbiosis and recurrent candida would continue to hold her back along with others yet undiagnosed.

Dietary research had increasingly drawn us to the nutritional foundation of all health, and being confronted by the excess of supplements Alice was required to take this more natural approach made more sense. It's fair to say there was something of urgency about certain areas of dysfunction in Alice that required high dose supplementation and bio-identical hormones for her adrenals and because of all these allergies there were obstacles to simply eating right, but a recurring theme in a study of healing arts holds that nutrition and gut health is the key. When you look to healing with nutrition you soon discover the Gerson Therapy, a very powerful, age old nutritional therapy commonly used to heal cancer and other degenerative disease. This is where we were at when cancer caught up.

A fashion rules each age, without most people being able to see the tyrants that rule them.

Albert Einstein (1879 -1955)

A Family Affair

Condition of electron deficiency explains why measures that increase electron availability like magnetized waters, lemon juice, negative ion generators, standing by water falls, standing by the ocean surf, use of electron rich antioxidants, consumption of electron dense foods (fresh vegetables and vegetable juices and essential fatty acids like fresh flax oil) help some people with chronic degenerative conditions and cancers get better.

Dr Steve Haltiwanger, The Electrical Properties of Cancer Cells

Alice's aunt Evelyn had been through conventional cancer treatment 12 years earlier in 1999 and if you do the research you find it perfectly normal that in most cases cancer returns, in sweeping waves. There's the first wave that die in the weeks and months following treatment. Then the second wave known as 'the cured' who make the 5 year 'cured' date but don't quite make 10 years. Evelyn was one of the lucky ones as she hadn't had chemo, only what they call 'radical' surgery (butchery) and she was going to make it to the final phase. She was vegan and that may have helped but the standard processed vegan diet is actually harmful to health in the long run. Evelyn's story is quite telling in that she was treated in London, at a hospital considered by the drug experts to have the best breast unit in Europe at the time. Keen to grab this moment before it passed the hospital invited her to stand as an example to other potential patients/customers who were going through the conventional approach and might need some jollying along with the help of a cancer survivor.

Through this experience Evelyn, along with a dozen fellow 'survivors', volunteered to mentor hundreds of other breast cancer patients. A striking similarity in the story of these patients was the use of chemotherapy. It may of course be purely coincidental that one of the effects of chemotherapy is cancer, but over the course of the 5 years drifting into 10, every single one in Evelyn's group had cancer return typically in the bone or brain. At ten years Evelyn was the only one in her group still here but her continued survival depended on deciding for herself what to do next because soon after she reached that milestone, among the cured, the cancer was back in view.

She originally had a Ductal Carcinoma in Situ (DCIS), a benign non-invasive pre-cancerous lesion. The orthodox consider it a type of breast cancer but it's a very unconvincing argument and others do not consider it as such. This is one of those medical mysteries of which there are many. What is clear is that if ever there was an example of something best left alone this is it. Whatever label it is given the DCIS does not readily or necessarily develop into cancer, particularly if the environment in which it formed is adjusted to pro-life and anti-cancer. It is largely because of the increased use of mammograms that DCIS are more commonly being diagnosed and an opportunity opened up for more product sales and services where they aren't needed. It's broken down by David Icke as 'problem, reaction, solution' or the psychopath signature. They create a problem for us to react to and then they offer a solution which we readily gobble up. We're like piggy in the middle. Typically the solution they offer doesn't solve the problem but they get to sell a load more solutions on the back of the problems, be it bombs, legislation or drugs.

In this case it's a whole mess of junk. As is standard operating procedure, they loaded on the fear and soon got their permission to hack at this DCIS blemish in their cancer survivor, and everything around it. Everything! Not once did anyone suggest a lifestyle change instead to see how that helps. But if you need a new breast, no problem! Solution: silicone implant. A kind of mad scientist booby prize. That technological breakthrough sprung a leak soon after it was inserted, emptying its toxic innards into their human guinea pig. The bag of gack our experts replaced the faulty implant with also then leaked, only the second one caused gangrene and more misdiagnosis that very nearly killed this survivor. Having dodged that bullet she was duly rewarded soon after with a diagnosis for spleenic marginal zone, a spleen/blood cancer. She had been one of the lucky cancer survivors who made the 10 years, just, and who are used to make the ortho-docs look like heroes, but her luck had run out and the ortho-docs were waiting. With more short-term solutions!

Bounced from one medical expert to another in 2012 they each read from the script about how they needed to act and act urgently or she would die a silly woman. They may well have assured her once that she had been cured by their genius but that was old science and things had moved on a long way since 1999 (cancer at least) and now they wanted her spleen before any further medical curing would be discussed. This would facilitate a more precise grading of the new, improved cancer. To be clear, so they could tick their boxes plot a chart and pick some poisons they demanded physical possession of her spleen. But she had witnessed first hand the slippery death slope this aggressive, irreversible medical intervention leads down, having almost died from the last few and Alice had not let up from the day of diagnosis about the need to get a grip of this situation. Dog with a bone come to mind.

The quacks didn't help themselves with their increasingly frantic behaviour. Resistance they almost find sweet, if they get you to change your mind, but dig in and they can get desperate. The more this patient resisted the ortho madmen's demands for her organ, the more intense the bullying and blackmail became. Doctors throwing wobblies? Bring it on! She had been openly laughed at by one doctor for mentioning she was going to do coffee enemas. Refusing their superior expensive medical knowledge they see as a sign of a poor education and a lack of understanding, but choosing a natural therapy instead is an insult. As punishment they told her no spleen no blood test results. They tried to get her to have more CT scans *to see what was going on inside*, to scare her with their findings, but she was digging in. These were all big hints that she had to get away from these lunatics and the only place to turn was to Alice.

Bedridden and drawn to this dream of healing, Alice had long since filled her head with the various available options for actually curing cancer and had been desperate to save her aunt from a system she knew was in a critical condition itself and in no position to care properly for others. Alice knew this cancer thing would be back whatever they said about cures and was well prepared.

Listening to Charlotte Gerson talk about the Gerson Therapy and its ability to cure not only far advanced cancer but most other diseases using nutrition at its core was an enticing revelation. Not to mention her father the great Max Gerson and the attention to detail he had perfected over many years. No agenda, nothing to gain just direct honest inquiry and simple, logical advice based on years of clinical research at the bedside. For **over 90 years** Charlotte has witnessed her father's protocol healing terminal cancer patients and she was on a mission to make it known. How do we dismiss these generations of knowledge and thousands of testimonials? We could only wonder at the potential this lifestyle therapy had on so many levels.

Evelyn eventually trusted what Alice was teaching her about 'Gerson', as I will refer to The Gerson Therapy, and couldn't avoid the fact that the principles of cellular nutrition and detoxification make more sense than chemo. Within two months Alice had her booked into the Gerson clinic in Hungary (a feat in itself as there are limited places and many applicants) for two weeks of coaching while we arranged local supplies and set up a clean water system and so on. For the next three years she and her partner did the full Gerson Therapy. This involves detailed repetition and it's <u>all</u> you do if you are to do this properly.

The Gerson Therapy is the best known so called 'alternative' approach to treating cancer and has been utilised by the open minded, the free thinkers for over 100 years. Gerson is for those who have identified the difference between treatment and cure; between the promise of improved treatment sometime in the future and the recovery of health.

Gerson puts cancer control into the hands of the patient. It's a common claim that anyone claiming a cancer cure is a quack out to fleece the victim. This claim is typically made by a cancer industry that has for decades consumed incredible sums of money on the promise of a cure just around the corner, while delivering false hope in treatments that do the opposite of cure. Gerson, on the other hand, is a self-help process for which the Gerson Institute and its practitioners gain little in the face of cynicism and insult. The Gerson Therapy has proven itself over and again since the 1920's capable of achieving remarkable results. Even if this happened only once, it is an approach that should be thoroughly investigated by anyone genuinely wanting to find answers, yet this has never happened. I will return to Gerson and see how Evelyn gets on later.

Divide and conquer is the motto and as long as people continue to see themselves as separate from everything else they lend themselves to being completely enslaved. The men behind the curtain know that if the people realise the truth of their relationship to nature and their personal power the entire manipulated zeitgeist will collapse like a house of cards.

Zeitgeist the Movie

Trust Grandma!

It is unnecessary to understand the whole life in its minute biological particles and effect – but it is necessary that, for the problem of therapy, the entire sick human organism be attacked in its totality, especially in degenerative diseases. It would be a great mistake to apply the therapy only as far as we understand the corresponding biological reactions or as far as they can be proven in animal experiments. In particular, in degenerative diseases and in cancer, we should not apply a symptomatic treatment or only one that we can fully understand; we need a treatment that will comprise the whole body as far as we know or can imagine it.
Dr Max Gerson (1888 – 1959)

Soon after in early 2013 Alice's grandmother had a stroke. She was 91 and full of fun and Alice and her were very close. Two weeks earlier Gladys had been injected with the latest flu vaccine, a precursor to a demise which I hear an awful lot and which I find deeply suspicious. You will see why as we make our way through our story. Over the next five weeks Alice and I spent our time between her gran's flat and the hospital.

Gladys couldn't feed herself and was struggling to remember things, she was frustrated and words were now coming out comical and reconstructed and it was hard not to laugh every time she spoke! She could laugh at herself and had no idea we were laughing at her anyway! It was equally rewarding as she responded to stimulus as it was difficult watching her lose the battle. We were five weeks in a hospital surrounded by very poorly people before we lost Gladys. Dearly departed Gladys was dead but she would be back shortly and she wouldn't be alone.

I'd had drenching night sweats for some months through this period which I put down to an infection I got from spending all that time around dying people. But Alice remembered that the same thing had happened a year earlier. I also now had some unexplained weight loss. My weight had long fluctuated and high energy has meant it never sits on me for long. This wasn't just one of those things, it was an indicator that something was seriously wrong. This sweating wasn't just hot in bed type sweat, more like been-under-water-fully-clothed got to get up now and change everything type wet. Alice often chuckles at the sheer speed at which I would leave the bed in the middle of the night the instant I woke in the dreaded bed bath. It wasn't funny at the time though because she had done some research and she had an idea of the possible cause, and I wasn't sleeping. But then came the most curious clue in the form of our dearly departed Gladys and her long passed husband Morris, who confirmed for us the cause of my night time bathing.

It's April 2013 and Alice had been re-living the last few weeks of her gran's life pawing over photos, reading letters, listening to the Andrews Sisters and Glenn Miller as Gladys had when she grew up. In some way she was looking to blame herself for not doing enough to keep her gran here a little longer. Truth is Gladys was way past her sell by date and was ready to go and Alice did everything she could to make her life as comfortable as possible, in spite of her own difficulties.

This was reflected in the curious experience Alice had this night in late April when Gladys reappeared.

We're in bed and I am asleep. Alice isn't sleeping, as such - she's more hanging out with Gladys and her granddad Morris who have appeared on the scene. The four of us, Alice recalled in the morning, were in a cancer hospital, best of friends chatting away and having a blast. Now I'd never met Morris but Morris was holding my hand and talking to Alice and telling her she should stop fretting about Gladys, who is clearly fine, and that she should focus her energy on me. He expressed his deep gratitude for us looking after Gladys.

Alice is tuned in and switched on in so many ways and she was a little baffled by this experience but was deeply affected by it. The following day for the first time in weeks Alice didn't listen to any old music. Well that was some good news! I like the Andrews Sisters but all day? Every day? One week later I found lymph nodes in my neck. I pointed this out to Alice and she pieced it all together in an instant! From that moment on the focus has indeed been on me!

She called my GP immediately and booked me in. The doctor told me to wait six weeks and come back. Before I knew it the sweating had come back and lymph nodes had appeared in my armpits and groin. With no sign of these lumps regressing I was eventually passed onto the conveyor belt and an urgent trip was booked to theatre for Keith. Only me in denial at this stage and still hoping this meant I was going to see a movie but of course it was the operating theatre and this was for real.

Front row seat for me at this show. A few days later I attended for a short stay as an outpatient and the excision of a swollen lymph node from my right collar. Curiously the surgical procedure was quite pleasant if anything. And thank you for anaesthetic. I lay there with a towel over my face so that, as the surgeon reminded the nurse, "he can't see what I am doing to him". Hmmm, I probably didn't want to be reminded of what he was doing to me but too late now! This is like that moment when the plane starts along the runway and you realise that no matter what your instinct is saying you're flying! The tray of tools was placed onto my chest and I chatted to the nurse to my left about gardening. Before we had got to discussing greenhouses my gland had been excised, dissected and sent off for testing. Before I knew it I was sewn up and back home to await the results.

A few days later I was called back to see the consultant who had referred me for this procedure in the first place. This is that worst life moment for most of us but we were way ahead by now and had figured out what was coming. We'd had the grandparents pop by and the obvious symptoms, but we also noticed about five minutes before I was called in for my appointment a Macmillan nurse had gone in the consultation room. That was the final clue and we knew it. It's not their fault, but death follows them around like a grim reaper in the shadows.

We both knew what was coming but you still need to hear it. In that instant life officially changes. Everything is suddenly going to be different to your forever plans.

That said, our dream was to be together and to make the world a kinder place and this was the big one laid out on a plate! For this particular specialist this was all rather matter of fact as he told me bluntly I had an "incurable" form of blood cancer. He neatly softened that blow by offering to refer me to another specialist who he assured me would have "plenty of treatment available". These are enticing words where cancer and drug therapy is concerned and we should pay close attention. A treat on the face of it is quite comforting. If they called it a trauma we wouldn't load up our loved ones. A treat could be something to look forward to and *plenty of treatment* sounds almost mouth watering and implies that a cure doesn't really matter. Thing is, we could treat cancer with raw sewage or orange squash but what of the final outcome? That's all that matters. Chemotherapy doesn't cure cancer, as the millions of chemo treated patients who die soon after being treated clearly prove. Decades of a war on cancer at a cost of trillions, and the best options are expensive and more likely to kill.

We live in a world where the rich can buy islands, governments and spaceships but all the money in the world is only going to buy the same crappy cancer treatment from the agents of death. And even then you don't want much of it!

Unless we shift ever so slightly our view of the world to where we have real cures!

Often with this type of cancer, known to spread slowly but inevitably, the patient is left to watch and wait until intervention is necessitated by blocked organs for example. This way survival time progresses more naturally and isn't hastened by carpet bombing the immune system. Once intervention begins the clock is ticking as the immune system can only take so much medical intervention. I was advised to wait but wasn't planning on waiting for this thing to get worse without doing something. I never expected to be a cancer candidate and Alice was rattled too as she says she always saw me living to a ripe old age, with her. Funny enough she might yet be right! Arriving home from hospital later that day I set up a coffee enema. This is a key element of the Gerson Therapy, a lifestyle shift that would be the centre of my world for the next few years. Yet still the plot would thicken as Gerson would fail to cure me and the root cause of my cancer would be revealed.

My lymph node pathology report recorded:

> *Immunohistochemistry shows follicular structures... with B-cells spilling out into the interfollicular tissue... overall appearance are those of low grade follicular lymphoma. In addition, some black pigment is present within the lymph node. The cause of this is not certain but it might represent black tattoo pigment and it would be worthwhile checking whether the patient has any tattoos in this area.*
>
> *Material from this case has been referred to King's Hospital for an expert opinion... and has been reported as follows: "The lymph node architecture is effaced by confluent neoplastic follicules predominantly composed of centrocytes and occasional centroblasts. There is extracapsular spread is seen. (sic) There is also black pigment seen suggesting Tattoo.*

Diagnosis right neck lymph node (excision) Low grade follicular lymphoma (WHO grade 1-2).

At the final count, aside what could be seen under my skin and the wet bed B symptoms, my diagnosis was confirmed by a combination of lymph node biopsy reports from histology and microbiology, plus three CT scans. A second biopsy revealed my bone marrow to be "bubbling over" with cancer and a further lymph node needle biopsy reinforced the mess my body was in. However it was described, it was all going to get a whole lot worse before it got a whole lot better.

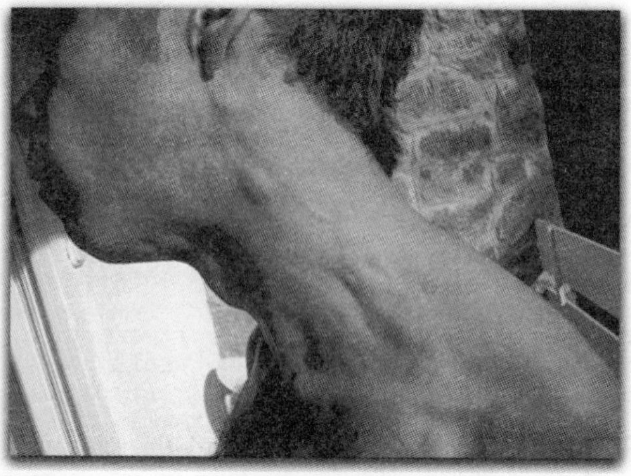

Early stages. Non-Hodgkin's lymphoma is increasingly common and we now have evidence of why this might be.

My haematologist (blood specialist) asked me early on what I thought about tattoos being involved in my cancer. I think it likely. Officially they don't know what causes most cancers so pick on our genes, but no one's really interested asking too many questions beyond that in case the truth comes out and the truth is shocking. I am and I found an even more interesting explanation that took me back to an original cause of my cancer way back at the beginning of my time. For some reason ink was lodged in my lymph system, and maybe in everyone who has tattoos? We have hundreds of lymph nodes making up an elimination organ for filtering out waste. Tattoo ink is composed of poisonous materials any fully functional entity would want rid of. I last had a tattoo 13 years previous, suggesting my lymphatic system had been clogged up for some time but I don't believe this to be the cause, only a contributing factor.

In previous years I had read up on cancer and chemo and cancer cures and cancer politics and conspiracies and had formed my opinions, but you don't have to read that much before distinct recurring themes come up. The main one of course is that cancer is considered confusing and incurable. Another says chemo is helping patients live longer. Then there is the confusion surrounding the purpose of treatment, and the question of the urgency with which this process is initiated. The average patient expects treatment to start soon after cancer is discovered, it is *believed* to be urgent, *believed* to be the only way and *believed* to be curative. Studies invariably reveal that the majority of cancer patients feel they did not get the full story from their doctors and have no idea if their chemo is meant to be curative or palliative. Some patients are given chemo to help them feel as though something is being done and indeed some patients are happy with this. Others may get some symptom relief but of course palliative ultimately equates with short lived.

> *Advanced cancer patients commonly have misunderstandings about the intentions of treatment and their overall prognosis. Several studies have shown that large numbers of patients receiving palliative radiation or chemotherapy hold unrealistic hopes of their cancer being cured by such therapies, which can affect their ability to make well-informed decisions about treatment options.*
>
> *[One] study looked into the expectations of patients with incurable lung cancer from palliative radiation therapy, and found that 64% did not report understanding that the treatment was not at all likely to cure them. This study also found that 92% of patients with inaccurate beliefs about radiation therapy also had inaccurate beliefs about chemotherapy.* [4]

The problem stems from doctors' inability or unwillingness to communicate the reality to their patients, since doing so would pour scorn on the cancer research narrative about improved treatments and patients living longer thanks to all that research.

Success of most chemotherapy is appalling...There is no scientific evidence for its ability to extend in any appreciable way the lives of patients suffering from the most common organic cancer... chemotherapy for malignancies too advanced for surgery which accounts for 80% of all cancers is a scientific wasteland.

Dr Ulrich Abel. 1990

[4] http://onlinelibrary.wiley.com/doi/10.1002/jmrs.188/full

It's not the animals. It's you!

Our cancer research is misdirected, inefficient and inadequate. We have almost as many people living off the disease as dying from it. The government spends billions on cancer research but at the same time allows known carcinogens in our processed food, subsidizes cigarettes and continues to develop new radiation, surgical and chemotherapy techniques when burning, cutting and poisoning have already proved largely unsuccessful. Physicians have not been trained in preventative medicine and, not having experience or knowledge of preventative medicine, they continue the outmoded but orthodox approach of treating symptoms rather than the entire body.

Dr Richard O 'Brennan, Coronary? Cancer? God's Answer: Prevent it!

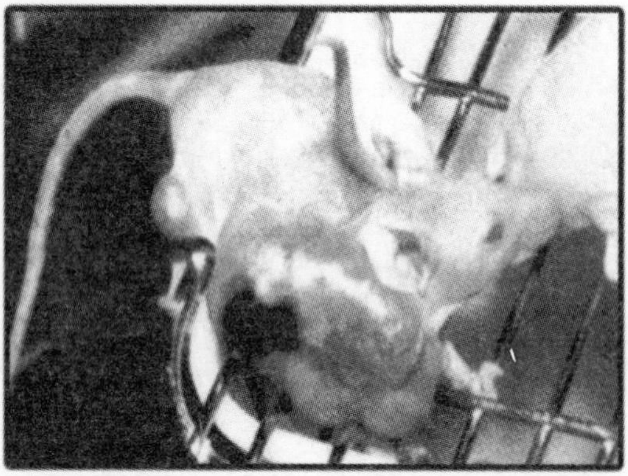

Animal experiments are another recurring theme and their role is confusing too. There's one school of thought which says that lab animals have been the saviour of humankind, but that's not what the evidence says. This was personal to me long before I discovered a direct link between experiments on monkeys and the cancer growing in me. There is a clear cycle of profit and in a few rats anything can be proven or disproven depending on who is paying for the results and these creatures form the foundation of the orthodox medical vision. But when it comes to actually healing another species, the science of vivisection is a little too simplistic and much too crude. Embedded in the claim of necessity is the implication that this desperate drive for cures is so crucial and complicated that other living systems are needed, without which we can never understand. And of course no one would inflict horrors if it weren't essential to do so. What kind of sick monster would vivisect another being!

We believe these people are just like us and so wouldn't do terrible things to others, but they aren't and they do.

A vast interlocking interdependent industry has built up providing a wide variety of differing strains of rats and mice and beagles, some designed to grow cancer like they grow hair, there are strains that grow no hair, then there are the cage and feed manufactures, the transport companies and specialised vehicles, the surgical instruments and restraining devices and endless wicked torture tools and all manner of associated sundries. We used to protest outside one of the businesses that took its piece of this pie from disposing of all the corpses used in the nearby lab. It's not all doom and gloom though; there's money to be made from recycling dead animals and sick people.

Essential medical research they call it. Business is what it is. And the animals are products from which to return the best profit possible, as we all are. Cancer, viewed as a group of more than 100 different diseases and caused by as many factors, has become highly lucrative, lumped into one broad-spectrum treatment package with the large variety of animal models keeping it all circulating.

An alternative to testing on other animals would of course be to test on humans, which is easy when we move away from the toxic drug model. Like I did! I decided that the dog on the sofa was not perhaps the best model for me to use to heal my body and instead did some study on me and what do you know! Oh and by the way I'm going to add in an interesting story about that very dog and his simultaneous cancer journey, which didn't turn out as well as mine but may nevertheless be of help.

Rats and mice are the favourite tool for proving nothing very much about human health. They are compact, docile and easy to handle and they aren't very human like, which is another good reason we should care. They have created all manner of mice to research and profit from, such as the Knockout mouse. This poor soul is a patented genetically modified being and there are hundreds of versions of them.

They use them to study the role of genes by knocking out existing genes and replacing them with others that don't belong so that researchers can "infer their probable function." The 'genius' who came up with this idea got a Nobel Prize. The people at Creative-Animodel boast that of the 106 Nobel Prize awards in Physiology or Medicine, "94 were directly dependent on animal experiments." But what became of all these prize worthy discoveries? You might well ask.

These kindly souls have all manner of animals for sale and boast:

> *The development of animal models played important roles in every aspect of clinical research. From diagnostic to treatment of disease, from efficiency to safety test of new therapy, animal models were used in all steps of medical research. Here at Creative Animodel, we provide the best and most comprehensive service in animal models. Our service includes but is not limited to genetically engineered model creation, animal models of disease, preclinical services, xenograft model creation, and genotyping.*

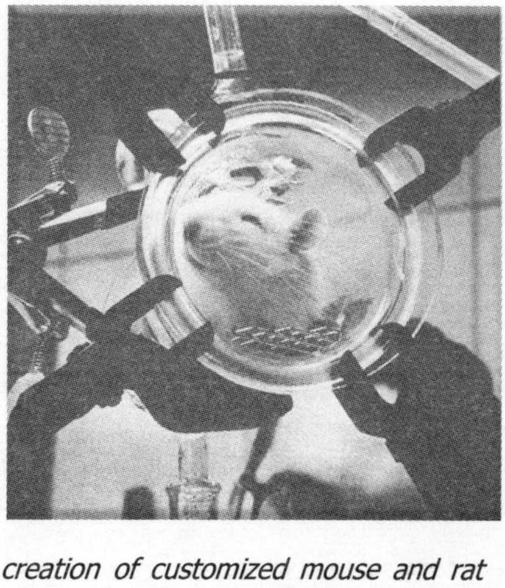

> *We offer full service for design and creation of customized mouse and rat strain. We provide animal models and preclinical service for common and uncommon human diseases. Moreover, our diverse xenograft models*

of hematological malignancies and solid tumor are cutting-edge research in the fields. And we also have genotyping service that are fast, accurate and affordable. Our service and models have assisted researchers in both academic and clinical area all over the world to faster and better achieve their goals. [5]

Pick a disease and they'll fix up some designer mice and ship them to you. They have a 'Knockout repository' of 249 varieties, each afflicted with some dysfunction or other for dysfunctional disease researchers to try and fix. Typically when they've done with these miniature 'disease models' the scientists move up through the species and when their idea of science shows what they see as potential (to turn a profit, publish a paper or win a prize) they then go on through the process of multiple clinical trials using increasing numbers of human victims, every one desperately hoping the horror stories of animal torture and of cutting edge scientific research and of ground breaking medical developments has some meaning for them.

All of this 'cure seeking' takes years and countless lives so you would imagine there has to be something significant in it all, but as we are learning things are seldom as they appear. What this recycling of ideas is doing is taking us further away from the simple natural path that has served humanity and the rest of the natural world for all time, and into a bit of a mess.

Alzheimer's is a graveyard for expensive drug tests. One study showed that between 2000 and 2012, 244 compounds were tested in 413 clinical trials. Only one was approved for use, a failure rate of 99.6 percent. Cancer drug tests fail at 81 percent. In at least one case, a potential Alzheimer's drug test was stopped because it appeared the drug could potentially kill subjects, showing how little is known about potential treatments even when testing has already begun. [6]

Hooray for the animal tests! A little investigation and it becomes clear that the answer to human ills does not and cannot rest with these crude primitive theories. And it isn't just that they haven't been able to find any cures but they are actively suppressing them and it has become much more sinister than just harassing the opposition as we shall see. Seriously folks the world is not the place we think it is and it's time we came to terms with this.

Innovators are rarely received with joy, and established authorities launch into condemnation of newer truths, for... at every crossroads to the future there are a thousand self-appointed guardians of the past.
Betty MacQuitty, Victory Over Pain: Morton's Discovery of Anesthesia

---

5 https://www.creative-animodel.com/

6 https://www.insidescience.org/news/failure-upon-failure-alzheimers-drugs

The Original Organic Hand-Crafted Cure

I see in Gerson one of the most eminent geniuses in the history of medicine. Many of his basic ideas have been adopted without having his name connected with them. Yet, he has achieved more than seemed possible under adverse conditions. He leaves a legacy which commands attention and which will assure him his due place. Those whom he has cured will now attest to the truth of his ideas.
Dr Albert Schweitzer, Nobel Laureate who was himself cured of TB by Gerson.

Max Gerson was a German Jew living in Germany at that time. He was also a very bright man and a doctor and he had a strong instinctive desire to help people. This combined is a heavy burden for one man to carry in modern human society and sure enough Gerson soon had everyone out to get him. Not just the SS but also fellow doctors and the very medical profession he was governed by, because he was curing people! This sounds ridiculous I know and trust me I have experienced *that* reaction from people when they hear such claims, but the truth is stranger than fiction and as ever it only takes a brief spell of homework to confirm this. Gerson had courage and he was motivated to build upon what he discovered. Max Gerson is my interpretation of a hero. To be clear the Gerson Therapy did not cure me, but the Gerson principle of detoxification and nutrition is the foundation of an anti-cancer environment whoever you are and whatever you think you know and it will forever remain my foundation.

On this foundation we have built something equally awesome.

Nearly 100 years ago Dr Max Gerson out of personal desperation discovered a way to cure his own crippling migraine headaches that would floor him for long periods. His peers were firmly of the view he would simply have to live with them, but this was his life and that wasn't a viable option. Exploring all possibilities Gerson read medical papers relating to diet and illness written by those who had gone before him and through a process of eliminating foods from his own diet, experimenting upon himself, he began to identify aggravating factors such as salt, fat and chemicals and managed to cure his illness with nutritional management.

This learning process had started for Max Gerson when he was a child, observing with curiosity how the worms in his grandmother's garden would evacuate the soil onto which she had applied newly marketed chemical fertilisers and make for old ground which was still organic and poison free. Now there's a thing, eh! We look at a worm and think it is just a worm but that simple instinctive reaction makes worms smarter than the human experts and their business buddies! It struck Gerson that maybe, just maybe, the plant life and the other life would have a similar issue with these products as the worms had and from that simple observation great things grew.

Later on, observing himself he would notice changes in his urine prior to a migraine attack and how it was mostly clear of waste. Two or three days into an attack it would become cloudy, thick and dark and with an elevated sodium content. This intrigued Gerson and caused him to realise in time that sodium was being retained in cells and was detrimental. Once the detox had passed he felt well again and once he had eliminated aggravating factors such as salt and sausages he never suffered again with migraines.

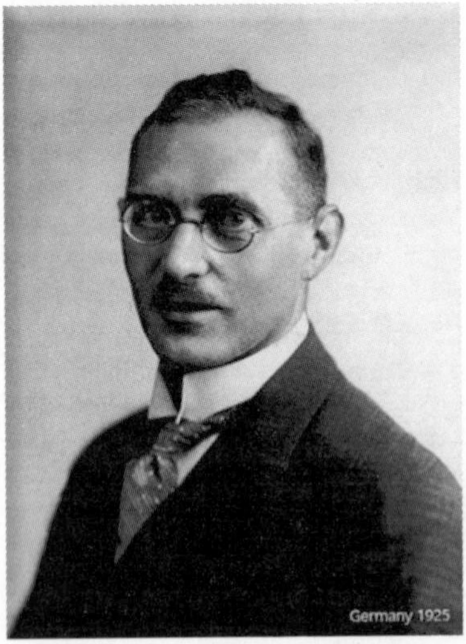

Lupus vulgaris is a skin disease also considered a no-cure area for conventional medicine, but Gerson had stepped out of the box and changed all that single-handedly. Intrigued by the realisation that one of his patients who had tried his elimination diet as a migraine treatment, and succeeded, had additionally observed his long-standing lupus symptoms dissipate. Gerson investigated further. This area was not his speciality and was difficult to fathom but he had surpassed all the specialists and the disease had gone and there wasn't a dead mouse in the house.

Over time, experimenting on willing human patients who had been written off by the medicine men, Max Gerson grew more and more confident he was onto something big. The conclusion of his research could be replicated with every ailment he investigated and what he and his methods have proven, time and time again since the 1920's, cannot reasonably be denied. They are denied of course because human beings seem to be living in denial but the proof as they say is in the pudding. Can we really dismiss all these cured 'incurable' Gerson patients as coincidences? Thousands of them? We do love a coincidence theory to explain away an anomaly or something we don't want to hear or want to think about.

Gerson was a physician whose field was internal and nervous system disorders, so to be treating people with skin disorders and indeed curing them was frowned upon by the medical authorities. Given that Gerson had been curing the incurable one might feel it purely academic that he hadn't been trained to specialise in treating the symptoms of lupus, but this technical detail would form the basis for the official objections to his achievements and guide an attempt to stop him. But Max Gerson was more a humanitarian than a box ticker, he had already achieved two firsts and he was on a roll.

In acknowledgement of successfully treating an incurable skin disease outside his remit, Gerson was hauled before the regional Medical Association - a panel of nine fellow physicians. You'd think he'd have been invited for an award given what he achieved, but as we are discovering it doesn't work like that. "Dr Gerson, you have been accused of a gross breach of medical ethics. As a specialist you are only permitted to treat diseases specified on your nameplate, and none other". They then went on to castigate him for "openly and blatantly" treating this skin disease and warning how it went against all the rules and regulations. This may have been

Europe 100 years ago but this is standard operating procedure and suffocates innovation in healthcare to this day.

Max Gerson was a free thinker and thankfully that's now on the rise again as we awaken from our collective slumber. The foundation of all the healing protocols are based on what this one man pieced together. He responded to his accusers:

> *Gentlemen, I see you have done your research thoroughly, so I cannot, nor would I deny that I have been treating lupus vulgaris. It would be foolish to attempt to deny that lupus is not a skin disease, for it is quite clearly that. However you have not mentioned the contents of the article that I wrote, which demonstrates that **I have cured this disease, not just treated it.***

Gerson proceeded to lecture his accusers about Nobel Prizes awarded to one physician for simply developing a treatment for lupus vulgaris and another to a microbiologist, Dr Robert Koch, for discovering in 1882 the microbe that causes lupus and other tuberculosis conditions. Yet no one offered a cure until Gerson arrived on the scene. The role of microbes in cancer and the cures hidden therein come back to us later in our story and will one day soon haunt the wider medical profession.

Gerson stood his ground and spoke his mind:

> *Today I stand before this panel accused of unethical medical behaviour for having succeeded where so many others have failed before me. I am fully aware of the consequences of being found guilty by the Association, yet I have no fear of your verdict. On the contrary, I would consider it a great honor to be punished or even imprisoned for being the first physician to find a successful treatment for lupus vulgaris.*

That's the attitude!

Gerson's achievements were well known in medical circles and in the communities he served he was something of an urban legend and his accusers were aware that punishing this man would make of him a martyr and that they wouldn't look good. The board had been cornered by an intelligent, articulate and unrepentant Dr Gerson and when they reconvened having weighed up the facts, the tables had turned full circle and the lights had come on.

> *Dr Gerson, the Association congratulates you for your outstanding success in treating lupus vulgaris. We encourage you to continue this aspect of your practice and the excellent research associated with it. The article you gave us leaves us no question as to your high degree of integrity and truthfulness. You will have no further difficulty from the Westphalian Medical Association regarding medical speciality... The hearing is adjourned.* [7]

---

[7] Excerpt from Dr Max Gerson: Healing The Hopeless, Howard Straus

Still no recommendation for a Nobel Prize, but better than all the prizes, awards and accolades that self important people share around each other, Gerson had free reign to use his initiative. Had they voted to punish him or lock him back in the box, the knock-on effect would be a death sentence for thousands of patients, as has become the norm in the intervening years.

Gerson's reputation was put fully to the test in the early 1930's in the first clinical trial of its kind studying this concept of nutrition and the curing of medically incurable disease, in this case tuberculosis. The conclusion of this trial involving 450 patients was simply astounding and is unlikely to ever be matched. This one factor alone stands as a wake-up call and should cause us pause for thought. We will compare later with the best of today's cancer drug clinical trials and get a real feel for how far ahead Gerson was 100 years ago, without the wealth of industry and the might of nations.

It is interesting to note that this trial was almost abandoned due to the actions of one of the nurses assigned to care for the participants. Gerson was absent for a time during the trial and some of the patients had begun to relapse. In his autobiography Master Surgeon, Professor Sauerbruch explains what happened:

> *That afternoon, a nurse called me to an emergency case: a patient had a severe post operative hemorrhage.*
>
> *I hastened along corridors and down stairs and did what was necessary. Pensively, I was strolling back along the corridor near the lupus ward, when I saw a nurse, the fattest nurse in the building, carrying an enormous tray loaded with sausages, bowls of cream and jugs of beer. It was four o'clock in the afternoon, hardly the time for such a feast in a hospital. In amazement I stopped and asked her where on earth she was going with all that food. And then the whole story came out.*
>
> *"I couldn't bear it any longer, Herr Gereimrat", she explained. "Those poor patients with skin TB. The stuff they are given - no one could eat it!"*
>
> *She was astonished when I dashed her tray to the ground. It was one of the occasions when I completely lost my temper.*
>
> *Every day at four o'clock, when no one was around, she had been taking the patients a nice appetizing, well seasoned meal.*
>
> *I sent a telegram to Dr Gerson, asking him not to open the letter I had written him. [with regard to abandoning the failing study]*
>
> *We were back at the beginning again, and from that moment we took extra precautions in guarding the lupus wing. In comparison, a prison would have been a holiday camp.*

> *Soon Dr Gerson proved right. Soon nearly all our patients recovered; their sores disappeared almost under our very eyes.*
>
> *In this experiment involving 450 patients, only four could not be cured by Dr Gerson's saltless diet.* [8]

The take home message from this impressive example of how it can be done is clear. Nutrition is crucial in the treatment of disease and in the promotion of disease.

People often invite that "surely a little won't hurt?" as they will us to risk further disease. A rational proposal that we consume something we don't want, like cheese, chocolate, wine or a piece of that lovely wedding cake, but no thanks. These are someone else's desire, I have my own. Would we offer granny a nice bag of chips if she was told to avoid fat? Or a couple of fags to help granddad deal with his emphysema? I was a happy vegan but not so healthy, now I'm happy and healthy and vegan. I no longer have cravings for anything unhealthy and manufactured and should I, I'll be the one to choose my poison. These small details matter when trying to heal but we can be a little more flexible with food in the absence of disease. If we want to we can get away with the odd bit of toast, but why risk the pleasure of the artificial flavours becoming a habit and a little bit too convenient? And how long does it take before doing the wrong thing catches up and the piece of toast turns into a fried breakfast just once a week and at weekends and special occasions?

Early on, in spite of his successes with migraines, lupus and then allergies, kidney disease, arthritis and more, Gerson hadn't even considered that cancer could be cured nutritionally. When the idea was proposed to him he was dismissive and considered it crazy. In 'A Cancer Therapy – results of 50 cases' in which Gerson summaries 30 years of clinical experience and fully documents 50 cases of cancer patients sent home to die who he recovered and sent home cured, he explains how he only discovered it was possible to do this because his first experimental patient had begged and bullied him to try and save her life with his method.

It is a funny story, he recalls:

> *When I was a physician for internal diseases in Bielefeld in 1928, one day I was called to see a lady. I asked her what was wrong with her but on the telephone she didn't want to tell me. So I went there, a little outside of town. Then I asked her 'What's wrong?' She told me she was operated on in a big clinic nearby and they found cancer of the bile duct. I saw the operation scar. She was running a high fever, was jaundice. I told her, 'Sorry, I can do nothing for you. I don't know how to treat cancer. I have not seen the results, especially in such an advanced case where there is no longer the possibility of operation.' So, she said, 'No, doctor, I called because I saw the results in your treatment of tuberculosis and arthritis in various cases. Now, here is a pad and you write down a treatment. On that table over there is a*

---

[8] From Dr Max Gerson: Healing the Hopeless – Howard Straus

> *book, and in that book, you will be good enough to read to me aloud the chapter called 'The Healing of Cancer'.*
>
> *It was a big book of about 1200 pages on folk medicine and in the middle there was that chapter. I started to read. That book was edited by three school teachers and one physician. None of them practiced medicine. So they put together that book. I read that chapter. In it there was something about Hippocrates who gave these patients a special soup. I should like to tell you, we use that soup at the present time! That soup from that book, out of the practice of Hippocrates - 550 years before Christ! He was the greatest physician at that time, and I even think the greatest physician of all time. He had the idea that the patient had to be detoxified with the soup and the enemas and so on.*
>
> *I read and I read but finally I told the lady, look because of my tuberculosis treatment physicians are opposed to me. Therefore I'd like not to treat you. Again she insisted, 'I'll give you in writing that you are not responsible for the outcome of the treatment and that I insisted that you do so.' So with that signed statement I thought, all right, let's try.*
>
> *I wrote down the treatment. It was almost the same which I used for tuberculosis patients which I had worked out in the University of Munich with Prof. Sauerbruch. After the work at the University Clinic the treatment had been established and had been found effective. I thought it may well be effective in cancer too. It is always written in the scientific books that tuberculosis and cancer are both degenerative diseases where the body has to be detoxified. But this latter thought was written only by Hippocrates.*
>
> *I tried and the patient was cured! Six months later she was up and around in the best condition. Then she sent me two other cancer cases. One of her family members with a stomach cancer where it had been found during an attempted operation that there were metastasised glands around the stomach - also cured! And I had to cure then, against my will, a third case. I expected to have still more opposition from the medical profession, the third case was also a stomach cancer.*

Gerson freely admitted he didn't understand fully what he was seeing and tells of the next six cases he treated in Austria after leaving Germany, all of which failed:

> *The sanatorium where I treated my patients was not so well organised for dietary treatments. They treated other diseases by other methods and didn't pay much attention to diet. So, I attributed the failures to that.* [9]

In time he treated thousands of patients, many who had been sent home to die; hopeless cases with advancing cancer. Some he allowed to live with him, treating for free, observing and curing. "Cured", insists Gerson repeatedly as he goes through

---

[9] From Dr Max Gerson: Healing the Hopeless – Howard Straus

his patient list in a broken German accent. "Sent home to die. Cured! Sent home to die. Cured!"

Max Gerson was an innovator and there's no telling what he would have achieved with one of those cancer charity blank cheques. It is interesting to me, knowing what I now know, to see just how close Gerson comes throughout his career to joining the next piece of the cancer puzzle. The previous passage is from a lecture he gave in 1956, in which he draws attention to what Hippocrates thought about a link between TB and cancer. That link is a simple microbe. And that is where we will be focussing our attention. Alternatively, we can continue to feed the greedy monster waging that long-lost war on all those tumours.

Good luck with that.

So, coincidence or conspiracy Max Gerson like many others have been dragged over the coals and had their lives made very difficult for being that little bit too smart. And their innovation ignored. Not disproven. Unapproved by those with control of the approval process. There's a world of difference. The Holiday Inn won't approve the Ritz Hotel to its customers. That would not make the Ritz a crappy place to stay. It's all about the competition, innit? The opposition. The people who will take your money if you send them your customers, breaking the first rule of business. Of course they don't approve!

Chemotherapy is highly approved of and has the market (cancer patients) flooded with the stuff. And in the minds of those delivering these products of death that's exactly how it's going to stay. This, in spite of the fact they don't cure cancer and no, they don't go through the much acclaimed super science double blind placebo trial testing process to see if chemo patients would do better or worse with no chemo. Believe it or not drug makers most often dodge testing these vile products to this scientific placebo benchmark. Instead new drugs and vaccines are tested against each other in a kind of creepy battle to the death, with the odd sugar pill thrown in and the science thrown out. Because the placebo reveals the truth they have sought to eliminate it.

There is no financial incentive and nothing to be gained for the market holders to compare their broad chemo catalogue with any other treatment or therapy, a new idea or even against nothing. Any chink in the armour would mean death to the status quo, and this modified testing system where the poisons always win looks for all the world like a loophole plugged.

The purveyors of these chemical products of fearsome reputation are playing a dangerous game using their made-up rules to market mostly useless, mostly dangerous drugs, and no one else is allowed to compete. They will inevitably win because the game is rigged, so we stop participating or we keep on dying.

Max Gerson established from studying the research of others and from his own clinical observations with live patients and the process of disease, that the human body is perfectly capable of fixing almost anything if given the right conditions. Drugs don't do that.

Gerson's first three successes in the treatment of cancer occurred in 1929 and it has never stopped, it just isn't publicised. With the politics of Germany in the 1930's Gerson and his immediate family were soon fugitives and would spend the coming years dodging detention. Next stop Austria then France, the UK and finally America.

Soon established and back in business by 1946 Gerson's reputation had carried him into the US Senate. In a once in a lifetime opportunity he was invited by a sympathetic senator to present proof of his concept to the US policy makers, who controlled a one hundred million dollar cancer war chest. This was 26 years before the war on cancer was officially launched and they're still attacking tumours and losing! In breaking this new ground Gerson made his case loud and clear. He lined up more cured patients and more documentary proof of his brilliance than would be necessary to convince a jury, but that wasn't going to wrestle this pot of gold from the pharmaceutical interests with all their talk of patented cancer cures just around the corner.

In spite of the testimony of the living witnesses and Dr Gerson himself, the Pepper-Neely Bill which sought funding for further research into the first proven cancer cure in history was defeated by a mere four votes. Deciding votes were cast by senators who were also medical doctors, funny enough. Medical doctors treat disease with drugs and they do very well thank you very much, they do not seek to heal.

And as such another deeply significant moment in history was recorded as Bill S.1875 was set aside and the future direction of cancer funding was diverted to pharmaceutical drug production.

Max Gerson died in the US in 1959.

And the rest is history, albeit not confined to. The Gerson Therapy has been revitalised by youngest daughter Charlotte in recent years and saves lives in spite of mainstream medicine. Charlotte at the time of writing is well into her 90's. Ever courageous and well informed she grew up close to her father who she adored, as did his patients. Charlotte hung out with her father from a young age and lent a hand in the care of his patients so witnessed firsthand the implementation of his ideas and the remarkable progress he made with those incurables sent home to die.

We are told 1 in 2 of us are now destined to get cancer in the near future and most will die from the effects, this often means malnutrition or infection brought about by the toxic, cancer causing treatment that target the tumour and kill what's left of the immune system. Meanwhile doctors are taught virtually nothing about nutrition, and the micronutrient building blocks of life, let alone the phytonutrients, while at the very best they encourage patients to eat five servings of fruit and vegetables each day, grown in cancer causing poisons. The perversity is, of course, that we know about the food link when dealing with hyperactive kids, osteoporosis, type 2 diabetes, scurvy, heart disease and even cancer and we know pesticides cause cancer. If it is a diet of chemical grown food and a course of chemical treatment that takes your fancy then that is what you should do and you'll get plenty of encouragement.

Just enthusiastically we encourage each other to go to the doctor when health issues arise. But do we even stop to ask to what end? We should. I did as I was pressurised by others to do as my doctor advised, but the only response I received was to be told "they know best". Really? If all else fails we can try to cling to such dire predictions of 50% with cancer, imagining we will be one of the lucky ones, but that would be to assume someone else will do the caring for our loved ones if they happen to be in the other 50%. This is about all of us.

I got home from being diagnosed in August 2013 and the first thing I did was break open a new bag of coffee and brew up a coffee enema on the bathroom floor. For pain or ill-ease I invite everyone to consider the bum hole as first port of call. If we consider that everything is upside down and that shovelling all that stuff down the other hole, as we do, isn't really helping us achieve longevity, why not! Coffee enemas are safe, effective and essential in healing. I've done thousands since that date and the word is spreading, as personal hygiene takes on new meaning and this simple cleansing act finds its place as we come to terms with the real possibility of healing. We'd also purchased a decent juicer and were already setting up at home having begun to establish a Gerson household with a view to repairing Alice. The cupboards were cleared of all the processed rubbish and chemical cleaning products, the aluminium cookware replaced by stainless steel and glass and the enema buckets prepped and ready for action.

Enemas were good enough for Florence Nightingale and the Egyptians and even Hippocrates was tweeting, but the experts of today and a billion hangers-on think they know better. They don't. Next to cannabis oil there is nothing more valuable and non-toxic for pain relief. Coffee enemas were actually in the arsenal of modern medicine and officially advocated within the orthodox medical bible, the Merck Manual, from the late 1800's until the late 1970's after which they were deleted from the public record. The hippie herb can't be patented either and would put a big chink in the armour were it legalised. Almost as soon as the coffee goes in the positive effects are felt. I cannot foresee a time when I stop using them and to the average Gersonite this is as normal as having that bottle of wine.

Twelve to fifteen minutes lying on the right side allowing a litre of warm specially prepared organic coffee to stimulate one's bile and rinse one's liver is a jolly good idea. This in itself is useful downtime in the hectic schedule and becomes more of a treat than an effort. Much more helpful and normal than the dose of radiation that they use to look inside us! I started on the bathroom floor with a pillow, a book, an enema mat or towel, rubber gloves and instant access to the toilet. The toxic elimination event can be a matter of urgency, but I've handled it well and soon moved to the sofa for my coffee breaks. Even had occasion to answer the postman en route to evacuation, much to Alice's amusement. I haven't discussed this with the postman. I'm happy to but there's a time and a place.

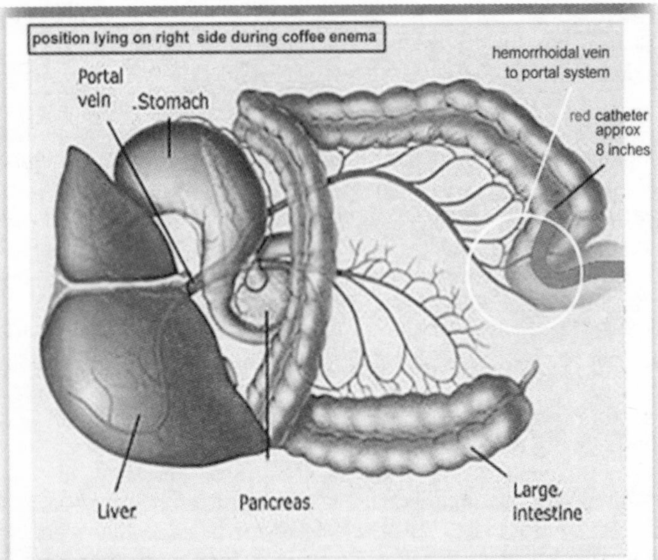

why 6-8 inch insertion of catheter? The distance from anus over the bump where the hemorrhoidal vein is located is 5-6 inches. Its important to get past that so the coffee absorbs into the vein system which begins past that point. **why lie on right side?** This lets gravity do its job. The purple veins are on the right side of the colon. This position facilitates the caffeine getting to the liver quickly. Its very important to use the soft red catheter NOT the hard tube that comes with the enema bucket.

We changed our water supply to reverse osmosis and distilled, we use 3% food grade hydrogen peroxide and vinegar for cleaning. It was a steady shift to a fresh start.

Natural therapies such as Gerson and our more evolved creation are comprehensive. Holistic. Wholesome. Coming at it from all angles. The whole story is *most* important! Ours is a lifestyle therapy which requires a whole new way of thinking and tuning into the natural rhythms rather than fighting with them. Traditionally the aim for 100 years has been to kill the bad cancer cells forming the tumours and the more aggressive the cancer, the more aggressive the kill. This is a fully documented disaster. The modern orthodox proving ground is the randomised double-blind placebo controlled blah blah blah, a medical test designed for chemical drugs with a sole purpose to block a pathway, kill a disease or replace a nutrient. Such a simplistic test cannot cope with something as sophisticated as whole body healing with multiple variables. Our way requires distilled water for daily enemas brewed as we might a fine wine, organically grown nutrient dense meals, pulped juice, nutritional supplements, magnetic pulsing, blood cleaning, ozone water and a complete shift in thinking lasting a lifetime. No drugs, no doctors, no vaccines, no junk food.

Of course there are no studies! It would be foolish to think it possible to pretend to squeeze all this into such a limiting, pill centric study designed over decades to streamline drug distribution.

We have seen the remarkable outcome of one early clinical test of nutrition. Here's another hint at what it can do in this retrospective review recorded on PubMed:

Five-year survival rates of melanoma patients treated by diet therapy after the manner of Gerson: a retrospective review.

OBJECTIVE:
Compare 5-year melanoma survival rates to rates in medical literature.

SETTING:
Hospital in Tijuana, Mexico.

PATIENTS:
White adult patients (N =153) with superficial spreading and nodular melanoma, aged 25-72 years.

INTERVENTION:
Gerson's diet therapy: lactovegetarian; low sodium, fat and (temporarily) protein; high potassium, fluid, and nutrients (hourly raw vegetable/fruit juices). Metabolism increased by thyroid; calorie supply limited to 2600-3200 calories per day. Coffee enemas as needed for pain and appetite.

MAIN OUTCOME MEASURE:
5-year survival rates by stage at admission.

RESULTS:
Of 14 patients with stages I and II (localized) melanoma, 100% survived for 5 years, compared with 79% of 15,798 reported by Balch. Of 17 with stage IIIA (regionally metastasized) melanoma, 82% were alive at 5 years, in contrast to 39% of 103 from Fachklinik Hornheide. Of 33 with combined stages IIIA + IIIB (regionally metastasized) melanoma, 70% lived 5 years, compared with 41% of 134 from Fachklinik Hornheide. We propose a new stage division: IVA (distant lymph, skin, and subcutaneous tissue metastases), and IVB (visceral metastases). Of 18 with stage IVA melanoma, 39% were alive at 5 years, compared with only 6% of 194 from the Eastern Cooperative Oncology Group. Survival impact was not assessed for stage IVB. Male and female survival rates were identical for stages I-IIIB, but stage IVA women had a strong survival advantage.

CONCLUSIONS:
The 5-year survival rates reported here are considerably higher than those reported elsewhere. Stage IIIA/B males had exceptionally high survival rates compared with those reported by other centers.[10]

---

[10] https://www.ncbi.nlm.nih.gov/pubmed/9359807

So it *does* work! The Gerson Therapy does cure cancer.

Curiously, perhaps, when you look for evidence of the efficacy of the better well known and most profitable cancer drugs you find something equally interesting. We hear an awful lot how chemo is "helping patients to live longer". They all make this fantastic claim - Macmillan Cancer Support, Cancer Research UK, talking heads, politicians, medical students, the repeaters. So I go to see how much longer patients are living thanks to chemo, and oh my goodness!

First thing you find is that term "living longer" is cruel and subjective and so precarious in this circumstance it is often highlighted by a decimal point conveying the extra days one might live. And crucially there is no placebo baseline for comparison so the claim is false anyway. What we find when these study statistics are unravelled, and account has been taken of the various adjustments that are made to refine participants in these not so random trials, what we are left with at best is an additional 4 or 5 weeks of life. More like drugged to death! And even then there's wriggle room on whether the cancer treatment alone can be credited for these bonus days of dying. It is equally questionable that the poisons killed people quicker than no intervention at all! One trick that shows up time and again in these 'randomised' trials funded by industry, is the editing out of weaker patients who for example may be unlikely to survive to the end of the trial either due to age or disease status or whatever, leaving only a selection to participate. This is not random and is not representative of how it works in the real world and as such improves the outcome, or makes the drugs look a little better than awful.

In the real world the disease process is barely affected by these drugs, without getting into the side effects they cause. But the sucker punch comes for many once the cancer treatment has failed and the oncologist reveals the open secret about there being "nothing more" they can do. The average cancer patient has been led into a false sense of hope and now there's no way back. All of the cancer experts and all the doctors know that the ever weakened human body can only take so much before the chemo wins.

Medical students traditionally learn more about the practice of gradual disclosure than about nutrition. It's what I see as the trickle feed trap door and as the truth is revealed the vast majority of cancer patients will experience that terrible sinking feeling in the hands of their chemotherapist. Isn't false hope exactly what orthodox medicine accuses the competition of? The people they call quacks. The people who guided me back to health. That makes me a "quack lover" apparently, which I think is preferable to being dropped through a trap door, but each to their own!

Back in our world at the end of 2013 Alice is in limbo and I have cancer. Grandma has been and gone again. We are no longer squatting and have a rented flat on the south coast, so far south we can hear the waves on the beach. We have seagulls and storms and it is ideal for healing. And best of all, our neighbour's dog soon adopts and moves in with us. Taz was loved but he wasn't previously allowed on the sofa or the bed, but we do things differently and the dog loved that. In fact he ran around in circles and wee'd himself in excitement the first time he was told to jump on the bed! We are also in a lot just now and he likes that too. This dog was another gift.

A month after my diagnosis we spent two weeks at the Gerson clinic in Hungary, thanks entirely to dear friends who covered the £5,000 cost and to who we are eternally grateful. Knowing what I know now I wouldn't spend the money that way. There is another Gerson clinic in Mexico. None here or in the US due to the laws in place to stop people healing with non-toxic protocols. Open up a Gerson clinic in the land of the free or some place that the people "never, never, never will be slaves" and the authorities will shut you down. It was a nice experience but with hindsight I wouldn't have gone, but then how would I know it wasn't necessary? The cost is not excessive, all things considered, and from such an experience comes the real possibility to heal. But the principles of food preparation are easy to understand and advice is available closer to home, from where we are in a much better place anyway to monitor our own progress using the latest technology. Regular Gerson practitioner reviews add to the bill, and with the benefit of that hindsight and a flawed personal experience I think money is better spent on you nearer home. We actually did a better job of sticking to the long-established Gerson rules than we were taught to do so at the Gerson clinic, where we found corners being cut.

Late in 2013 I had the pleasure of experiencing signs of the healing reactions that accompany the healing process. As the immune system gains strength it begins to dump the accumulated toxins buried deep in the cells and organs. Early on in his experience Max Gerson lost patients through this process as the toxic dumping was too much for them to handle, hence the utilisation of coffee enemas. These things freak out the closed-minded medicine men, who are more prone to probing the anus of patients with cameras and fingers, but have been used to detoxify the liver and as pain management for many years. When used in conjunction with organic juices to maintain a healthy balance of electrolytes, 5 or 6 enemas can be done in a day. These healing reactions, or flare ups, vary greatly but occur once the body has the strength to begin dumping toxins and while they might not be pleasant, they are typically short lived, mine extending for 72 hours on occasion and a very encouraging indictor of the unwanted leaving.

Dr Gerson was achieving cures in a matter of weeks 100 years ago and was close at hand to monitor the progress of his patients. Nowadays this monitoring has to be done from a distance and the situation is far from ideal. This is why it is important that we gain the courage to choose our treatment not have it chosen for us. We aim to be our own doctors with them working for us, not against us, doing as we say not as Big Pharma says. Ultimately, collectively we need to take back control of the medical system so it works for people not profit. Today the Gerson Institute advise that it can take two or three years or more to achieve healing and I would apply that equally to whatever path we choose and with whatever cancer. That we can heal at all is mind blowing, but the added time it now takes and the extra elements may be in part due to the increased toxicity we have to deal with today and the increasingly denatured food which contains fewer micronutrients and other elements, such as sulphur and magnesium, which are especially important. It is also perhaps unhelpful that the Gerson Institute isn't moving with the times.

With Alice coordinating this project from her bed, researching, ordering supplies and so on, I did the other. It was hard going in the beginning but we figured it out and made it an exciting and pleasurable experience. We had many offers of physical help but that can create its own issues, so we opted to do it our way for the most part. Led by Kerry and Maria, my cancer campaign teams' online fundraising efforts evolved in unison so we were able to actually pay for this project. There were gigs lined up, auctions, sponsored all sorts and friends dipping into their pockets. You find out who your friends are when you need them and ours stepped up in droves, including many we have never even met. Our gratitude is more than words and I hope this book will serve as some reward.

These are good people and we have a good team; how could we fail?

Ha! Failure was a possibility but we seldom discussed it and it seemed less likely the more people rallied to help us, the easier this new lifestyle became and the further toward the mythical two-year benchmark we got. However! Unbeknown to all, there was always a bigger story building, something quite unbelievable.

For all the work we put in over the next two years, Gerson couldn't catch my cancer and it continued to spread. By the August of 2015 we had trashed our plan to cure me with Gerson and went back to the drawing board. I didn't change how I feed myself or stop the enemas but I desperately needed to kill some cancer. I cannot be sure why Gerson didn't do it for me but I don't think it helped matters that five months in, at my second review, my Gerson practitioner reduced my protocol. From a present moment perspective this reduction was a relief for us as it released some of the daily intensity and some cost, but it was surely too soon.

Further to this, for the few weeks prior to diagnosis we were able to count seven lymph nodes in my neck and five in my groin. Then in the June of 2013 I had one surgically removed from my right collar which confirmed cancer. In theory that should have left me with one less lump of cancer to deal with but we actually noticed a distinct rise in the number of tumours over the coming months, which we seemed to have gained some control over until my protocol was tweaked and off it went again on an unstoppable spread. It is our view that the biopsy sped it up.

My very visual tumours were both a blessing and curse throughout this experience. While it has been useful to be able to monitor them myself at home, waking every morning to see these things in the mirror or feel them when I stroked my neck, shaved or washed under my arms, it also meant there was no escaping the reality facing me. Especially when they noticeably grew. This growth was ever so subtle but you know when it's happening and it is very intimidating and just knowing it's there is stifling. The idea of more people living longer with cancer sounds to me like such a retarded compromise and not something we should be getting excited about. Living with cancer means you will die because of cancer or the treatment and if you let the crazies loose on it that will come much sooner than their cure.

And on the 8th day God created Big Pharma
(to fill in any gaps)

Perhaps the greatest obstacle that frontier scientists are unprepared for but inevitably face is political - the tendency for human systems to resist change, to resist the impact of new discoveries, especially those that challenge the status quo of the scientific establishment...

"Science" has become institutionalised and is largely regulated by an establishment community that governs and maintains itself... in recent times there has been a narrowing of perspectives resulting in a growing dogmatism, a dogmatic scientism. There is arrogance bordering on worship of contemporary scientific concepts and models... taught in our schools in a deadening way which only serves to perpetuate the dogma.

Strangely, the contemporary scientific establishment has taken on the behaviour of one of its early oppressors: the church. Priests in white coats work in glass-and-steel cathedral-like laboratories, under the rule of bishops and cardinals who maintain orthodoxy through mainstream "peer review".
Beverly Rubik, PhD., director for the Center for Frontier Sciences at Temple University, Philadelphia

Chemo was an option for me to buy some time as we drew up plan B, in spite of my intense distrust of the entire pharma product; I would use it to my benefit if I needed it. Chemo is the easiest cancer question to figure out in cancer research and from this I quickly concluded long before I got to the 11th hour that chemo would always be my last resort and you will see why. My position was ever thus regarding the dreaded pharma drugs as can be seen in a TV interview, if that's what you can call it, in 2007 on the BBC's HARDtalk with Stephen Sackur, when he asks the inevitable...

SS: *Do you use drugs yourself?*
KM: *Well fortunately I've not needed to, no. But I would do, I wouldn't have any objection.*
SS: *You wouldn't?*
KM: *No.*
SS: *If for example you or a close family member or friend developed diabetes, you wouldn't have a problem using insulin?*
KM: *It's not a case of well this has been tested on animals so you're not entitled to use it. These products would have been developed without the animal testing.*
SS: *... blah, blah... [something about my] principles ... so you would be prepared to use it?*
KM: *Well of course I would if I thought it was going to do me some good. I'd certainly use alternatives first and there are many more efficacious alternatives on the market rather than pharmaceuticals, which are doing people an awful lot of damage.* [11]

---

[11] https://www.youtube.com/watch?v=nrNd_OSiDuQ

Principles! Now that is funny! That was 2007 and I have to say it shows more foresight! Not him. I agree with me and I am now able to document two deeply personal experiences that weaved themselves into this story after I started writing it. Also priceless. One was a voluntary participation with the pharma poisons and the other involuntary and I have nothing good to say of either outcome, except they add great impetus to my story and deserve my gratitude for the experience. Helpfully in both cases we get to see the real worth of the best of the best the ortho-docs have on offer and it ain't pretty. I have taken my research to the fullest extreme, in keeping with my perceived persona.

In what could be compared to a tribe making a land grab or a rapist claiming ownership of his victim, comes the idea that having a principled objection to the medical sacrifice of animals automatically makes anything tested on animals the exclusive property of those who do the deed or don't care, and denies all access to those who speak up. The animal tested products are mostly unsafe, ineffective and deadly anyway, long after the animals have been tortured by them. The animal is a distraction, like a freak show. And if the animal is to be credited with every human ailment temporarily relieved, then the animal is to blame when it all goes tits up and the patients keel over. So no one gets punished, except the animals, but who benefits? Clearly the drug makers, the guilty, but do we the consumers really benefit in some way?

I've studied the subject and it is perfectly clear to me that the odds of a cure using chemo are close to zero. A cure to me means not dying with or of cancer. A cancer cure in conventional thinking is typically 5 years symptom free but with a recurrence almost inevitable and anticipated. The clock may begin ticking when treatment starts or when treatment finishes and the 5 years no cancer 'cure' may be 2 years, depending on who you ask. We refer to this moment in time as being in the "all clear" or "in remission." We associate the all clear like a freeway or clear road: full speed ahead with the pre-cancer social life and eating the same food, like it never even happened. That makes us look and feel like we overcame, defied death and got straight back to normal, repeating the same cancer causing behaviour over and over. The same patterns that created the cancer environment and caused the tumours to grow. Repeating the same patterns may paint a pretty life picture but the picture will be the same and we didn't really do anything to positively affect our own destiny. Einstein referred to it as a definition of insanity, though it could equally be described as convenient.

But however we describe it this is the reason why most cancer comes back. They can get us into remission (by blasting to death loads of cancer cells) but they have not a clue how to keep us there (by stopping them re-growing), only we can do that by changing our ways and rebuilding our own broken defences. Such is the futility of simply seeking the death of some cancer cells as a solution, as the goal posts have been moved we are now hearing increasingly of victims left in partial remission, like a bit of a hair cut. Which means the treatment didn't treat all of the tumour let alone every cancer cell. But still "remission" is thrown around and it paints a prettier picture than really is. Partial remission is most often defined as at least a 50% reduction in measurable tumour, which means that up to 50% of the tumour and probably 50% of the cancer remains and all of the reason the cancer formed in the first place. Forget all the fancy phrases I think we'll simply call that a failure. Everyone will soon be in remission following chemo no matter what the response to their overdose of poison. This is another way to create an illusion of progress and something this profession excels at.

I have a place for the word cure back when it belongs, where there is no cancer and will be no cancer. I served a repossession order on the quacks and have recovered the word cure for those of us who want to keep it real!

I also got dragged kicking and screaming into mainstream medicine and its data dumps such as PubMed and the Lancet and The National Institute for Clinical Excellence (NICE), The Journal for Clinical Oncology, Oncology Times, Medline and a whole mess of others. There are a lot of them and many want paying silly money to allow us to view their science papers, which I find incredible and frustrating, so you'd think there must be a lot of medical progress in there worth us paying for, eh? You'd think! These places can be pretty dull for those of us wired another way, but needs must and for my purposes it became very useful. I began looking for evidence, hints, leads, anything that might be useful against cancer, or the opposite. Cancer is after all where the vast medical industrial complex invests its vast resources and so it should be easy to prove what they say.

It was very much in my interest at this point to find evidence of efficacy so I might be able to save my own life. For that reward I would be happy to admit I was wrong about the ortho-docs and their drugs. But alas!

The first thing that strikes you when exploring these peer reviewed scientific journals is the proliferation of studies in which some new but mostly old cancer drug or combinations of such are being 'blind' trial tested not against a placebo (the proverbial sugar pill) but instead against each other, yet they still label it placebo. This is like building a house without foundations or like two football teams playing only against each other throughout the season to prove they're the best in the world. And it's deceptive.

However we compare it, what is clear is that something got switched in the science lab while we were out to lunch and few seem to have noticed. But I noticed and I think it matters. Pattern recognition is a staple of science and repetition is crucial but only when you pay attention and apply the findings.

I get the value of antibiotics, life savers, and look how they're messing that one up! Antibiotics eat through the cell wall of bacteria to kill them but the bacteria are evolving and the antibiotics can't get in. Antibiotics are over prescribed in humans and are used like feed in intensively farmed animals. Many versions such as Isoniazid, Chloromycetin, Clindamycin, Kanamycin have had to be withdrawn for killing people. Anaesthetics are a wonder drug comparable to none. This was brought home to me as I lay in the dentist chair early into my treatment when cleaning up my mouth of toxic mercury. Those fillings have to be removed and replaced with safer material. During this I was trying to focus on anything other than what was being done to me by these two masked figures working around a bright light with various tools inside my mouth. I couldn't feel anything in the way of pain thank you anaesthetics, but I really wanted to be elsewhere. Rather than count sheep (into the back of a van) as we might to try and sleep, I lay there and went through the alphabet looking for the rest of the list of wonder drugs.

Seems we all got stuck around A and even then I am reminded that the recovery from a general anaesthetic can be like living with an illness in itself and how many recovering patients are warned of the devastating side effects that can follow such as depression, which for some can be deep, dark and long lasting? And perhaps worst of all misunderstood. After that it's mostly an alphabet soup of disasters too many to name and creating far too many victims to count. I have compiled a list in the next chapter nonetheless. Look at it! Are we insane? Organic fruits and vegetables don't kill people! I have been generous and listed the multiple chemotherapy drugs under C as one cock up and vaccines get minor league listing that they don't deserve either. And this is only a small selection of an ever expanding list. How is it possible with such a stringent, highly advanced scientific testing system to get it so terribly wrong so often? No, it isn't just clumsy or a coincidence, they are deliberately screwing with us. Once withdrawn from the market in one country these death delivery systems are often re-branded and sold to other nations. What kind of monster would do that? The damage they do this side of death can't really be quantified and no one is really counting that toll.

But some of us are adding things up.

If we approach the cancer problem from a more practical viewpoint – the clinical side – based on the concept of totality, we learn two things: firstly, we have to live near nature, according to our natural development. Secondly, science cannot help us to solve the deep, underlying cause of cancer.

Dr Max Gerson 1949

Exhibit A
- the weapons of mass destruction -

The further a society drifts from the truth, the more it will hate those who speak it.
George Orwell (1903 -1950)

Alredase caused liver toxicity and death.
Avandia led to increased risks of heart attacks and death. GlaxoSmithKline settled 11,500+ law suits with more pending.
Clofibrate for the prevention of heart attacks. It was banned after it had been shown to cause heart attacks and death by cancer. I guess that does juggle the heart attack statistics! A decade long study by the World Health Organisation (WHO) reported that men taking the drug were 25% more likely to die of a broad range of disorders, including cancer, stroke, respiratory disease (and heart attacks) than those who got a placebo.
Chemotherapy has caused cancer and death in countless millions.
Chloramphenicol an antibiotic which caused aplastic anaemia leading to death.
Clioquinol was alleged to cure an upset stomach. Turned out to be neurotoxic caused 1000 deaths, 30,000 blinded or paralysed and was responsible for creating yet another new type of disease called SMON (a severe disease of the nervous system).
DDT - an insecticide and potent neurological poison, causes paralysis, chronic weakness, muscle wasting, brain damage, cancers, infertility, miscarriages, nervous system, liver damage and death. DDT is implicated with the rise in polio.
Digitek killed hundreds in its first 3 months.
Domperidone - dozens killed, hundreds suffered heart attacks.
Duract - a painkiller, withdrawn in 1998 after one year, leaving 68 dead and many with liver failure.
Eraldin caused blindness, death.
Flosint caused death.
Fialuridine caused liver failure, death.
Flamanil caused loss of consciousness.
Gemtuzumab caused deaths.
Ibufenac for arthritis, caused death from liver damage.
Isprotenenol killed approximately 3,500 asthma sufferers.
Ketorolac caused haemorrhage and renal failure.
Lotronex a drug for treating irritable bowel syndrome. Lotronex has been linked to at least five deaths, the removal of one patient's colon and other bowel surgeries.
MEL/29 caused cataracts.
Methaqualone caused severe psychiatric disturbances leading to at least 366 deaths, mainly through murder or suicide.
Methysergide for migraine. Max Gerson cured migraine nearly 100 years ago with nutritional manoeuvres. This chemical treatment also offers a risk of fibrosis, a scarring of the organs which may be serious and, in some cases, fatal.
Nomifensine withdrawn due to serious adverse effects, such as death.

Opren Eli Lilly failed to report 26 UK deaths from Opren to the Food and Drug Administration, when it was seeking an American licence. The widow of one man who died told how:

> *The drug caused his hair to fall out, his kidneys became infected, dried his toe nails and finger nails on both hands and feet, burst two toes on the left foot which never stopped discharging till his death... he couldn't even bear the weight of a sheet on his feet. It is only those of us who have witnessed the sufferings from this drug who can tell of the agonies it produces on the human body.* [12]

There were thousands of victims like this one and many more deaths.
Orabilex caused kidney damage with fatal outcomes.
Osmosin killed 20, many more seriously harmed.
Oxyphenbutazone caused bone marrow suppression and Stevens–Johnson syndrome.
Phenacetin - a painkiller found to block the kidney functions, destroy the kidneys, cause kidney tumours and destroy the red blood corpuscles.
Phenformin caused 20,000 deaths.
Perhexiline was withdrawn from the market in the 1980's due to the emergence of 'unwanted side effects'. Perhexiline is once again being revived in Australia and New Zealand and is trickling into Europe.
Pemoline caused liver failure, the need for organ transplant and death.
Posicor for blood pressure. Lasted one whole year and killed at least 100.
Prenylamin caused sudden death.
Pronap and Plaxin tranquillisers killed tons of babies in South Africa.
Primados caused miscarriages, cerebral palsy, brain damage and children to be born without limbs. The details of which medical experts have covered up for years but the tide is turning. Scottish MP Graeme Morrice is in the fight for clarity:

> *It is beyond comprehension that doctors were encouraged to hide or destroy documents which proved that certain drugs caused adverse reactions.*

Propulsid - a heartburn drug approved in 1993. This is a long-term survivor with 7 years of death to its name. Withdrawn in 2000 after killing at least 300.
Raxar - an antibiotic that lasted 2 years, killed over a dozen. Withdrawn in 1999.
Redux - a diet drug killed over 123 people in just over a year and caused heart-valve damage in countless others. Withdrawn in 1997.
Reserpine to reduce blood pressure, shown to increase the risk of breast cancer, cancer of the brain, the pancreas, the uterus, the ovaries and the skin and is infamous for causing nightmares and depression.
Rezulin for diabetes, survived 3 years withdrawn in 2000 linked to 91 liver failures and 391 deaths.
Rimonabant caused suicide and depression.
Stilboestrol (DES) to prevent miscarriage in pregnant women. Created a vaginal cancer in hundreds of female offspring and can also affect the genital organs of the male offspring. Damage from DES can extend to the third generation too and who knows where it will end, if ever.
Sibutramine - an appetite suppressant caused heart attacks and stroke.

---

[12] http://hansard.millbanksystems.com/commons/1988/mar/17/opren-settlement

Thalidomide - another wonder drug that caused thousands of deaths and deformed thousands of children. We were assured such a tragedy would never be allowed to happen again. Never! They blamed the animals, claiming the ones they used hadn't been the right ones, but they were going to make sure that loophole was secured by many more animals! Science would soon be super scientific; billions of animals would go through hell so everyone could live happily ever after, free of all disease and danger. Children would be safer in the doctor's hands than at home with mummy. Thalidomide was a product of the 1950's and was a clear sign of things to come. All the death drugs in this list and many other doctor-induced diseases went through those animals. In fact we are in the midst an epidemic of expert-induced cock ups, in animal and human alike.
Troglitazone was withdrawn after 3 years after causing at least 63 deaths and other life-threatening liver injury in patients:

> *I believe that the company... deliberately omitted reports of liver toxicity and misrepresented serious adverse events experienced by patients in their clinical studies.* [13]

Trovan - an antibiotic that caused liver failure and death. It was first tested on multiple animal species by Pfizer and on 200 Nigerian children, eleven of whom died in the trial five killed by Trovan and six by another antibiotic it was tested against! Others suffered blindness, deafness, brain damage and meningitis.
Tienilic acid caused hepatitis, liver failure and death. SmithKline pleaded guilty to hiding data related to toxicity while seeking drug approval and to 14 counts of failure to report adverse reactions and 20 counts of selling a misbranded drug. No one responsible was imprisoned or even called derogatory names.
Tolcapone caused liver toxicity and death.
Vivisection is the crime of our time and the cause of more death and suffering in more earthlings than all the drugs and poisons combined. In fact animals are the excuse they use to produce killer drugs.
Vioxx caused between 55,000 and 500,000 deaths in the US alone from heart attacks and strokes. In a class action in an Australian court in 2009 involving over 1000 victims it was revealed in internal email exchanges that Merck staff had drawn up a hit list of doctors known to be critical of Vioxx and had plotted to discredit and "neutralise" them. [14]
Vaccines - pick a number. We are going to inquire of vaccines shortly. There is no adequate official record keeping and the boast of benefit is widespread, but vaccine damage is up there with chemo and vivisection – the three biggest achievements of orthodox medicine after making money.
Zelmid caused Guillain–Barré syndrome.
Zipeprof for coughs, caused severe neurological damage at high doses, seizures and coma.
Zomax 14 dead etc.

This little list represents countless millions of people. The antibiotics Cipro and Levaquin alone account for thousands of direct fatalities and are stacking up

---

[13] Janet B. McGill, an endocrinologist who had assisted in the Warner–Lambert's early clinical testing of Rezulin, wrote in a March 1, 2000 letter to Sen. Edward M. Kennedy (D-Mass.)

[14] https://aftermathnews.wordpress.com/2009/04/27/vioxx-maker-merck-and-co-drew-up-doctor-hit-list/

countless more victims with serious, long lasting 'side effects' yet are still in use. Statins, pick a number. We would also do well to remember that both the passive drug and vaccine side effect reporting system is widely accepted as a failure and recorded reports reflect only between 1 and 10 percent of the actual side effect occurrence. In reality we are talking about millions more victims annually over and above the reported fallout. Every poison thoroughly tested on animals over many years and certified safe and efficacious. Efficacy is the end point of many clinical trials and determines only whether a product produces an expected result under ideal circumstances, such as in a controlled clinical trial. Efficacious drugs reach the market. *Effective* is not the same thing and this is much more important to the patient and will be determined by the outcome in the real world, and we can see how well that pans out!

It's all a bit of a joke but it isn't funny. I started to regret listing these examples once I realised how many there were so stopped. New cancers, dead animals and dead people aplenty but cures are not so easy to find and it is crystal clear from a quick glance through the chemist shop window why this is.

The significance placed on the use of a placebo in the drug trials cannot be overlooked or understated. First of all it tells us there is a clear understanding in the medical world of the power of the mind. That our knowledge may be more powerful than all of the pharmaceutical test substances in the world is encoded in the design of the clinical trial, where the truth must be hidden (blinded) from participants so not to influence the outcome. Isn't that interesting? We are most certainly being kept in the dark and not just about the flavour of the old sugar pill! We know the outcome of using these drugs by now whatever the trials purport to show, but this tacit acknowledgement of something superior gives us something incredible to work with. Our mind creates the world we inhabit and that is a pretty powerful tool because when we open our mind to all possibilities, all possibilities become possible.

Placebo therefore plays only a secondary but significant role as a secret inert substance to measure against the active test substance. It's the yin and yang. But once we apply the power of our minds to the question of health we can do away with the need for testing all this stuff to treat disease symptoms.

Cancer Research UK (CRUK) (appropriately: crook) is littered with these sense/science-less drug studies. Sometimes there are four or five toxic drugs in the mix being tested against each other in just one trial alone and the outcome is never good. These trials are loaded at every level and it isn't just the cancer drugs. Crucially they do the same with the vaccines, the wonders of modern medicine right, the saviour of all mankind? You wish!

As I was, you too may be a little unnerved by the expanded definition of the simple sugar pill. Placebo is no longer likely to be something simple, harmless and benign, what was traditionally a test substance that has **no** pharmacological effect administered as a control in testing experimentally or clinically the efficacy of a biologically active preparation. Most medical 'placebo pills' today are highly toxic and just as likely to be as deadly as the test substance itself.

It's a sham. For example:

> ***Phase III tests are randomized and double blind and involve the experimental vaccine being tested against a placebo (the placebo may be a saline solution, a vaccine for another disease, or some other substance).***[15]

Some other substance? What the Fcuk is that? But this is not science! What is this? An insult to our intelligence is what. Don't ever forget this confession. It was once the mark of what they call science that these trials could calculate how a new test substance compares to doing nothing and from nothing we have a baseline everyone can compare to and can build upon. Not any longer. This pick and mix of poisons in which a chemical drug or combination of such are compared to one another, or to a multiple of other chemical drugs that have often already been on the market and passed through millions of now deceased victims is surely the definition of quackery? And how do we assess the cause of side effects under such circumstances?

I don't want to bore you but a flavour for these trials is important so we know where they're at and we can see why we need to be somewhere else.

The NCI and ACS have embarked on unethical trials with two hormonal drugs, tamoxifen and Evista, in ill-conceived attempts to prevent breast cancer in healthy women while suppressing evidence that these drugs are known to cause liver and ovarian cancer, respectively, and in spite of the short-term lethal complications of tamoxifen. The establishment also proposes further chemoprevention trials this fall on tamoxifen, and also Evista, in spite of two published long-term European studies on the ineffectiveness of tamoxifen. This represents medical malpractice verging on the criminal.

Samuel S. Epstein - The Politics of Cancer

15 https://www.historyofvaccines.org/content/articles/vaccine-development-testing-and-regulation

Exhibit B
- the coded confession -

Chemotherapy combinations can significantly raise the risk of secondary tumors, especially nonlymphocytic leukamias... Nitrogen mustard, vincristine, prednisone, and procarbazine for the treatment of Hodgkins disease yield leukamia rates up to 17 percent... Radiation further increases the risk of leukemia.
Dr Leonard DeVita, Cancer: Principles and Practice of Oncology

Neoplasm/neoplastic is an abnormal growth.

Oncogenic - *giving rise to tumors or causing tumor formation; said especially of tumor-inducing viruses.*.[16] **Oncology** is the orthodox medical discipline most associated with shrinking and creating cancer tumours.

Complete Response/Remission (CR) - The disappearance of all visible signs of cancer for **at least 4 weeks**.

Partial Response/Remission (PR) - Cancer has shrunk by **at least a third** (or 50% depending who you ask) with no sign it has grown elsewhere in the body **for 4 weeks.**

As the science has progressed and numbers better juggled, patients fresh out of chemo with tumours remaining under 10mm in size may now be considered in 'complete remission', whereas prior to this cancer treatment data re-evaluation patients with this residual cancer stockpile would be considered in partial remission. Does it really matter? Not to you and I as life will still be cut short, but as we find through Roland Bammer's book 'MR and CT Perfusion and Pharmokinetic Imaging' there are the standard benefits in fiddling with statistics. This they call 'Response Evaluation Criteria in Solid Tumours' and while it sounds like meaningless waffle it matters to some.

> *Pharmaceutical companies will greatly improve operational efficiency across many line functions (particularly clinical, statistics, data management and imaging). Pharmaceutical company interactions with clinical research organisation partners will be more efficient and consistent and will reduce the time and cost of image review charter development.* [17]

But there will be no less cancer.

Progression Free Survival (PFS) is the length of time **during and after** treatment that a patient lives with the disease where it does not get worse. Or the length of time before it starts growing again.

---

16 https://medical-dictionary.thefreedictionary.com/oncogenic

17 MR and CT Perfusion and Pharmacokinetic Imaging: Clinical Applications - By Roland Bammer

Especially during treatment one would hope to see no signs of disease progression at all, but this is not always the case and cancer may just as likely keep right on growing. Calculating either from the date of diagnosis or the start of treatment leaves the door wide open to making things look better than they actually are. In my case I could have been diagnosed a year earlier than I was as I did have symptoms in 2012 and treatment would not start until 2015 so three years of no treatment could theoretically be added to my 'survival' statistic and who's going to argue?

Disease Free Survival (DFS) - the period when there is no recurrence of cancer.

Event Free Survival (EFS) - is the period of time when there appears to be no cancer growth.

Overall Survival (OS) - the length of time that patients lived from **either** the date of diagnosis or the start of treatment.

Median Survival - refers to 50% alive at the mid-point of a trial.

Objective Response (OR) - some sign of tumour shrinkage.

Cytotoxic - is a substance that kills cells.

Metastasis - This is a cancer that has spread; cancer cells leave the main tumour and pass through the blood to settle elsewhere. This can be facilitated by a needle piercing the tumour and releasing material or by surgical incision or simply by a lack of adequate treatment or by further suppression of immune defences with massive doses of cytotoxic agents.

Cure/cured - This is a tricky one and the only one in this list of confusing terms you would ordinarily want to aspire to, but in the murky world we're swimming through even a cure isn't all that clear. In the broader sense it means to restore health but that's not how it's being used. In the world of orthodox cancer treatment a cure represents a period of time with no sign of disease. At the cut-off, typically 5 years, a cure is granted and the patient is sent away to fend for themselves. And defend we must! It is entirely possible to maintain this survivor status and turn it into an old school cure, but we are required to be fully engaged in the process.

Disease Progression - means it is spreading. Although even this can be confusing and may be calculated thus:

> *20% increase in the sum of longest diameters of target lesions compared to smallest sum longest diameter recorded. [sic] In addition, the sum must also demonstrate an absolute increase of at least 5mm. Unequivocal progression of non-target lesions, or the appearance of new lesions is also considered progression. Unequivocal progression means the patient has overall status of*

> *progressive disease at that time point.* ***Modest increases in the size of one or more non-target lesions is usually not sufficient.*** [18]

See what I mean, in the crazy world of drug treatment multiple tumours growing in a cancer patient is **not** a sign of disease progressing! Go science!

Relapse - it's back.

Refractory - is a hard or impossible disease to manage; resistant to orthodox methods of treatment. Ultimately this is how most cancer will end up, unless you deal with it a different way.

Peer Review - Some people who have been trained in the manner you have read something you write and give you a pat on the back. If you stray from what is seen by them as 'the normal way of thinking' and suggest in your publication that any of the research or findings of you or your peers has been misguided, you won't get your thing reviewed. This is how science gets stuck. Wider society is also peer reviewed. Persist and you may be defrocked.

Meta-analysis - is a mathematical statistical compilation of multiple study results.

Apoptosis - is programmed cell death. It's a natural thing, a good thing to induce.

Efficacy - determines whether an intervention produces the expected result under ideal circumstances. This is unlike 'effective' which is real world. Test drugs will be described as efficacious at the conclusion of a clinical trial but will typically provide a more honest outcome in the real world.

Placebo – this is well dodgy. To most of us a placebo is an inert substance that has no pharmacological effect and is given merely to fool a patient who supposes it to be a medicine. But most clinical trials have replaced the 'sugar pill' with toxic drugs and have really muddied the waters. Most double-blind placebo trials today are fraudulent.

The all clear - this is fake news and represents the ultimate in false hope. Think about that brief moment you are free to cross over the main road as the green man beeps and the traffic stops. Your cancer doctor is the little green man and you have the all clear until he shows up flashing red.

Most of these descriptors are utterly meaningless when aiming for long-term disease-free survival, which most of us are. All this is is a lesson in how to compartmentalise an illusion. They say a lot but they've got very little.

---

[18] http://www.focus4trial.org/centres/recist-response-definitions/

Trial & Error

We have to bear in mind that there are still some unripe cancer tissues in the body, or hidden cells in glands or lymph vessels or necrotic tissue, after the large tumor mass has been absorbed and are no longer palpable. *These immature cells do not respond as fast as the ripe cancer cells. This is the reason why benign tumors, scars, adhesions, etc do not respond as rapidly as the ripe, fully developed cancer cells.*
Dr Max Gerson - A Cancer Therapy 1958

Some, very typical, waffle-edited clinical trial findings from CRUK. My **bold**:

- 363 women used. In this trial, the researchers were comparing a combination of doxorubicin and docetaxel versus doxorubicin and cyclophosphamide for patients on pre-surgical chemotherapy.

With the combination of doxorubicin and cyclophosphamide, the cancer **responded** in 61 out of every 100 women treated (61%). In just 17 out of every 100 women (17%) who had this combination, all signs of cancer had disappeared when their breast was later examined.

With doxorubicin and docetaxel, the cancer **responded** in 70 out of every 100 women treated (70%). And with this combination, breast examination showed that all signs of cancer had disappeared in 20 out of every 100 women (20%). The length of time the cancer disappeared for was of no interest.

- 51 children used. The goal was to assess the best dose of erlotinib to treat children with brain tumours and discover more about the side effects of erlotinib in children. No mention of a cure or living longer or quality of life.

The research team concluded that they had found the best dose to give children and young people, and that erlotinib was "safe" to use for this group of patients. They suggest that it is **looked at further in other trials, possibly in combination with different drugs.**

- 52 patients. This trial looked at fludarabine, cyclophosphamide, and mitoxantrone with or without rituximab. The aim of the trial was to see which combination of treatment was better for CLL (chronic lymphocytic leukaemia) that had either not responded to other chemo treatment, or had come back after the treatment.

The trial team concluded that adding rituximab to fludarabine, cyclophosphamide and mitoxantrone improved the tumour **response**. **They suggest this should be looked at in larger trials**.

- 45 children used. This trial looked at using high dose chemotherapy and a stem cell transplant for children who had a neuroectodermal tumour that had come back following treatment.

After a follow up period of nearly 7 and half years, 37 of the 45 children had died. The trial team concluded there was little benefit in giving high dose chemotherapy to children whose tumour had come back.

- 41 people used. This trial was looking to see how well the combination of alemtuzumab (Mabcampath) and methylprednisolone worked for CLL.

After having alemtuzumab and methylprednisolone, 8 people were later told they needed a transplant using bone marrow or stem cells from a donor. The average length of time that the people in this trial lived after treatment was just under 2 years.

The researchers think that this drug combination helped people with CLL but may need to be improved. I say it probably helped them to die and it can only be improved!

- This trial recruited 130 people who had already had treatment for peripheral T cell lymphoma (PTCL).

The research team looked at how well romidepsin worked and found that the lymphoma

Went away in 19 people (15%)
Got a bit better in 14 people (11%)
Stayed the same in 33 people (25%)
The lymphoma either got worse, or the trial team wasn't able to do the study assessments in 64 people (49%).

The most common side effects other than cancer growth were feeling or being sick, infection, the loss of blood clotting platelets, fatigue and diarrhea.

The trial team somehow concluded that romidepsin was a "useful" treatment for PTCL that had not responded to treatment or had come back after treatment, and didn't cause too many side effects. Useful for who?

Roll up, roll up! More cancer patients needed for more dead end drug trials!

There is no enthusiasm in this half-hearted pretence at building on something that's shattered at the foundations and has been since the introduction of chemotherapy in the middle of the last century. Millions upon millions have already died prematurely after taking these drug treatments while hundreds of thousands of hopeful cancer patients are used in these trials, none of which set a goal to restore immunity and health, and all too often the conclusion is to do more trials of the same failed drugs!
When we hear that this or that new drug has "shown promise" in these clinical trials and is helping patients to live longer, we might well ask compared to what and for how much longer are they living? There are still a few trials in which patients are merely observed or given the once popularised placebo or dummy drug, but these are much more the exception than the rule and typically the contest today is drug v

drug, with the placebo a redundant reminder of a simpler time. We can learn from this that the drug pushers fear the outcome of their products up against the true placebo of leave well alone.

Were you asked if the goalposts should be moved away from benign placebo to a poison combo? And to what end? And who benefits? And does this not undermine the entire foundation of the current medical gold standard for drug testing proof of concept against that placebo baseline?

The medical literature is loaded with these toxin-challenge clinical trials and you could spend months trawling through them all, but I wouldn't bother because it's really quite sad. I keyed the word placebo into the search box on the CRUK clinical trial database and got 21 hits for completed trials, with a further 3 trials pending, two of which are to test drugs for use on customers once the first round of drug treatment has failed and cancer has returned. This group represents a market so lucrative the industry runs clinical trails for products of failure! To compare, in the CRUK database with regard to drug v drug trials there are over 300 trials recorded for lymphoma, lung cancer, and breast cancer alone, not to mention all the other cancers. Another 150+ trials are pending to test drugs against drugs. No testing of nutrition against the drugs, no new ideas in the mix, just drugs. This is an incredible revelation and it gives us a clear indication of the modus operandi and should alert us to question the very foundation of our medical system, propped up as it is by drugs.

Doctors are obligated, as are we all, to first do no harm. But how is that even possible when applying the current medical standard of using one drug or a multiple, each of whose side effects involve death? And where no safe alternative is permitted!

And look at this. Five of those 21 so called placebo trials are nothing of the sort. Digging deeper we find they instead involve a concoction of drugs with a placebo jumbled into the mix, perhaps so they were able to include it in their placebo list, and bulk it out a little? That's 3 drugs to one group of test subjects, 2 drugs + the placebo thing to the other group. Who benefits? I keep asking but it's always the drug makers. I mean, what is the point? It's like the vegetarian who eats fish! The sixth drug trial in the list of 21 showed some promise if you need a drug to give you an erection after surgery. I kid you not.

And in the best of the remaining 15 CRUK placebo trials, (I'm not certain we can trust even this list is honest since the placebo has been so heavily infiltrated, but we're giving the benefit of the doubt because it isn't clear these few aren't genuine and we should examine just what it is their placebo trials do achieve), coming in at number 2 is a drug that achieves no more than 12 weeks of extended life over the placebo group (including side effects). And at the top spot is a drug achieving just over 16 weeks versus placebo in its controlled trial setting (plus side effects). This is the best of the best. Some tout it as a glimmer of hope. I don't think so. In the mix of these expensive experiments we also have a whole mess of damage done to participants who were hoping they were going to be part of a cure, such as secondary cancer or "developing a hole in the wall of their bowel (perforation or fistula), or serious bleeding (haemorrhage)". We also see reports of the all important tumour shrinkage (response) and calls for more fancy trials, but is that it?

Decide for yourself here they are, the best of the best CRUK's token placebo driven clinical trials.

- 941 men used. Atrasentan did not help to stop prostate cancer growing for the men in this trial. But many of the men stopped taking atrasentan earlier than they should have due to side effects. They found the cancer had spread to another part of the body in 267 men who had the "dummy drug" (placebo?) and 227 men who had atrasentan. But this difference was no bigger than could have happened by chance, in other words, it was not 'statistically significant' and that seems to matter more than the lives of patients.
- This trial used 1,195 men with advanced prostate cancer who had already been failed by the chemotherapy drug docetaxel. 797 men had abiraterone + prednisolone tablets each day, 398 men had a **dummy drug +** prednisolone tablets each day. The researchers found that in this trial the average length of time men lived was just under 16 months in the abiraterone group and just over 11 months in what they call the placebo group. This is their best result.
- 1,421 men used. In this trial zibotentan did not help men with prostate cancer and was stopped early after a review by the committee that monitors the safety and design of the trial (the data monitoring committee). This was because early results suggested that it was very unlikely this trial would be able to show that zibotentan would be of any benefit for men with prostate cancer.
- In this trial the research team found that erlotinib did help stop the cancer growing in some people tested on **but that it didn't always help them live longer.** When the research team looked at the results in 2010, they found that a year after starting treatment the cancer had stopped growing in 4 out of every 100 people (4%) who took the placebo and 9 out of every 100 people (9%) who took erlotinib. They looked at how many people were living one year after treatment and found that it was

  24 out of every 100 people (24%) who had erlotinib and developed a rash
  10 out of every 100 people (10%) who had erlotinib but didn't develop a rash
  18 out of every 100 people (18%) who had placebo

  The people who developed a rash lived, on average, just over 2 months longer than those who had the placebo. And the people who didn't develop a rash lived, on average, just over one month less than those who had the placebo. The research team concluded that having a rash is a sign that the treatment is **working,** and that people who do not get a rash within in the first 4 weeks of taking erlotinib should stop treatment.

This stuff makes my head spin.

- 450 people used. The trial team found that oesophageal cancer took longer to start growing again in people taking gefitinib. Seven weeks for those who had gefitinib, five weeks for those who had the dummy drug. Two whole weeks of living longer with cancer!

- 90 women used. We learn that exemestane can **affect** Ductal Carcinoma in Situ (DCIS), but celecoxib does not. So, the researchers conclude that exemestane **may help to treat some** DCIS patients. They suggest it should be **studied further** as an alternative to tamoxifen for preventing DCIS coming back or developing into invasive breast cancer.

- 1,522 men used. The research team found that dasatinib and docetaxel did not work better than docetaxel alone for prostate cancer that was no longer responding to hormone therapy. The research team looked at how long it took for the cancer to start growing again after the men started treatment. They found, on average, it was **11.8** months for men who had docetaxel + dasatinib and **11.1** months for men who had docetaxel **+ placebo**. They also looked at how many men in each group had died, and found it was 452 men who'd had docetaxel + dasatinib, 462 men who'd had docetaxel + placebo.

- 1,299 people used who had non-small cell lung cancer that was stage 3B or stage 4. 649 of them had paclitaxel, carboplatin and ASA404. 650 had paclitaxel, carboplatin **and a dummy drug.** The researchers found that the number of people whose cancer responded to the treatment was about the same in both groups. On average, people in both groups lived for about 13 months.

- 1,090 people used. The trial team found that motesanib with carboplatin and paclitaxel **didn't help** people with advanced non-small cell lung cancer live longer. The researchers found that the average overall length of time that people lived after treatment was 13 months for those who had chemotherapy + motesanib, 11 months for those who had chemotherapy **+ a dummy drug.**

- 723 women used. A third had fulvestrant and anastrozole, a third had fulvestrant **and a dummy drug**, and a third had exemestane. The researchers looked at the average length of time the women lived without any signs of their breast cancer getting worse. Researchers call this progression free survival. They found it was about 4½ months in the group who had fulvestrant and anastrozole, about 5 months in the group who had fulvestrant **and a dummy drug**, about 3½ months in the group who had exemestane.

  They also looked at the average length of time women lived overall and found it was about 20 months in the group who had fulvestrant + anastrozole, about 19½ months in the group who had fulvestrant + **dummy drug** and about 21½ months in the group who had exemestane. These results show that there does not appear to be a difference between the 3 groups that is significant in statistical terms. The researchers concluded that for post menopausal women whose breast cancer had stopped responding to aromatase inhibitors, a combination of fulvestrant and anastrozole was no better than either fulvestrant or exemestane alone.

Makes me dizzy, and nauseous.

- This could perk me up. 583 men used. The trial team concluded that having tadalafil once a day after prostate surgery did help men maintain their erectile function. It's nice, because quality of life is seldom considered! But why the need for such a drug to be trial tested instead of say the Gerson Therapy?

Here's why.

'The Weekend Pill', as it is known, has a much wider market than a minority of cancer patients. It got the name for its superior staying power over market competitors such as Viagra. But it has status in our story because we are told it is needed to help patients harmed by cancer surgery. Doctor-induced in order to treat a symptom of cancer. Cancer that could be treated without the need for surgery were it not for vested interests testing such drugs in place of therapies that don't have life changing side effects.

- 88 people used. The trial team found that EPA was safe and that it reduced blood flow to the cancer cells in the liver **but didn't reduce how much or how fast the cancer cells grew.**
- 1,513 people used to test a cancer vaccine. They found those who had tecemotide for **non-small cell lung cancer** lived an average of 25.6 months. And those who had the placebo lived an average of 22.3 months.
- 265 women used. 136 women had olaparib and 129 women had a dummy drug. **The researchers looked at how long it was before the cancer started growing again.** More women in the olaparib group had side effects such as sickness, tiredness (fatigue) and a drop in the number of red blood cells (anaemia). Most side effects were described as mild, but 41 women in the olaparib group and 12 women in the placebo group had to have a break in their treatment due to side effects. The trial team found that on average, women who took olaparib had a longer time without any sign of their cancer coming back than women who took the dummy drug. Doctors call this an improvement in progression free 'survival'. In March 2012 the researchers published the results in a scientific journal where it was noted that the overall length of time the women lived (whether or not their cancer gets worse) was similar between the 2 groups - they now refer to overall 'survival'. These researchers are **now looking to see** whether there are patients in the study with certain types of ovarian cancer **where there might be a difference** in overall survival between the 2 groups.

Seriously, this is what they do day in day out with your money while making fantastic claims about surviving cancer.

- 920 people used who had non-small cell lung cancer that was stage 3B or stage 4. Everybody taking part had already had chemotherapy, but their cancer had continued to grow or had come back after treatment. 460 people had docetaxel + ASA404, 460 people had docetaxel **and a dummy drug**. The researchers found that the number of people whose cancer responded to the treatment was about the same in both groups. On average, the length of time people lived after treatment was about the same in both groups. The trial team concluded that in this study, ASA404 **did not work any better than the dummy drug and the trial was stopped early**.

- 330 people used. Everyone taking part had medullary thyroid cancer that had spread outside the thyroid gland and continued to grow and couldn't be removed with surgery. The research team looked at how long it was before the cancer lump got any larger. They found on average it was just over 11 months for those who had cabozantinib and 4 months for those who had the placebo. When they looked at the number of people whose cancer had not got any bigger a year after starting treatment, they found it was nearly half of those who had cabozantinib (47%) and fewer than 1 in 10 people who had the placebo (7%). **They then looked at how long people in each group lived for. They found there was no difference between the two groups, but they will continue to look at this.** The people taking cabozantinib of course had side effects, and some of them were classed as serious. A small number of people in the cabozantinib group did have some serious side effects such as developing a hole in the wall of their bowel (perforation or fistula), or serious bleeding (haemorrhage). The trial team concluded that cabozantinib helped stop medullary thyroid cancer growing, and could be a useful treatment for this rare cancer.

- 7,154 women used who all had an increased risk of developing breast cancer, mainly because of their family history. This trial showed that tamoxifen does reduce the risk of developing breast cancer for women with a high risk and that this effect continues after they stop taking it. Half took a tamoxifen tablet and half took a dummy drug every day for 5 years. In 2014, 22 years after the trial started, the research team looked at how many women in each group had developed breast cancer. They found it was 251 out of 3,579 women (7%) in the tamoxifen group 350 out of 3,575 women (10%) in the placebo group. **The research team worked out that for every 22 women who took tamoxifen, 1 less woman would be diagnosed with breast cancer after 20 years**. They looked at the number of women in each group who died from breast cancer and found it was 31 in the tamoxifen group, and 26 in the placebo group. They also looked at the total number of women who had died from any cause and found it was 182 in the tamoxifen group, and 166 in the placebo group. A difference that could be due to chance and it was not statistically significant. They also looked at how many women developed womb (endometrial) cancer. They found it was 29 women in the tamoxifen group, and 20 in the placebo group.

- 939 people used. The trial team looked at the average length of time that people survived on pemetrexed chemotherapy with non-small cell lung cancer before it came back (progression free survival). **They found it was just over 4 months for people who had pemetrexed and just under 3 months for people who had placebo. This apparently showed that maintenance treatment with pemetrexed "helped to reduce the risk of the cancer coming back"**. These results were considered **statistically significant**. **The researchers looked at the average length of time that people lived after starting treatment (overall survival). They found this was nearly 14 months for people who had pemetrexed and 11 months for people who had the placebo.** [19]

Nearly 12 weeks of living longer with cancer thanks to all that world leading cancer research. Now we're rockin'! There are a couple more of the same in this CRUK "placebo" trials list but you get the picture. Can't you just sense how desperately close they are to a cure? Will it be sooner or later?

They focus an awful lot on breast cancer and this is what they have achieved. Pancreatic cancer gets much less attention and is notoriously bad for responding to orthodox treatment and why? It's a classic case of failing to ask the right questions.

The Lancet:

Pancreatic cancer: are more chemotherapy and surgery needed?

Pancreatic cancer is curable only in a small minority of patients with localised and resectable tumours, which accounts for only 5–10% of the cases, and only 10–20% of patients survive more than 5 years after surgery. With such bleak figures, every attempt made to improve the survival rates of patients with pancreatic cancer should be welcomed. This is the aim of the ESPAC-4 trial published in The Lancet.

These results open the field to several questions. Can an increase in chemotherapy cure more patients in a cancer considered for more than 60 years to be chemoresistant? Do the figures from the ESPAC-4 trial at 5 years really represent patients cured of pancreatic cancer? How can we now improve the survival of patients with pancreatic cancer further? ***Do we need to give patients more surgery or more chemotherapy?***

First, the paradigm of pancreatic cancer as a chemoresistant tumour has been largely undermined in the past 5 years. In the metastatic setting, oncologists can now choose between diverse monotherapy or a combination of gemcitabine, fluorouracil, nab-paclitaxel, oxaliplatin, irinotecan, and liposomal

---

19 https://www.cancerresearchuk.org/about-cancer/find-a-clinical-trial/clinical-trials-search?search_api_aggregation_1=placebo&f%5B0%5D=field_trial_status%3A4396

irinotecan. This means there are more chemotherapy drugs available for pancreatic cancer than for colon cancer.

A meta-analysis of adjuvant trials in pancreatic cancer published 10 years ago showed that adjuvant chemotherapy gave patients only an extra 3 months of median survival time, without offering a cure. *So does the addition of capecitabine to gemcitabine in the adjuvant setting of pancreatic cancer really translate into more patients being cured?*

... the number of patients alive without disease at the end of the analysis was 80 (21·8%) patients in the gemcitabine group and 93 (25·5%) patients in the combination group; an ***absolute improvement and likely cure rate of 3·7%.*** *This means that roughly we need to treat 25 patients with the combination of gemcitabine and capecitabine* ***to save one more life****. Of course,* ***this further adds to the other gains*** *achieved with the previous ESPAC trials as discussed by the authors.* ***As for cure, more follow-up is needed to ascertain that this is the case and not only prolongation of survival. No patient has yet crossed the 5-year survival boundary.***

So, even if modest, these figures are encouraging in a disease with such high mortality and clearly establishes the combination of gemcitabine and capecitabine as a new standard of care in the adjuvant setting of pancreatic ductal adenocarcinoma.

How can we further improve these results in the future? There is clearly a need for some kind of biomarker that could guide the choice of treatment or even surgery. The results of several other large adjuvant trials with new drugs or a combination of drugs are also ***eagerly awaited*** *and* ***it is likely that more chemotherapy will translate into more patients being cured. But again, this will be only for a small subset of patients with pancreatic cancer who received surgery****.*

More surgery is therefore clearly needed if we want to cure more patients, but more surgery means the possibility to offer surgery earlier in the disease evolution, and as a consequence more often. [20]

A likely cure rate of 3.7%! That's a 96.3% failure rate. An awful lot of dead people and still they claim to be saving lives! This is the cutting edge of an old theory that begun trying to cure cancer by removing the tumour with surgery and failed then added radiation and failed so mixed in chemo and failed so tried more chemo and failed again. Here they discuss going back to surgery and chemo, and more of it! Recycling is a good thing but not always. This revolving cut - burn - poison policy mixes well with that of the industry whereby drug company bosses in the middle of this mess move in and out of government jobs and back to industry – setting the rules, exploiting the loopholes.

---

[20] http://www.thelancet.com/journals/lancet/article/PIIS0140-6736(17)30126-5/fulltext?elsca1=etoc

US oncologist turned healer Dr Nicholas Gonzales [21] demonstrated consistently the curing of pancreatic cancers with the non-aggressive support network of nutrition, detoxification and supplementation. His cure rate is outstanding with patients living 5, 10, and 15 years and longer than the chemo'd. The Gerson Institute records less impressive success with this cancer but still out shine the tumour bombers by a mile. Just what would happen if all these unpronounceable poisons were tested against a home-grown therapy that works better? Like mine. How could it possibly do worse?

This is not just in the cancer field this is pretty much all there is wherever you look in orthodox disease management. If you're looking for a breakthrough, or a cure, for something revolutionary and healing, for some scientific discovery… then, err, well, there ain't. The whole thing is a bit of a disaster but this is where the established order has parked up. I can't quite make it sound like those TV adverts with the excited cancer patients just out of chemo and happy with their oncologist' claims and their tumour's response, but it's good to get two sides of a story.

Quack: an ignorant, misinformed, or dishonest practitioner of medicine

No doubt these misunderstandings and dashed hopes have driven many cancer patients and their families into the arms of quacks. Haydn Bush
https://www.merriam-webster.com/dictionary/quack

[21] http://www.dr-gonzalez.com/index.htm

A Motive Masquerading as a Treatment Revolution

The directed research practices and other activities of the National Cancer Institute and of the American Cancer Society have been scandalously counterproductive in the conquest of cancer, in spite of the billions of dollars expended. The cancer establishment is closed to new approaches and ideas, thus creating a self-perpetuating system with no clear objective even remotely in sight.
Dr Robert E. Netterberg & Robert T. Taylor - The Cancer Conspiracy

The latest revolution in cancer treatment, we are led to believe, has come in the form of a range of wonder drugs known as monoclonal antibodies: the mAbs. This is what they call targeted therapy. Immunotherapy, even! Now that is funny. If immunotherapy sounds enticing or like it supports immunity then the advertising is working, but these products are notorious for crippling the immune system to the point of no recovery. The only mechanism we can rely on to give us a genuine, old school cure and they trash it!

These mAbs are genetically engineered chimeric mouse/human hybrid creations. Also known as xenotransplantation other mammals may replace the mouse but they prefer mice. Transplanting genetic material from one species into another is fraught with danger and it is not just cancer patients the mAbs are aimed at, the mAbs like the vaccines have an increasingly broad target market.

MAbs are designed to recognize and attach to specific proteins on the surface of cells. Each mAb recognises one very particular protein and are each designed for different cancers. This range of products fill in the gaps between chemo sittings with a view to keeping the cancer suppressed, the patient 'maintained'. But they have to be withdrawn in due course as things get really, really serious and what's left of the immune system collapses, at which point there's nothing left to hold back the cancer (or any infection) and it is now you may become informed there's nothing 'more' they can do to you and you are told to go home to get your affairs in order. Perhaps you could pick up a pamphlet about legacies in the foyer on the way out of the hospital and consider leaving cancer research anything you have left when organising your affairs. The mAbs keep the market flowing as they extract as much out of each customer as possible for as long as possible while doing nothing to actually enrich or extend lives. Clearly, in endlessly inviting the public to pledge all available savings in legacies at the end of life, there is little expectation of a breakthrough in cancer research anytime soon.

Depending on your cancer, if you survive chemo and the mAb attack, they may next offer an even more powerful chemo mix which requires they first suck out bone marrow stem cells (they prefer to "harvest" them) in an extended hospital stay. I was told later as I was lured into their trap that I would be an ideal candidate, as I was young and fit and up for the extreme challenge of the high risk procedure that they reserve for the difficult cases as "worth the risk". Your stem cells are kept safe while they flood your body with a death defying round of chemo and maybe a hit of TBI (total body irradiation) until literally the point of death, in the hope of finally getting every last cancer cell. Survive that and they shove your (or someone else's) bone marrow back in, (or trickle it back in through a hole in your chest if you prefer the sound of that) with a glimmer of hope it will form a brand new cancer-free you. If you make it through that lot and don't succumb to infection along the way you will be thoroughly exhausted and may spend years recovering, if you are lucky. It is a very costly procedure at anywhere between £300,000 & £750,000 a pop and it is brutal and it still isn't curative, not even close! [22]

- *In patients who receive an allogeneic [someone else's] bone marrow transplant as treatment for acute myelogenous or lymphoblastic leukemia, chronic myelogenous leukemia, or aplastic anemia and who are free of their original disease two years later, the disease is* ***probably cured. However,*** *for many years after transplantation, the mortality among these patients is higher than that in a normal population.* [23]
- *Allogeneic bone marrow transplantation (BMT)* ***may be curative*** *in patients with follicular non-Hodgkin's lymphoma,* ***however, the impact of this therapy on long-term survival, disease progression and functional status is less clear.*** [24]

You have to love the spin. Cured but no idea for how long? The prognosis for surviving a BMT is clear for all to see. The studies tend to monitor the fallout at one year and then two years after treatment and by year three it becomes clear it's time to stop the study as relapses and secondary cancers and infections take their toll. First stop maybe surgery, then chemo then the mAbs maybe more chemo then the bone marrow and more chemo and see them out with some mAbs. What we fight we strengthen and this war is a long lost cause.

These are the top global selling cancer drugs for 2013, the year I was diagnosed [25]

1. Rituximab/Mabthera
2. Bevacizumab/Avastin
3. Trastuzumab/Herceptin

All mouse made mAbs.

Let's start with **number 3.** Arguably the most popular.

Who hasn't heard of **Herceptin**, also but not so well known as **trastuzmab**. This is used on people with breast cancer, oesophageal, gastric cancers and it's very good for business. In this case, the HER2 receptor is the target of the drug but it also damages a gene called erbB2, which is intimately connected with heart and lung function. Heart failure and lung disease are direct effects of this drug, leaving many

---

22 https://www.medigo.com/blog/medigo-guides/bone-marrow-transplant-cost-guide/

23 https://www.ncbi.nlm.nih.gov/pubmed/10387937

24 https://www.ncbi.nlm.nih.gov/pubmed/15491292

25 https://www.medscape.com/viewarticle/826649

patients with only a choice of how they would like to die, assuming, as I don't, that they have been fully informed of the real risk.

There has been significant hype around this drug especially over its application in breast cancer. In 1998 the US government's FDA (Federal Drugs Adminstration) fast tracked Herceptin's approval based on some shoddy phase II trials, the first of which saw 9 out of 37 patient tumours respond to this + cisplatin and remain progression free for approximately 8 months. In another such trial there were 5 tumour responders out of 43 patients. This lasting a few short weeks before 100% of the trial participants were in deep trouble. A really terrible performance you might think yet the mainstream media (MSM) went on a frenzy and dutifully jollied along public opinion.

> In the New England Journal of Medicine, Jo Anne Zujewski of the US National Cancer Institute wrote: "In 1991, I didn't know... we would **cure** breast cancer... in 2005, I'm convinced we have".

*Breast Cancer Is '**Cured**' By Wonder Drug, Says Doctors*
(Sunday Times, London)

*Breast Cancer **Curable***
(Daily Times, Pakistan)

> A lead researcher in the UK and head of the Breast Unit at the Royal Marsden Hospital, Professor Ian "quack quack" Smith, came out with the outrageous claim that, "This is the biggest treatment development in breast cancer, in terms of the magnitude of its effect, for at least the last 25 years, perhaps as big as anything we've seen".

'Miracle' drug giving real hope in the fight against breast cancer
(Belfast Telegraph, Northern Ireland)

*Drug Touted As **Cure** For Breast Cancer*
(Associated Press)

Gabriel Hortobagyi of the MD Anderson Cancer Center announced that "This observation suggests a dramatic and perhaps permanent perturbation of the natural history of the disease, and may even be a **cure**".

***Miracle Cure** for Breast Cancer at Half the Price*
(Daily News & Analysis, India)

These proxy advertising campaigns are super successful and cheap as chips. This one was made real by two breast cancer patients fresh out of treatment gracing the TV screens. Trusting in miracles and happy with the all clear you too could be like them, on Herceptin. Alive! So persuasive was the lie that desperate cancer patients cheated by the fake news staged protests calling for Herceptin to be shared widely. Some women sold their homes to get hold of this precious gift from the gods of good drugs.

But of course when we read beyond the promotional headlines things start to look a little less like they sound and one might not be quite so keen to leave everything for the drug pushers just yet.

In the following trial, funded by the drug maker (Roche/Genentech), we begin to discover how unlikely their wonder drug really is.

They went all out to test whether their drug was better used by patients for two years or just one year. For the makers of course two years would be better but for the drug takers most likely not. They experimented with over 5,100 women with HER2 positive early stage breast cancer. I'll edit out the waffle and leave the essentials but if you wish you can read it for yourself and much more of the same.

They observe:

> *The standard of care is 1 year of adjuvant trastuzumab, but the optimum duration of treatment is unknown.*
>
> *The HERA trial is an international, multicentre, randomised, open-label, phase 3 trial comparing treatment with trastuzumab for 1 and 2 years with observation after standard neoadjuvant chemotherapy, adjuvant chemotherapy, or both in 5102 patients with HER2-positive early breast cancer.* ***The primary endpoint was disease-free survival****. We recorded 367 events of disease-free survival in 1552 patients in the 1 year group and 367 events in 1553 patients in the 2 year group.*

They discover that:

> *2 years of adjuvant trastuzumab is not more effective than is 1 year of treatment for patients with HER2-positive early breast cancer. 1 year of treatment provides a* ***significant disease-free and overall survival benefit*** *compared with observation and remains the standard of care.* [26]

Their interpretation of significant is not mine. I was seeing 'statistically significant' appearing all over the place yet the survival of patients in the studies I was looking at was anything but significant, so I looked it up. Wikipedia's page agreed with my observation:

> *The term... does not imply importance here, and... is not the same as research, theoretical, or practical significance.*

And at the end of the day actions speak louder than words and these fancy phrases do not maketh good medicine. It's all part of the deception and is much more common than a cure in the world we are exploring here.

---

26 http://www.thelancet.com/journals/lancet/article/PIIS0140-6736(13)61094-6/fulltext

How is 367 out of 1552 whose disease had not started to grow again a good thing? There's no mention of what happened to other 1,185 who weren't experiencing disease free survival, but we can probably figure it out. They also found that adverse events were more common in the patients having 2 years worth of Herceptin. Yeah, like, duh!

Larry Norton, M.D., deputy physician in chief for Breast Cancer Programs at Memorial Sloan-Kettering Cancer Center in New York said, *The problem is that not only are there questions that these trials can no longer answer, such as long-term toxicity associated with the addition of trastuzumab, but also that we are never going to know... I think we are going to have to follow the patients who have been treated with adjuvant Herceptin very, very carefully. In terms of long-term effects and sites of metastasis, the story is not closed. There are still many unanswered questions.* [27]

Within 2 years at least 15 women had been killed directly by the drug, many others adversely affected and none cured, yet there it is right up there with all the other poisons on the World Health Organisation's List of Essential Medicines, as one of the most effective and safe medicines needed in a health system.

No matter the obvious indicators that these drugs are junk, they persist because this is about wealth not health. In this trial to

Evaluate the Efficacy and Safety of First-Line, Single-Agent Trastuzumab in Women with HER2-Overexpressing Metastatic Breast Cancer

they start with 114 patients. And find:

> *The objective response rate was 26% with seven complete and 23 partial responses.*

Remember an objective response is some sign of tumour shrinkage. Some shrinkage means you know right away the cancer is still going to get you.

> *CONCLUSION: Single-agent trastuzumab is active and well tolerated as first-line treatment of women with metastatic breast cancer.* [28]

I didn't do maths very well at school and fractions and percentages mess with my mind, particularly the way these people use them to confuse, but this miracle cure seems to have left us after one year with just 39 out of 114 patients with smaller tumours leaving the rest with the same cancer they started with or more. So it just as likely makes cancer grow? But it's well tolerated! How many times do you have to use this stuff on people before accepting failure?

---

27 https://academic.oup.com/jnci/article/98/5/296/2522045

28 http://ascopubs.org/doi/full/10.1200/JCO.2002.20.3.719

Even the ultra medical Lancet can see through this:

> *The best that can be said about Herceptin's efficacy and safety for the treatment of early breast cancer is that the available evidence is insufficient to make reliable judgments.* ***It is profoundly misleading to suggest, even rhetorically, that the published data may be indicative of a cure for breast cancer.*** [29]

Tons of animal experiments all the way through to human trials and rather than something that heals what we have are deadly side effects and more questions. No doubt more trials should be able to help assess if we need a new improved mAb or maybe a DEEb or two would be able to get at the problem? I made up DEEb by the way, but a DEEb would still do better.

The following statistical analysis of two of these Herceptin research papers published in the New England Journal of Medicine in 2005, is equally revealing. The studies are authored by dozens of doctors and referencing 4500 Herceptin treated patients v chemo and other controls and appear on the face of things to show something positive, if you can call it that. But deeper it's just more deception. [30 31]

The three-year disease-free survival rate was proposed as 75.4% for those on chemo and 87.1% for those on Herceptin. So, statistically speaking around just 12% more of the Herceptin users were helped to remain disease free for 3 years. I thought this a pretty poor accolade for Herceptin, especially after all that fake news got my hopes up, but found there was no need to worry, on paper at least, as they employ statisticians who can help when this happens. Biostatisticians, don't you know, and these guys are critical to the smooth running of this toxin supply line. They calculated instead not a mere 12% miracle but a **50% reduction in disease coming back after 3 years**. But how? You might well ask. Well it seems they simply subtracted 75.4 and 87.1 from 100 returning 24.6 & 12.9 respectively, which somehow becomes a 50% improvement! See how that works, half of 24 is 12 which of course equal 50%. Now that is a miracle!

This isn't a joke and it isn't funny. It's a slight of hand meant to deceive and something that occurs often in these expensive, go nowhere trials. The calculations were described by the tumour bombers as "simply stunning", a sentiment I agree with. So what about actual life expectancy? We know by now this isn't going to be good news, right? Don't worry, there's good coming out of all this. In one of these trials comparing Herceptin to doing nothing, death rates after one year "were not significantly different" with just over 2% dead in the untreated group and just under 2% in the Herceptin group. A significant number of women in the drug group were

---

29 Editorial Lancet 2005; 366: 1673. https://www.thelancet.com/pdfs/journals/lancet/PIIS0140-6736(05)67670-2.pdf

30 https://www.nejm.org/doi/full/10.1056/NEJMoa052122,
https://www.nejm.org/doi/pdf/10.1056/NEJMoa052306

31 http://www.healthy.net/Health/Essay/Herceptin_more_hype_than_hope/873/1

also reported to have suffered severe cardiotoxicity, which doesn't sound like something you'd want grandma to have added to her cancer.

But they don't care. Late 2010 the FDA granted approval for Herceptin in combination with cisplatin and either capecitabine or 5-fluorouracil (5fu). Insiders refer to 5-fluorouracil as "5 feet under", so that might give us a flavour for how well this is all going to turn out. The approval was based on results of a single international multicenter open-label randomized clinical trial of 594 patients who were randomly assigned (1:1) to receive either trastuzumab+chemo or chemo alone. The trial was closed following the second interim analysis, after 167 deaths had occurred in the group receiving trastuzumab+chemo and 184 deaths of patients on chemo. An updated survival analysis was done after 227 deaths of patients on trastuzumab+chemo and 221 deaths of patients on chemo. With just about everyone dead and little hope for the survivors, the analysis demonstrated median survival of 13.1 months for patients receiving trastuzumab+chemo and 11.7 months for patients receiving chemo alone.

They have thrown everything at this problem and sacrificed billions and that's the choice they offer. No effort is ever made to offer better ways of surviving and by the time you calculate the difference between those decimal point death dates your drug expert appointed survival time will have elapsed. Trastuzumab is on the WHO List of Essential Medicines, as **one of the most effective and safe medicines** needed in a health system. [32]

It's all a bit sick. Where are the long-term results? Where are the non-drug studies? Most importantly where are the cures? We may well ask and keep asking and if the answers don't add up, go find our own answers. Given they have been doing this for decades and given it takes 5.8 billion in investment and 10 years or more to bring a new drug to market and with 95% of experimental medicines failing to be both safe and effective in humans, this is clearly as good as it's ever going to get. [33]

> *It is surprising that although trastuzumab has a great affinity for HER2...* ***70% of HER2+ positive patients do not respond to treatment. In fact resistance to treatment develops rapidly, in virtually all patients.*** [34]

Bevacizumab, aka **Avastin,** comes in at **number 2** in the best seller hit list. This is another monoclonal antibody. How does this one do, do you think? Must do better because it's number 2.

Gross sales globally in 2013 $6.75 billion. [35]

---

32 https://en.wikipedia.org/wiki/Trastuzumab

33 https://www.manhattan-institute.org/pdf/fda_05.pdf

34 https://en.wikipedia.org/wiki/Trastuzumab

35 http://www.medscape.com/viewarticle/826649

Pretty good so far.

But that's it! The rest of the story follows the pattern and it's a struggle to find anything good to say.

It can be used for lots of cancers, but is that a good thing? When used on renal/kidney cancers this mouse mix up does ok on progression free survival but not so good at helping with overall survival.

Phase III trial from Pub Med:

> *Median Overall Survival was 23.3 months with bevacizumab plus interferon and 21.3 months with interferon plus placebo. Patients receiving postprotocol therapy including a tyrosine kinase inhibitor had longer median Overall Survival (bevacizumab plus interferon group: 38.6 months; interferon plus placebo group: 33.6 months.* [36]

On pharmafile:

> *In a blow for Roche, NICE has turned down its cancer drug Avastin because of 'too many uncertainties' over cost and efficacy. NICE has now said that, although median progression-free survival with bevacizumab plus capecitabine was 2.9 months more than with capecitabine alone, it was* ***unclear*** *whether that meant an improvement in overall survival.* [37]

Cancerconnect.com:

> *The combination of Avastin and paclitaxel significantly improved progression-free survival. Median survival without cancer progression was 11.8 months among women treated with Avastin and paclitaxel and 5.9 months among women treated with paclitaxel alone.* ***Overall survival, however, was similar in the two groups.*** *Median overall survival was 26.7 months among women treated with Avastin and paclitaxel and 25.2 months among women treated with paclitaxel alone.* [38]

The International Journal of Cancer Research and Treatment:

> *Bevacizumab leads to a gain of about two months in terms of OS [overall survival, in Non-Small Cell Lung Cancer]. Therefore, it is not clear whether it is really appropriate to choose such an expensive treatment burdened by many side-effects to gain a rather small clinical benefit. Adverse events most frequently observed during treatment with bevacizumab include hypertension, nephrotic syndrome, bleeding, gastrointestinal perforation, heart failure and neutropenia. [One] randomized phase II trial... in 2004 showed a high rate*

---

36 https://www.ncbi.nlm.nih.gov/pubmed/20368553

37 http://www.pharmafile.com/news/172260/nice-rejects-avastin-breast-cancer

38 http://news.cancerconnect.com/addition-of-avastin-doesnt-improve-overall-survival-in-metastatic-breast-cancer/

> *(9.1%) of severe pulmonary hemorrhage, fatal in some cases. The use of bevacizumab is related to some adverse events, such as bleeding, thromboembolism, hypertension and proteinuria.* [39]

In this clinical trial known as GOG240, sponsored by the National Cancer Institute (NCI) and run by the drug maker, two questions were posed: 1) whether topotecan+paclitaxel was superior to cisplatin+paclitaxel and 2) whether the addition of bevacizumab to either regimen improved overall survival.

Creative or what!

> *Patients with advanced, recurrent, or persistent cervical cancer that was not curable with standard treatment who received the drug bevacizumab (Avastin)* ***lived 3.7 months longer*** *than patients who did not receive the drug according to findings from a large, randomized clinical trial. These results were released, based on an interim analysis, in Feb. 2013, and updates were presented as part of the American Society of Clinical Oncology annual meeting in Chicago on June 2, 2013.*
>
> ***The study met its primary endpoint of demonstrating improved overall survival*** *in patients who received bevacizumab,* ***which also means that it delayed the chance of dying from the disease.***
>
> *Patients treated with chemotherapy alone had a median survival of* ***13.3 months*** *while those who received chemotherapy and bevacizumab had a median survival of* ***17 months.*** *This survival difference was* ***highly statistically significant****. Progression free survival, meaning that after treatment the disease did not worsen, was* ***8.2 months*** *for those who received bevacizumab vs.* ***5.9 months*** *for those who received chemotherapy alone.*

Jeff Abrams, M.D., clinical director of NCI's Division of Cancer Treatment and Diagnosis said he thought this was "welcome news".

Would he welcome this news if his daughter had cancer?

"Delayed the chance" of dying from the disease by 3.7 months and increase the chance of death! So are they lying or just not telling the truth? You have to love the decimal point! Like it matters. Maths again... Just how long is .7 of a month anyway, enough time to get your affairs in order? Avastin is of course on the WHO list of the most effective and safe medicines. When you add up all the patients in these experiments and look at the outcome invariably it is nothing short of tragic. Everyone an individual, just like you and me with loved ones each hoping against hope that the outcome will be a cure.

---

[39] http://ar.iiarjournals.org/content/34/4/1537.full

Remember what Max Gerson achieved nearly 100 years ago in clinical trial using nutrition against incurable disease. And he went on to cure terminal cancer using the same successful method, and no side effects! Shhhh!

In this NCI drug recycling trial they go on to report:

> *Patients receiving bevacizumab experienced more side effects than those who did not. These side effects were consistent with side effects previously known to be associated with bevacizumab and included hypertension, neutropenia (a low white blood cell count), and thromboembolism, or formation of blood clots. Quality of life during the trial was also measured and there was no significant difference reported by patients between those who received bevacizumab and those who received chemotherapy alone.*
>
> ***The findings in this clinical trial are important because they are likely to change clinical practice and provide an opportunity to improve outcome** in patients with recurrent cervical cancer who have previously had very limited treatment options.* [40]

In this clinical trial we get side effects to die for and death in abundance, and we are left with an inevitable opportunity to improve the outcome. Orthodox cancer research is imprisoned and is going nowhere very, very slowly.

Finally, in at **number one** in the cancer drug best seller list is **rituximab.** Will this be their opportunity to improve the outcome?

Don't hold your breath.

Rituximab was initially used for non-Hodgkin's lymphoma and chronic lymphocytic leukaemia. I was personally assured by my Macmillan nurse that this wonder drug had "revolutionised" lymphoma treatment and that would appear to be the current party line. But has it?

Gross sales in 2013 globally $7.78 billion.

You can see why they like it!

Rituximab or Rituxan is of course a genetically engineered chimeric mouse/human monoclonal antibody, which destroys both normal and cancerous B cells that have the CD20 antigen on their surfaces. Officially classified as immunotherapy, it is nothing of the sort. Trust me! It's an immune suppressor. It attaches to and kills healthy B cells as well as malignant cells. It has been categorised as less damaging than chemotherapy since it does not kill all immune cells only the B's. That isn't a

[40] https://www.cancer.gov/news-events/press-releases/2013/gog240

good thing by the way it's just not as lethal as it could be in the short term but the impact on immunity is very difficult to reverse unless you do what I did.[41]

The U.S. patent for the drug was issued in 1997 and expired in 2015. Rituximab was approved initially by the FDA and the European Medicines Agency for relapsed or refractory low-grade or follicular CD20+ B-cell non-Hodgkin lymphomas, i.e. those that have come back once chemo fails. But once in use and its market was established it was extended to include first-line treatment for low-grade lymphomas as well as the more aggressive subtypes such as diffuse large B-cell lymphomas. And then it was extended further to be used as maintenance for all manner of cancers and for other illnesses. One day soon perhaps it will be available for everything from varicose veins to migraines, or as an alternative to multi-vitamins? Why not!

According to Reuters Health in November 2005:

> *New treatments incorporating immunotherapy have significantly improved overall survival of patients with follicular lymphoma.*

Oncology Live:

> *The Rituximab Revolution... has **revolutionized** the treatment of B-cell malignancies, with **huge improvements** in **survival** rates... **real success**... **remarkable responses** and **substantial effects** on patient **survival**.* [42]

Considering that lymphoma patients on current treatment can live for several years anyway and can even remain stable for 2-3 years or more with no treatment at all, there could not possibly be enough data on this new stuff to claim it significantly extends overall survival. And what the studies actually demonstrated was that the 4 year progression free survival (PFS) was increased from 48% with chemo alone to 61% with rituximab+chemo (R-CHOP: **C**yclophosphamide, **H**ydroxydaunomycin/ doxorubicin, **O**ncovin/vincristine, **P**rednisolone).

This does not provide an increase in overall survival it merely shows a 13% increase in progression free survival which is a passing phase that soon passes and when it has passed the cancer returns quicker with less resistance thus cancelling out any short-term gains.

Maintenance rituximab treatment in the UK has become the current 'standard of care' yet this stop gap use of a useless dangerous poison is controversial even in the inner circle of haematology, where they know it does not extend life, it destroys immunity, the only thing keeping you alive, and it ramps up the cost of treatment.

2013: According to Oncology Live 'Rituximab's Success Fuels Interest in New Agents'. This is in reference to the pharmaceutical industry interests, but the

---

41 http://www.medscape.com/viewarticle/826649

42 http://www.onclive.com/publications/oncology-live/2013/april-2013/targeting-cd20-rituximAbs-success-fuels-interest-in-new-agents#sthash.dswipS1d.dpuf

actual facts tell of how this latest wonder drug failed to deliver for patients so quickly and comprehensively:

When used as a single agent, close to half of patients fail to respond, and complete responses are seen in less than 10%. Most significantly, the majority of patients who do initially respond to rituximab treatment will eventually relapse. [43]

2014: Journal of Clinical Oncology:

End of Rituximab Maintenance for low tumour burden follicular lymphoma - there is no evidence (yet) that an aggressive maintenance rituximab strategy influences overall survival compared with first line rituximab without maintenance. [44]

2016: As the patent for rituximab expired after millions had been subjected to another unnecessary medical intervention, the same experts who claimed a breakthrough in disease maintenance started to declare maintenance rituximab as optional.

With long-term follow-up, MR [maintenance rituximab] did not influence OS [did not live any longer]. The PFS benefit was maintained. [did not live any longer] MR should be considered optional [worthless] for patients with indolent B-cell lymphoma. [45]

2017: *Maintenance Rituximab Failed to Improve Survival After Bendamustine/ Rituximab for Mantle Cell Lymphoma*

Undergoing maintenance therapy with rituximab after induction treatment with bendamustine/rituximab appeared to have no additional benefit compared with observation alone for older patients with mantle cell lymphoma.

According to Dr Friedberg, of the University of Rochester:

It is very unlikely that you will see an impact on overall survival, particularly because ***the observation group, if anything, is doing a bit better than the rituximab maintenance group****.*

These negative results with rituximab should have implications on studies of prolonged treatment strategies incorporating other novel agents, including very expensive novel agents as well. I think it

---

43 http://www.onclive.com/publications/oncology-live/2013/april-2013/targeting-cd20-rituximAbs-success-fuels-interest-in-new-agents#sthash.dswipS1d.dpuf

44 http://ascopubs.org/doi/pdf/10.1200/JCO.2014.57.8328

45 https://www.ncbi.nlm.nih.gov/pubmed/27351685

> ***should give us pause in the design of those studies to look at appropriate endpoints.*** [46]

Dr Bruce Cheson is a prominent orthodox lymphoma specialist, who believes rituximab maintenance to be:

> *... expensive, time-consuming and inconvenient. In each, randomised study, maintenance was associated with increased infections in the rituximab groups compared with observation groups.* ***Importantly, none of the front-line studies demonstrated maintenance associated with a prolongation of survival.***
>
> *There are toxic effects associated with maintenance rituximab including neutropenia, grade 3 and 4 infections, and a small risk of potentially fatal, progressive multifocal leukoencephalopathy... another concern is whether prolonged rituximab may compromise responsiveness to subsequent therapy.*
>
> ***One of the strongest predictors of inferior outcome was receiving rituximab in a previous regimen.*** [47]

Oncology Times report:

> *... the hospitalization rate is higher as well. Delayed complications of rituximab maintenance include late cytopenias, prolonged reduction in serum immunoglobulins, infections, reactivation of hepatitis B and C, and interstitial pneumonitis. The worst is progressive multifocal leukoencephalopathy, which develops in the setting of rituximab and is a uniformly fatal complication.* [48]

The killer blow delivered by rituximab is on immunoglobulins (IgG's). These are antibodies produced by our white blood cells and serve as a critical part of the immune system by identifying antigens and binding to them. We need our defences in order to defeat cancer. Without them we have no chance.

Dr Morton Coleman, a leading lymphoma specialist noted an:

> *"Astounding"* increase in infections with rituximab maintenance, with toxicity reduced in the control group compared with the treatment group. *"In randomized controlled trials, the neutropenia and infection rates are twice as high with maintenance therapy. In other studies, the hospitalization rate is higher as well".* [49]

Remember how obsessively, in order to stop infections, they flood the population with vaccines, yet cancer patients are given them as standard! He added that recovery from infection is often sluggish and incomplete, and large doses of monthly gammaglobluin are often required. More drug sales are always good for business but none of them heal, which is why they are good for business!

---

46 https://am.asco.org/maintenance-rituximab-failed-improve-survival-after-bendamustinerituximab-mantle-cell-lymphoma

47 http://www.medscape.com/viewarticle/741155

48 https://journals.lww.com/oncology-times/Fulltext/2012/03250/Point_Counterpoint___Should_All_Patients_with.7.aspx

49 https://journals.lww.com/oncology-times/fulltext/2012/03250/Point_Counterpoint___Should_All_Patients_with.7.aspx

> *After treatment, 39% (69/179) of patients had low levels of immunoglobulin. In this data set, rituximab administration was associated with a high frequency of hypogammaglobulinemia, particularly symptomatic hypogammaglobulinemia, among patients who received multiple courses of rituximab. Baseline and periodic monitoring of SIgGs is appropriate in patients who receive rituximab.* [50]

Rituximab is on the WHO list of the best drugs ever.

Junk is what they are but that is of no consequence for its pushers. There is a market and when a gap appears competitors race to fill it. MAb sales in 2016 totalled over $90 billion, around half of the total revenue of all biopharmaceutical products, and with 2,836 mAbs currently in development, things are looking good for our druggie friends. [51]

And that, ladies and gentlemen of the jury, is of course the motive. Greed.

Herceptin biosimilar brands are pouring out since the patent started expiring with Novartis rituximab biosimilar completing trials with advanced stage follicular lymphoma victims and others with rheumatoid arthritis awaiting marketing approval. Boehringer Ingelheim is neck and neck with its biosimilar rituximab following phase 3 clinical experiments in patients with rheumatoid arthritis, and Pfizer is bringing up the rear in earlier stage trials with its biosimilar rituximab in patients with rheumatoid arthritis, and phase 1 clinical trials in patients with CD20 positive non-Hodgkin's lymphoma. Other familiar names in the Big Pharma family in the running for a slice of the market, such as Merck, have dropped out due to difficulties with their trials. Ahh bless! They'll be OK. [52]

'Biosimilar' in Keith's dictionary reads: 'Different smell; same sewage'.

Early into my diagnosis I took along a copy of the following 2004 report from Clinical Oncology for my haematologist to comment on. I'm not sure what I expected from a man 25 years on the chemo gravy train but I had to ask since it was one of their own studies and he was trying to sell chemo to me as a good idea.

> *The Contribution of Cytotoxic Chemotherapy to 5-year Survival in Adult Malignancies.*
>
> *The debate on the funding and availability of cytotoxic drugs raises questions about the contribution of curative or adjuvant cytotoxic chemotherapy to survival in adult cancer patients.*

---

50 https://www.ncbi.nlm.nih.gov/pmc/articles/PMC4035033/

51 https://www.researchandmarkets.com/reports/4419867/monoclonal-antibodies-global-trends-in-the

52 https://seekingalpha.com/article/1757582-roche-impact-of-rituxan-patent-expiration-in-europe

We undertook a literature search for randomised clinical trials reporting a 5-year survival benefit attributable solely to cytotoxic chemotherapy in adult malignancies. The total number of newly diagnosed cancer patients for 22 major adult malignancies was determined from cancer registry data... in Australia and.... in the USA for 1998. The overall contribution was the sum total of the absolute numbers showing a 5-year survival benefit expressed as a percentage of the total number for the 22 malignancies.

Some practitioners still remain optimistic that cytotoxic chemotherapy will significantly improve survival. However, ***despite the use of new and expensive single and combination drugs to improve response rates and other agents to allow for dose escalation, there has been no change in some of the regimens used, and there has been little impact from the use of newer regimens.*** *Examples are non-Hodgkin's lymphoma and ovarian cancer...* ***Similarly, in lung cancer, the median survival has increased by only 2 months during the same period and an overall survival benefit of less that 5% has been achieved in the adjuvant treatment of breast, colon, and head and neck cancers.***

Results:

The overall contribution of curative and adjuvant cytotoxic chemotherapy to 5-year survival in adults was estimated to be 2.3% in Australia and 2.1% in the USA.

... ***it is clear that cytotoxic chemotherapy only makes a minor contribution to cancer survival. To justify the continued funding and availability of drugs used in cytotoxic chemotherapy, a rigorous evaluation of the cost-effectiveness and impact on quality of life is urgently required.*** [53]

This is devastating! That says chemo fails nearly 100% of the time if 5-year survival is the ambition. Chemo contributes in less than 3% of adults. You could stick pins in your eyes and be better off!

My haematologist had no knowledge of these findings or the ramifications and showed little interest. He was always polite and he isn't afflicted with an enlarged ego, which is very unusual in this setting, and he listened. He patiently browsed through the pages and handed it back to me (it was a copy for him but he did not want it) and concluded it was rather out of date. He assured us that the situation had improved greatly in the intervening 10 years, thanks mainly to the introduction of a new generation of wonder drugs. Remember the mAbs? Junk drugs. He told me not to worry about the chemo findings because the mAbs had arrived and this is what we had all been waiting for.

---

[53] http://www.clinicaloncologyonline.net/article/S0936-6555(04)00222-5/fulltext

There isn't a single genetically engineered mouse that has been used to produce a drug that cures a disease.
Kathleen Murray, director of Transgenic Service at Charles River Laboratories

Hooked on Radiation

According to some estimates, the radiation exposure a patient receives from a full-body CT scan is often 500 times that of a conventional X-ray and about the same as that received by people living 2.4 kilometres away from the centres of the World War II atomic blasts in Japan. [54]

I continued to attend hospital appointments while treating myself at home. I kept quiet about my private life because they really don't get it and some doctors become quite obstructive and obnoxious with patients who know better. My consultant wasn't a problem but others on his team became uncontrollably awkward when I said no, or asked why. One area of pressure I got was to have full body CT scans. They constantly wanted "to see what's going on inside" so my status could be updated. This is often done, this and other questionable procedures, simply for the purpose of ticking boxes.

Yet I was a patient who had numerous tumours that could be seen, touched and measured more accurately and safely than a CT scan.

And they want to do this repeatedly to sick patients. I went into this with eyes wide open yet still had three of these CT scans, including my eyes. I asked one of my cancer doctors (they constantly change so there's no continuity) how much radiation each scan was giving me and why it mattered to keep looking inside me as we knew my status and I had been scanned recently. She shuffled about and looked irritated that I was even questioning what they do as habit and had no idea except to claim my radiation exposure was "only a little" or as much as I'd get on the average holiday flight. This was one of numerous outrageously misleading statements I would hear as they sought to tease me into their cycle of poison. I responded by agreeing on condition she could assure me that radiation was now curative. That kind of ended that discussion and stopped her pestering me.

Ionizing Radiation and Cancer Risk

> ***We've long known that children and teens who receive high doses of radiation to treat lymphoma or other cancers are more likely to develop additional cancers later in life.*** *But we have no clinical trials to guide our thinking about cancer risk from medical radiation in healthy adults. Most of what we know about the risks of ionizing radiation comes from long-term studies of people who survived the 1945 atomic bomb blasts at Hiroshima and Nagasaki. These studies show a slightly but significantly increased risk of cancer in those exposed to the blasts, including a group of 25,000 Hiroshima survivors who received less than 50 mSv of radiation — an amount you might get from two or three CT scans.*

---

[54] https://www.newscientist.com/article/dn11827-ct-scan-radiation-can-equal-nuclear-bomb-exposure/

The atomic blast isn't a perfect model for exposure to medical radiation, because the bomb released its radiation all at once, while the doses from medical imaging are smaller and spread over time. Still, most experts believe that can be almost as harmful as getting an equivalent dose all at once. [55]

Radiation causes cancer and the more you have the greater the risk. Laboratory studies and the human experience for over 100 years have found that X-ray, radiotherapy and other radioactive materials initiate DNA mutation and can cause cancer to become virulent and aggressive. Destroyed tissue or tissue that has been damaged is a parasitic paradise. Dr Victor Richards tells us in 'Cancer - The Wayward Cell. Its origins, nature and treatment'

A recent controlled clinical study by Fisher and his colleagues (1968) suggests that routine postoperative irradiation therapy may alter the immunological responsiveness of the host to the extent that systemic or generalized recurrences occur somewhat more frequently than they might have if the patient had not been irradiated... Physical and chemical forces alter cell function, for experiments on the irradiation of cells showed that X-rays produced structural and functional changes.

To add to the ionizing radiation from the machine, fluorodeoxyglucose may be included with PET (positron emission tomography) scans. This radiopharmaceutical is used to help diagnose cancer and other diseases. In this investigation a radioactive liquid sugar with a sprinkle of fluoride is injected into your bloodstream where it spreads out and gives off energy in the form of gamma rays.

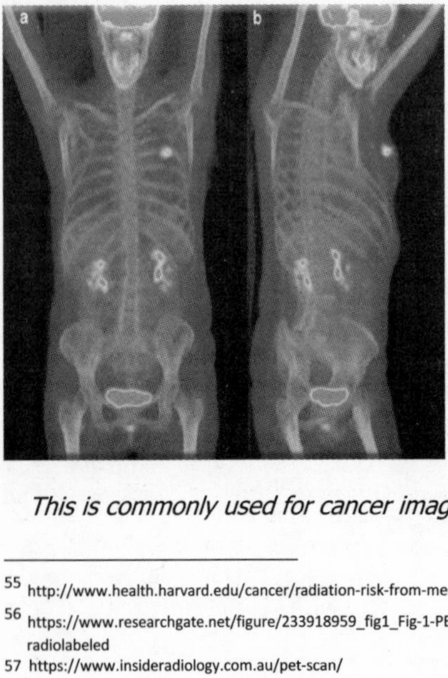

PET/CT scan of a patient with breast cancer. A trace amount of radiolabeled glucose (18 F-Fluorodeoxyglucose) was injected intravenously 1h prior to the scan. The CT scan enables the visualization of the anatomical structures such as the bone in grayscale. The color-coded image represents the distribution of the molecular tracer in the body. The radiolabeled glucose shows normal uptake in brain and elimination via kidneys into the bladder. At the level of the left breast there is an intense signal signifying the presence of hypermetabolic cells in the breast cancer. On the left (a) is the anterior view and on the right (b) is the right oblique view of a 3D reconstructed image. [56]

*This is commonly used for cancer imaging as **tumours need sugar to grow**.* [57]

---

55 http://www.health.harvard.edu/cancer/radiation-risk-from-medical-imaging

56 https://www.researchgate.net/figure/233918959_fig1_Fig-1-PETCT-scan-of-a-patient-with-breast-cancer-A-trace-amount-of-radiolabeled

57 https://www.insideradiology.com.au/pet-scan/

Not my words. I do say that cancer feeds on sugar and that cancer patients should be informed of this so they can decide if they want to eat cakes to raise funds for cancer charities or to encourage cancer patients to load up on fats and sugars to put on weight. CT and PET scans are often used together as according to our inside source on their own they're of less value.

> *The PET-CT combination allows any abnormality on the PET scan to be precisely located within the body, allowing for more accurate diagnosis of any problems.* [57]

They cause cancer, they aren't that accurate and they can't cure you anyway. And there's more to consider before we consent.

The gadolinium-based contrast agent used in a third of MRI scans has recently been found by researchers to carry a previously unseen risk to patients. Gadolinium is a heavy metal with unique paramagnetic properties. All the expert scientists in the orthodox medical system 'believed' for decades that this toxic compound they were injecting into sick patients was flushed out soon after and was therefore safe, but it is now known that some of the toxin remains trapped deep inside patients subjected to MRI scans, even in the brain.

The theory was:

> *Gadolinium... ions... are toxic, but bound to a ligand, they can remain chelated in the body and* ***are excreted intact.***

But an article published in the journal BioMetals in 2016 stirred up a hornet's nest by raising serious questions about this pseudoscientific belief in safety. According to lead author Moshe Rogosnitzky:

> ***Although gadolinium is bound to chelating agents designed to flush out the rare metal following an MRI, it has been found to deposit in the brain, bone, and other organs.*** [58]

Gadolinium was known to carry a higher risk for kidney damage (Nephrogenic Systemic Fibrosis) or NSF, a debilitating disease in patients with impaired kidney function, but it was not meant to be able to cross the blood brain barrier and damage that too. There is a broad view within this often-times backward community that toxins are generally safe and that nutrition is for wimps. Evidence now shows that all patients are at risk from this agent and these authors have called for urgent retrospective and prospective studies to assess the scale of harm caused by their reckless comrades. Will more studies confirm the truth, force a response and save lives? Don't be silly! Contrast Induced Nephropathy (CIN) is yet another creation of the quacks to add to the encyclopaedia of doctor-induced disorders. This doctor disease, they tell us, affects about 2% of recipients. Meanwhile, apparently radiologists are going to be more careful to recommend gadolinium contrast only

[58] https://link.springer.com/article/10.1007/s10534-016-9931-7

where it is likely to assist a better diagnosis. [59] Some progress, I guess, but when someone needs reminding to intervene only where necessary we should be on high alert. First do no harm guys!

And remember what happens when they do diagnose disease? They do all this to see how damaged your body is but at the end of the day they still can't cure what they see! Our grandkids will call this time in history the Barbaric Age when they hear what we did to ourselves in the name of diagnostics and disease management.

When epidemiologist Alice Stewart published her findings in 1956 questioning the orthodox science of X-ray scanning expectant mothers as a matter of course, on the basis that this foetal radiation exposure was causing lymphatic leukaemia in the children, she was cast out of the brotherhood and sent off to the duck pond, her career stunted.

Studying children who had died of cancer before the age of 10 she found they had been X-rayed twice as often in utero as the live children. A single X-ray was well within official "safety limits" but only a fraction of this was enough to double the risk of early cancer in children. Unashamed, it took until the late 1970s before the leading US medical institutions, followed by the British medical experts, began to recommend that doctors should no longer routinely X-ray pregnant women and only eventually did the practice end. Radiating unborn babies does seem really rather stupid, as does injecting them with aluminium and mercury, mouse and monkey viruses but this is all perfectly normal, as we shall discover.

Alice Stewart died in 2002 age 95 after fighting a long and often lonely battle with the medical priesthood to bring to light the dangers of exposure to low-level radiation. She later recalled, "They don't burn you at the stake any more, but they do the equivalent, in terms of cutting you off from your means to work." But it was too little punishment too late; she'd done her bit in forming a public understanding of this lethal X-ray technology, which she observed was "the favourite toy of the medical profession." And not much has changed as they continue to fire their ray beams around like we're some kind of target practice, oblivious, uninterested in the harm they do.

No amount of radiation is safe. Every dose is an overdose

George Wald, Nobel Laureate 1953

---

59 https://www.insideradiology.com.au/gadolinium-contrast-medium/

Open Mind - Open Heart

The secret of change is to focus all of your energy not on fighting the old, but on building the new.
Socrates (469/470-399 BCE)

I'm a big fan of allowing others to speak freely whatever they have to say. Free speech is free speech after all. It isn't regulated, controlled, limited or censored. That would be oppressive. We don't have to believe what we hear or agree with it, but it is helpful to have as many of the facts, the arguments and the opinions as we can get so we can make more informed decisions. Otherwise we are ill-informed idiots. As such I've given them a platform to do the talking and they have given us a clear hint at what's on offer in the cancer field.

There is still a perfectly valid argument for looking inside, or deeper when suffering disease and in the absence of an alternative then needs must. But not for the sake of it! Fortunately there are other options available which are much safer and more informative than the CT/PET/MRI scans, just not approved of by the current monopoly, reliant as it is upon this nuclear industry diagnostic gold standard.

This is VEGA Bio-Resonance, my favourite.

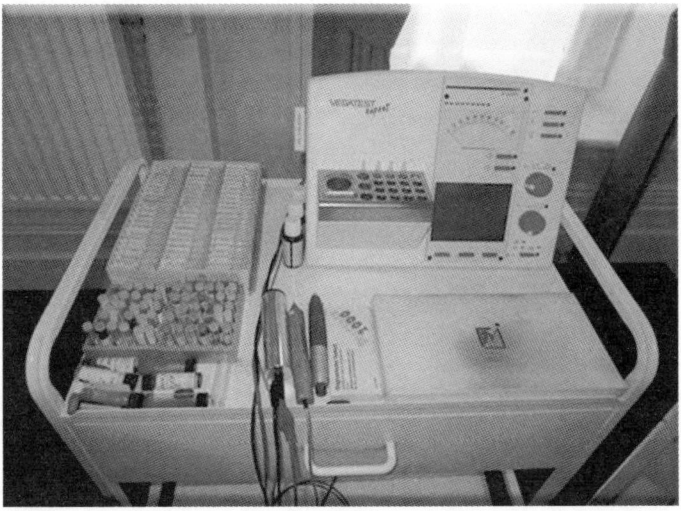

I have nothing invested in any of these products, only my health. This is what worked for me and I believe it holds the key. This is science at its best.

The VEGA diagnostic system is amazing and can identify everything from cancer to food allergies and has been pivotal in my healing. This is a finely tuned non-invasive physiological energy measuring computer, which tunes into subtle electrical signals down to the cellular level and identifies disharmony. We might equate with an instrument designed for reading the signature of an element on a celestial body 100 million miles away. This medical technology is simply brilliant and so bloody simple and so bloody obvious it's almost funny that we allow them to do what they do to us in the name of approved science.

By the summer of 2015 there were people around us we had been in touch with two years earlier heading towards full health on the Gerson Therapy, including Alice's aunt, while my situation was going in the opposite direction, yet I followed the protocol diligently. Aside the kitchen work, there are simple things we don't really consider normally such as charting vitals each day – blood pressure, temperature weight - and obtaining a copy of each NHS blood test or scan to be charted for Gerson reviews and our records. This simple act in the beginning was something of a campaign in itself as the ever present 'jobsworth' doctor's surgery receptionist – they are scattered throughout the community – would seek to deny me my blood test results, protesting that there were rules and that doctors were the keepers of information about my health and only they could agree to release my information. I don't think so! It took a few weeks but by the time I'd done being me a note had been placed on my file by my GP informing receptionists that I was to be given a copy of blood test results as requested. Aside the fact this was about me, my GP as a matter of norm seldom checked the blood work of his patients. He showed me as much one day as he pressed the down key to scroll through a long list of his unopened emails, explaining that he didn't have the time to read them all. He was polite, honest and helpful but he wasn't going to heal me.

I had wanted Gerson to work for me more than anything in the world and we invested everything in it but I have to say I'm pleased it didn't. A great many brave people have written their Gerson journey and the stories are as individual as cancer itself, but they are about the Gerson Therapy which is very well documented. But some of us need more and I can now add another more powerful option, one that pushed back a post-chemo recurrent cancer, something Gerson was not going to do for me.

The curtain came down on my official Gerson protocol when we tried to contact my practitioner at the Hungary clinic in the summer of 2015 as we were drawing up plan B. I wanted his advice on how to manoeuvre into and out of chemo if that was to be my next move. I wanted to ask how other patients were faring using chemo during Gerson and if he had any other updated advice. I knew that the standard advice is to do chemo if Gerson doesn't work (unless there is an urgency to intervene chemically first), the aim being to buy time by debulking a heavy cancer load and then get back to rebuilding immunity on full Gerson - 13 juices daily, 5 enemas etc. But we'd seen enough continued growth of a not-so-bulky disease through Gerson into a bulky one to know what to expect and we were already morphing my protocol.

Incredibly, everyone at the Hungary clinic was away on their summer holiday break at the time and could not be contacted. And that was the end of that. He did eventually check in to tell me what I already knew but we have had no contact since. A pretty poor show but every cloud has a silver lining and we make things better by recognising where we went wrong.

I can take a hint and didn't need telling it was time to move on. Now we were on our own again. I knew to reduce the number of juices and enemas during chemo for safety reasons, as this is a powerful detoxifying combination when used properly and to increase the therapy as manageable afterwards so not to force out too much chemo at once. All this information is available in books and via online Gerson Institute coaching conferences. The Institute remains the best resource for the Gerson protocol but they can't tell you what's best for you or how you will react as an individual or even what else you may need to heal.

Tumours had been growing all over my body and this subtle but steady growth was making me look more and more like a lizard every day. Although you don't really see it; it creeps up inevitably like that new housing development. We had invested everything in this process, and quickly excelled, at times there was no obvious growth and I experienced detox reactions, clear signs we were winning, but something wasn't right.

But what?

Gerson doesn't work?
Bad luck?
Something missing?
Charlotte Gerson's parked up her organisation where she feels it's safe?
It's a conspiracy theory?
Meant to be?

Max Gerson's therapy is an amazingly simple and effective route to health restoration and daughter Charlotte has brought it back from the dead with a passion, but it's flagging. Technology and toxicity have moved on, there are new ideas and new techniques but these are not being adopted and incorporated into what must become the Gerson Therapy. I dragged the principle into 2017 because I was forced to, but Gerson at present only do the 1930's version. In fact any attempt to speed things up or individualise the protocol is frowned upon. Indeed one may find oneself abandoned by one's practitioner if one wishes to tweak the therapy to suit one's own needs. I don't make this wrong for everyone and I would urge due diligence to the protocol if that is your choosing, but the advice from Charlotte Gerson is to continue ad infinitum drilling away with the standard protocol, to keep juicing, keep doing the enemas, keep taking the supplements your body may not need. "You must keep going", she demands, but that would have been the end of me.

You gotta let it grow, girl.

One of the most significant findings at this point was the apparent stress on my kidneys. Why were my kidneys struggling after two years of Gerson? VEGA had revealed this kidney stress but there is no point telling a GP about the wisdom of the magic box, you may as well be talking about aliens, so instead I asked mine for a blood test so he could find it! The test indeed revealed elevated creatinine which is a sign of kidney stress, but because it was down to me to monitor my blood work on behalf of my GP (something I was happy to do) I found it and showed him. We had a hunch this pressure on the kidneys was caused by bulging lymph nodes but curiously my relaying of this detail to my NHS cancer team elicited only more confusion. They told me blocked kidneys wasn't a common problem and was not likely anything to do with the lymphoma. I'm not sure how this happened but suddenly we were on the opposite side of this fence with me talking of cancer progression and considering chemical intervention and them not!

So I asked for a CT scan (my second), which did indeed confirm it was in fact the lymphoma, which was building up internally and blocking the tubes to my kidneys. I don't mind being wrong but now I really wanted to be wrong! Healing reactions typically cause tumours to grow before they shrink, which is one reason why Gerson is not recommended for brain cancers because there's little room for manoeuvre. This was not a healing reaction, however, this was steady growth and something needed to be done. Here my story begins to turn. The CT was performed on the Friday, first thing Monday morning the phone rang as we anticipated and feared it would. It was my Macmillan nurse, ever efficient, telling me chemo was needed and needed urgently. They always say that! But we saw the scan, the blood work, VEGA and the state of me and couldn't disagree. The pressure was on.

Medical science has broken the totality of natural laws in the human body to little pieces. It has studied and re-studied single processes and overestimated them. The symptoms of a disease became the main problem for research and clinical work. The medical theory of the old and middle ages to combine all parts in the body to a biological entity was pushed aside almost involuntarily, and finally became very far removed from our thinking. How such thinking of totality will help us to find the cause of cancer can best be seen in practical examples – not animal experiments – in the nutritional field of people who do not get cancer, and, on the other hand, of those who get it in greater or increasing amounts.

Dr Max Gerson.

Between the Devil and the Deep Blue Sea

To unleash the horrors of chemical warfare and the atomic bomb in the form of chemotherapy and cobalt radiation on the victims of a microbial disease is illogical.
Dr Virginia Livingston PhD (1906 -1990)

I hadn't expected this moment but I was prepared for it and I wouldn't have missed it for the world. I didn't really have much choice at this stage and I'd made my mind up and into a round of chemo was an easy transition. Helpful as it is for someone in my position with such a bad attitude toward chemo, the outcome was all I could have hoped for. I could have succumbed to the chemo as so many do; glorying in my predictions of its evil, and that would have only been a happy ending for those circling my wagon. But not this time, suckers! I did what everyone insists we must when we get cancer, but for me, and it was a very, very poor show. If you understand the cancer-treatment-disease-progression process then the significance of this unfolding story won't be lost on you.

September 2015 I went for my first chemo infusion over two days and then again every three weeks until I'd had six double doses of the mustard gas extract, Bendamustine and 5 hits of rituximab. R-Benda they call it. A few years earlier I was rescuing lab mice and now extracts of them were being injected into me. I'm not sure what to do with that but there it is.

Aside my obvious revulsion at this ghoulish turn of events in my life, it does neatly fail the test. From my viewpoint this was an in your face vivisection disaster and it's directly because of our obsession with this failed methology that better treatments are passing us by.

At the end of my first cycle we came away with this feeling of excitement but not about the chemo. Certainly not that! For starters I'd been in the hospital all day having had an allergic reaction to the rituximab infusion. Tickle in the throat is a first sign, got that, told myself it was nothing and for a while it was, but then itching starts accompanied by a rash and now we have a pattern building so they slow down the drip and add steroids; supposed to take one hour took nine. Nine long hours! By then I have no food left in my large rucksack and that is the worst thing of all.

It wasn't all bad. Before the day had turned irritating, to the bewilderment of the chatty cancer ward orderly, we'd been studying beta glucans as an immune support, partly to counter the internal chemical insult that he was regularly checking was going OK. This budding young medical gofer had some fancy notion that vaccines were for the immune support and couldn't understand why we would pay to import pills that hadn't been officially approved or recommended by my consultant. Bless. Beta glucans had been speaking to us through this curious couple of days and had shone a light. We were steadily getting a feel for what we needed to make sure this window of opportunity I was having injected into me wasn't wasted. Beta glucans were soon on order and would become part of the network of immune support elements of my new protocol.

Having chemo was a bit like I was cheating on myself and it didn't feel right. So to make up to myself I made a conscious effort to feed my soul with the solution at each chemo sitting. Our research was the main focus for my hospital appointments and Alice's too, and when she was laid up in bed for days on end paying the price for having pushed her luck on an earlier journey, she'd study. We were on a journey of discovery and we knew we were being guided and we felt ever confident that nothing was going to get in the way. More often than not if the appointment wasn't essential for Alice she would stay home and research and be loading me all day with my homework. I miss her when she's not there and we don't eat the food they provide in hospital and I knew there was a price to pay for the chemo so the only rewarding bit of my stay was the free internet. So while I was infused I searched for a way to cure cancer!

Every trip is an adventure, even for chemo, but Alice does struggle sitting for long and often struggles to get comfortable at night and can't sleep. Through those nights she can be found with her head in her iPad. Many mornings through the spring of 2016 I would wake to this extra excited creature next to me bursting with information to share. I'd say "Let me do my enema first then we'll talk", but you can't keep a good woman down and you can't shut this one up even when there's nothing to talk about! She had to get it out and would end up talking to me as I slipped my tube where the sun don't shine about the chemical structure of some element in periodic chart and its relationship with free radicals and how that can be used alongside ozone therapy; about cell membranes or lipid bilayers and the transport of biochemical data through the correct oils... "What?! It's half past four! Fuck off!" Little made sense until I'd dumped my enema, but gradually the day would dawn and clarity arrive and I could begin to understand where this might fit in.

When all was said and done my short-term chemo experience wasn't all that bad, but for one potentially life-threatening event or side effect as they call them, which had me admitted for two days attached to an antibiotic drip to bring down a persistent high fever. Over 4 days I'd tussled at home with a fever that reached 40C, hopeful it might reach the right temperature to kill cancer cells but not me. That's a tricky one to manage at home and I lost that battle, or didn't win.

We live on a road off the sea, a man-made wind tunnel that costal storms roar through horizontally to the point where you can't breathe if you face it and cannot get from one end to the other when it rages. Some joker built an old folks' home on the end of the road. They don't go out much or they say a prayer before stepping out on a windy day. I have escorted many down the road to safety over the years. Anyway 2am in a gale in the midst of my body over heating I stood out on the street freezing my nuts off trying to bring my temperature down from 40c. I could see the dog trying to hide in the sofa as I passed in case I tried taking him out! It was soon deeply unpleasant to be outside but it helped, along with drinking cold water, a wet flannel and a cold head shower. That was like being tortured while I should be fast asleep. My temperature did come down until later the next day when that cycle repeated and soon the realisation dawned that I couldn't control it so I took myself to hospital where I was fast-tracked to a ward to be wired to a drip with some urgency and held for two days.

The minimal combination of cancer drugs I was given, gross as they are, was the favourable choice of my haematologist and the least side effect laden. This combo is showcased as the cutting edge of non-Hodgkin's lymphoma disease management but it couldn't manage mine! It also leaves the nastier stuff for use later when the patient returns for another go once its effects wear off or to treat the transformation of the disease (into a more aggressive form) when that occurs. The negative effect of chemo et al are amplified as the dose builds and I had my eyes wide open and viewed the eventual outcome with enough scepticism to know never to return.

A couple of weeks prior to starting the chemo I was given an oral steroid, prednisone. This is an immunosuppressant. I had an immune stimulated cancer that was over producing white blood cells and the response to that one agent alone had a really dramatic effect on my tumour load in just a few days with minimal toxicity. I recall it shrank more than any other agent they used; Alice thinks the first cycle of chemo did more, but whatever. I can't fully explain this lack of toxicity but it clearly matters that we properly go through the detoxification process for a long-lasting effect. From my perspective only once I had gone through it properly did I heal. No detox, no heal.

This kind of response to the steroids from an immune cancer is almost instantly impressive but just like the chemo it is superficial and short-lived. Cycle one of treatment took some more off the tumour load and cycle two did a little bit more, but after that there was no obvious shrinkage and I was left with cancer. It was revealed to me after the first three cycles that this was quite a normal outcome and that there would probably be no more or very little shrinkage from the next three. This of course begs the question why! Why continue? This is a well understood complication in treating cancers with quick kill treatments - the slow growing sleeping cancer cells are unaffected. As in most communities and colonies, citizens will be found in all stages of development and as such the less mature, unseen entities can 'hide' from the poisons aimed at the more accessible. Only full immune restoration will overcome such obstacles. This is of course the same for all cancers, indolent or aggressive, where one remaining cell/microbe sabotages a cure, and explains why signs of cancer may remain following the chemo carpet bombing and is the reason why a cure is not a stated aim of the ortho-docs.

I was now in what they call regression. Or partial remission - at least 50% gone/left. I was a good responder! Whatever! Less cancer for a while is all it means. We were keen to hear the result of my next CT scan after the 4th cycle in the November and I have to say we were briefly encouraged when my haematologist entered the day ward during my 5th cycle three weeks later and announced that I "couldn't have responded better" to the treatment. I felt a little like I had achieved something, like getting a gold star at school or an award. Well done Keith! The other patients were excited too, but what of the all important pre-treatment aim to clear all sign of disease from my body? I could have responded better by having no sign of cancer, but this wasn't me. These scans soon after treatment capture the pinnacle of chemo's achievement when there is least likely to be any sign of cancer and when that false sense of security sets in. I see the almighty US military after they carpet bombed the jungles of Vietnam in the 1970's with their chemical weapons, obliterating all sign of the enemy. And then evacuating the country soon after: overwhelmed by the enemy.

The reality is I still had disease, the scan confirmed that and we could all physically feel it just under the surface bubbling away. I had taken in another big hit of radiation with what was my final CT scan and my immune system had taken a serious assault that took years to recover. The scan report suggested the cancer had a head start on my immune system, littered as it is with areas of cancer: "reduced... the largest measuring... decreased in size... the largest measuring... mild residual... improved in comparison... significant decrease in the size... nodes are smaller..." Piles and piles of cancer. Remember it takes just one cancer cell, here were billions.

This was more depressing than impressive and did not merit an award. On the positive I was no longer bulky to look at and the pressure was off my kidneys. I had been assured this treatment would get me to the point of no disease, temporary as that inevitably is, but under the surface it was more of the same and the best drugs there are against one of chemo's best *responding,* albeit incurable cancers, on which the industry was founded, had failed spectacularly in its first test and there was worse news to come. Chemo cycle one of the six sittings is always the most productive but from there on it gets at less and less of the cancer. I had bought a few months but I had a much more compromised immune system, as blood tests, VEGA and lingering viruses would later reveal. I was invited to have yet another CT scan after the final chemo infusion just a few weeks after the 4th cycle but I was having none of that and they duly agreed with me that it wasn't necessary because of the obvious disease signs I presented with. None of it is necessary!

And then came the kicker. My chemo inspired 'progression free survival' honeymoon would appear to last eight short weeks when perhaps the best recognised side effect of chemo - after hair loss - the rebound effect occurred and the cancer started noticeably growing again. As spring turned into summer my shadows grew larger as the lumps started to poke through my skin all over me. I was noticing Alice covertly eying my neck from different angles with a look of discomfort, and I knew why. She wasn't saying anything at first, just looking, squinting, hoping to make those shadows shrink. And she was living with the horror and disbelief that we could be back here so soon. She had noticed changes, the new growth, significant tiny lumps now poking through when I stretched, and they weren't there yesterday. Were they? We both felt that sinking feeling of an urgency but to do what? You can't do chemo again. Intravenous vitamin C was in our scope so was cannabis oil but where is all the money coming from and how long do we have to experiment? I wanted to try everything ASAP but primarily just what I needed! We bought a sauna blanket and a selection of supplements.

Meanwhile I landed one infection after another and found myself staggering through most of 2016 and beyond. It is part of the cancer treatment process that patients are loaded up with antibiotics and anti-fungal, anti-viral and anti-sickness drugs during chemo and beyond - life-long dependence once they get you on the mAbs - to keep infection controlled while the immune system is paralysed. These drugs further impair immunity and still the infections move in and often become an inevitable side effect or cause of death of their approved cancer treatment.

The likelihood of this cancer coming back is a given but this wasn't quite what we expected. Then again none of this was what we expected. It was central to my thinking that the foundation of two years of Gerson would give me a head start in overcoming the cancer and the chemo, but you live and learn and we were being jostled to learn fast. Early one morning in June 2016 I woke with a start and sprung to the mirror in the bathroom after I'd had the sudden realisation in my sleep that I had a tumour appear in my neck overnight. And sure enough there it was to my total horror, it was the size of a grape and it wasn't there when I went to bed. Such a rapid growth had never happened before and that literally scared the shit out of me. I felt quite sick! And that sinking feeling of an urgency to get on the toilet. The rest of the day was a challenge as I wondered how we were going to cope with a cancer that was bubbling over in my bone marrow and was now showing ominous signs. They do that, they transform into a crazy state. Then what?

As intimidating as it was to have the clock ticking, it hadn't fully transformed and with the benefit of hindsight this couldn't have turned out much better. As a side effect of trying to heal we were competing with the might and the organised chaos of orthodox medicine, and without knowing it we were tantalisingly close to unravelling the mystery of cancer while they were locked in secret experiments and manufacturing mice to test things on. This was all the more remarkable since the whole point of chemo was to buy time. Healing takes time. Had they suppressed my cancer for a longer period, even 3 or 4 years, as we anticipated, I would be in no position to boast of a rebirth and offer genuine hope to others. We wouldn't have felt such an urgency to search for something more, had my foundational work and continued adherence to an anti cancer lifestyle allowed my immune system to take over. It would look to outsiders like Gerson had failed and chemo had worked and the sceptics would be gloating that a cancer cure and a conspiracy theorist had been ridiculed, their ignorance satisfied by their gloating. Of course even in that event it could be argued that Gerson had made chemo work better or be less damaging but that idea would have the cynics in hysterics. Yet who ever asks a cancer patient what they are doing at home to assist their healing?

The clever scientists assume their poisons did it when someone lives a few years but what of the patients' own actions, the critical lifestyle choices, abstention and additions? Without considering immune support there's little point even participating in the search for health let alone claiming victory after a short-lived chemical bombardment of some cancer symptoms. Comprehensive scientific research doesn't leave out data, such as how someone fuels their daily existence and grew their cancer. Of all the social groups that make up our society, the people most likely to make changes in the way they live are those confronted with life-threatening illness. It's a commentary we hear over and over - an evolutionary opportunity we are all facing - we learn and we grow through our suffering. It's those subtle changes, those dramatic changes that change us internally and externally. This omission makes all hospital induced remissions, cures, recoveries or claims that chemo works simple anecdotes.

I don't know for sure yet but I suspect I will always be a statistical success in the annals of chemotherapy. Had it, survived it and thrived.

Anecdote: 'based on casual observations or indications rather than rigorous or scientific analysis' [60]

We were rigorous. From my earliest hospital appointments in 2013 we were firmly assured by both my consultant and my Macmillan nurse, that the mAbs had transformed cancer treatment and survival. They were an affable and professional team, kind and considerate and plainly excited by this breakthrough. But we had done our homework and when you do that you get to see not just what your experts hear from drug reps, cancer charities and the mainstream media but the less promotional material too. And the stuff they don't show us is always better. More rounded. Honest. And they were wrong. My guide was herself misguided. It's like Chinese whispers around the operating table! I was told by my Macmillan nurse (and consultant) that the chemo would get me to the point of no disease and that there was no reason why I shouldn't stay there for a number of years. She actually sat there looked me in the eye and told me there was "no reason why you shouldn't live a normal life". Well I had cancer for starters, that's a big reason. I was also assured that my bulky disease was no more difficult to control than any other yet none of this was true.

She was a consummate professional; flawless in her supporting role, high energy, dedicated and focussed and she ensured the process flowed seamlessly. She was all you could ask of a friend, but this charitable kindness seems to have morphed into something of a de-facto sales rep role for Big Pharma's product and only that product. Now don't get me wrong, I see the empathy and that innate human kindness in the work these people do and I see the desire to help others, but to what end? I envision a lollipop lady, who rather than guide the children over the road to safety is luring them into the Pharma's arms. There are many natural protocols and products which can heal any disease and are non-toxic, away from which Macmillan and its nurses are guiding people. I was given a lifelong free prescription card by my guide so I didn't have to pay for the drugs they anticipated I would need in future but I haven't used it. And I got a free car parking pass at the hospital where I was invited for radiation, chemotherapy and was sent away with fearful ideas. The free parking space was helpful but to what end? And why are patients and visitors made to pay to park anyway? I expect it to be free for everyone!

By the time you realise this treatment is anything but revolutionary you are caught in that trap and instilled with such fear that you will agree to just about anything the kindly nurse suggests, not that they offer any choice. Even the suggestion you might

[60] http://www.thefreedictionary.com/anecdotal

do nothing will be resisted. My Mac nurse would do this cajoling more enthusiastically than my consultant.

I later contacted Macmillan Cancer Support to query their advice and enquire of their role. They certainly don't promote themselves as sales reps for chemo but that was every bit my experience. Looking through the material they provide potential customers to browse as we decide our fate, and at their website, and visiting their London hospital there can be no doubt where their allegiances lie. There is no mention of any other way, only the usual treatment options provided by the Chemical Brothers. In a series of emails I asked why this is and was told they only promote approved methods. Of course they do but that doesn't make it ethical or right and it removes all hope.

Macmillan revolve around cake and coffee mornings, raising money and selling cookbooks loaded with sugar, salt and fat processed foods which they encourage cancer patients to gobble down to put on weight. I asked if this was a good idea given what we now know about the impact of this stuff on the human body and its relationship with cancer. I asked if, given that cancer remains incurable against this cock-eyed dietary advice, they would consider a different approach and broaden horizons. I asked if they thought the principle of eating five pieces of chemically grown fruit and veg a day to improve health were translated into Gerson advice about flooding the body with organic nutrients might do more than simply improve and instead restore health. I asked for the science to back up their advice. Macmillan's response? They abandoned me at the third email. I persisted and received confirmation in louder and louder silences.

I like the silence and I do hear it a lot once I start probing, but what if I were a patient who really did need their help, how would the silence help me then? I'd been impeccably polite in the face of indifference to my fate, and my deeply personal experience, and they had presented their case for the defence. I was able to reach a unanimous verdict, so I stopped bothering them. At least for the time being.

Left to figure it out for myself I have and I think they are in bed with the devil.

I did resume something resembling a normal life in the few weeks post chemo. Most memorable from that brief, intense moment in time while my cancer was out of sight and not visibly active came the realisation of just how easy it would be to forget the cancer was ever a problem and carry on as normal. And why so many of us do just that to our detriment. For some, this is the time they feel a strong sense of gratitude for having survived this thing we are taught to associate with a cruel crawl to death. This is the window of opportunity that spawns those who, with all due respect, do the grunt work to gather in the charity money to reward the cancer charities and the researchers for their heroism.

The chemo ended for me in December 2015 after six two-day sittings, typically taking no more than an hour each day plus the faffing around it. We are told it is still apparently holding off the cancer for a couple of months thereafter. I was being cajoled to start the 2 years rituximab maintenance (every 2 months) in the spring of

2016, or ASAP after the R-Benda and was being hassled to get hooked up to the bag of immune immobilising mouse DNA before it was too late for them to maintain me, but as with those awful double-maths classes **all** Thursday afternoon, I was elsewhere. I was told it was now all about keeping the cancer suppressed for as long as possible, but it wasn't suppressed it was growing. It was always growing and if I took their advice I would die an ugly death. I'd taken all I needed and bought myself some time to do some more theorising.

Besides which I had been mislead more than once and this was now as serious as cancer coming back and further treatment would ruin all chance of a natural cure. This was my life in the balance, but to Dr Fear PhD, a lady with all manner of letters after her name, (which I've changed) she was simply going about her business with little consideration of the consequences of her actions.

I'd had R-Benda which sounds quite benign alongside their chemo combo's such as 5FU (5 feet under), BACON, BOLD, CHOP, COP-BLAM, CyVADIC, Hexa-CAF, ICE, MOPP, Pro-Mace and ProMACE-CytaBOM... As macho as it all sounds it ain't no good. As I said, it was my firm intention to avoid this stuff altogether but once I'd changed my mind I took the minimum I needed and scarpered. I got out not a day too soon because the impact the mAbs have on its victims is more irreversible than cancer. It is of course possible to recover health after one round of chemo but two rounds would take something special. With no immune system there would be little hope of healing from anything. Doc Fear tried to sell the maintenance process as their "standard of care", which it isn't, and suggested that my disease "may" progress more quickly without irreversible chemical suppression of my defences. It may well progress more quickly with chemical suppression and as the rituximab research clearly shows it makes no contribution to overall survival, but she never mentioned that. She enthused how the infusion would be no big deal and I would be unlikely to feel "symptomatic" during infusions. Yeah! When I probed she brushed aside the inevitable outcome of her intervention by comparing the horror of cancer with her "lesser of two evils".

I was standing on that trap door with the inevitable about to happen. The experts had promised to remove all tumours and then I'd be in a great position for the wonder drugs to keep me there at the point of no evidence of disease (where I intended to keep myself of course) for approximately two years since around that point patients become resistant to rituximab and the suppression of B cells is considered too dangerous to proceed any further. But I was still in a disease state with it growing and my one big chance gone. There was no point; this was a broken arrangement with goal posts being dragged around all over the place. Only in the autumn I was being assured I would soon have no sign of disease but by the following summer my suitability for a bone marrow transplant had slipped into the conversation in place of the chemo pitch which was followed by the 'wonder mAbs' stories they had spun for months. We laughed in the car on the way home on reflecting how this brutal bone marrow event was suddenly being sold to us as a kind of special treat saved for patients who are "young and fit, like yourself" so may have a half a chance of surviving the gruelling procedure. It is typically in those of us who fail the first hit of chemo so spectacularly that they justify this high risk experiment because there's little they can now do with chemo to beat their first attempt, and so this is seen as worth the risk to try and make good the broken promise of much less cancer. I am young and fit and I'm intending to keep it that way.

There are many temptations in the chemo honeymoon period to celebrate, especially with the cancer expert's excitement ringing like an endorsement. We are essentially and officially granted permission to go back to socialising and drinking and take-aways and those convenient treats we spoil ourselves with to celebrate our survival. Don't waste money on vitamin C, treat yourself to a bottle of wine was the suggestion of my cancer expert, who is an unashamed chocolate monster himself, but I don't have those temptations any longer because I found out they create the environment for cancer so obviously I'm not going to do that again! White wine, white chocolate and a takeaway curry was my treat, but that was then. I instead chose cabbage, kale, carrots and longer dog walks over the downs and far, far away. The dog came too but sometimes he wished he hadn't! Plenty of sun and juicing, regular enemas and hypothesising. I got my bike out for some long overdue cycling sessions too and did a bit of running.

But I wasn't running for very long when that sinking feeling came over me, that well known cancer patient wave of terror. A clear sign that the experts have missed something! Ralph Moss PhD talks about this in Questioning Chemotherapy:

> *It is a **common observation** that patients sometime seem to have an accelerated growth of cancer after receiving chemotherapy. This impression is often denigrated by oncologists. However, it is given credence from a study of patients who relapsed after treatment of breast cancer.* [61] *Ninety-four out of 176 of these patients receiving chemotherapy after their relapse; the rest received endocrine treatment as a control.*
>
> *There were favourable responses in 23 percent in the group that received the standard chemo protocol but in 47 percent of the patients in the control group. In addition, the disease began to progress after 9 weeks in the chemotherapy group, but in 17 weeks in the control patients. **Clearly after relapse, chemotherapy patients did worse.***

Remember the foundation of science is replication. If something can be repeated in a specially bred mouse (often designed for the purpose) then everyone gets excited there may be a medical breakthrough brewing in the little human-like rodent. This 1987 review of the topic serves the science model wonderfully:

> *Cancer chemotherapy is currently undergoing an intensive reappraisal because of its **unimpressive performance against major common cancers.** There are a number of possible reasons for this lack of success; one... is that under some circumstances **anti-neoplastic drug treatment***

61 http://www.sciencedirect.com/science/article/pii/095980499390285N

> ***actually increases the malignant behaviour of tumours****. Investigation of this phenomenon shows that* ***drug induced modifications of the host, including immunosuppression and vascular damage, can indeed facilitate metastasis. In addition, new data are presented demonstrating that the direct action of drugs on the tumour cells themselves can have similar enhancing effects.*** *The possible mechanisms underlying such direct effects are discussed and* ***the ability of the anti-cancer drugs to cause mutations, amplify genes, and alter gene expression are considered. While the nature and extent of this facilitation of tumour malignancy is not fully understood, it is suggested that this possibility should be considered in the design of treatment protocols.*** [62]

The cancer treatment that kills! Over and over and over again. What happened to the great god of science we were assured would guide us to immunity from death? I don't pretend that I didn't know all this, but I considered I was in a good position and had a single minded determination to outsmart these fools. This cancer science can't even follow its own rules and seems to be in no position to outsmart anything, so what is going on?

These chemotherapeutic agents of the modern era kill as readily as they have always done and cure as rarely. In the so called Dark Ages doctors failed to cure using arsenic, zinc chloride, lead and mercury and all manner of wacky potions and poisons and there has been little progress from the fixation with poisoning to death. The chemo family of poisons came about by a chance discovery. Studying damage caused by mustard gas through the world wars, war leaders found its victim's bone marrow and lymph nodes had been suppressed by the poison. It is a proliferation of cellular activity in these areas that create blood cancers and this observation gave someone an idea. Control the proliferation and you have some control of the cancer, right? It's a theory. It doesn't work. Early lab experiments with one mouse yielded a few extra scientist-induced days of life for the lucky cancer-induced creature before the cancer re-grew. But high achievers these people are not and from that 'breakthrough' of a few days of life what we have today is entirely fitting. By the way that one mouse experiment could not be replicated. Yet they run with it and have the nerve to bang on about science! Certainly in the havoc they wreak with their poisons there is the all important repetition but I think that's missing the point.

Dr Thomas Dougherty was a Yale anatomist who is credited with the idea of injecting nitrogen mustard into mice burdened with scientist-inflicted tumours. In 'The Initial Clinical Trial of Nitrogen Mustard' by Alfred Gilman, (one of a vast number of these research papers we have to pay to view) Dougherty tells of this experimental breakthrough that got us to where we are today.

> *After just two administrations of the compound the tumor began to soften and regress.*

---

[62] https://link.springer.com/article/10.1007/BF00047465

That's it. The breakthrough! Within a month it was growing again. I did slightly better, maybe 4 weeks better than the mouse. Ha! Living longer thanks to medical research on animals!

> *We then treated the animal again and a regression occurred again, although it was not as complete as the first time.*

The animal lived 84 days. That is described in medical circles as

> ***A very remarkable prolongation of survival.***
>
> ***The only one of the murine lymphomas in which we got complete remission was in the original tumor in which we tried the compound... The very first mouse treated turned out to give the best result... in most of the murine leukemias, particularly those which metastasise readily, we frequently obtained no effect at all. I have often thought that if we had by accident chosen one of these leukemias... we might possibly have dropped the whole project.*** [63]

This is the foundation of the cancer empire of today, from which chemo has become the approved method of *treating* cancer, about which we hear a great deal of the life saving drugs and the animal testing that made life for humans on this planet even possible! Not such a great accolade is it, but this is what living longer with cancer really means. I think about my time living with cancer and that time went fast. A few weeks, a few months, a few years is not good enough. None of it's good enough. Whatever time is left is often broken into with follow-up appointments and more tests and worrying about it coming back. Cancer twice? In the vast majority of chemo treated patients! Isn't that another replication to take note of? As long as I can remember the rhetoric has been about a cure for cancer just around the corner. Or 5 to 10 years away. More lately they promise it'll be "sooner". What the fcuk does that even mean? Sooner than when? It's that vague science again, open to interpretation.

The tumour 'reaction' to a poison attack, as exciting as it was to see for the first time in the human trials that followed the death of that lonely mouse, only affects the tumour and not the cause of the tumour. And temporarily. And even then not the slightest consideration is given to the all important microbes now known to us as an intrinsic cog in the mechanics of cancer, living in the cancer cells unaffected by chemo, only made homeless, briefly. Just one cell falls sick in the "all clear" and in move the microbes and off we go again. They are so far from solving the cancer puzzle, it's laughable! This is being drilled home to us from all the cancer coming back. Tumour removal seldom restores the integrity of the immune system but restoring the immune system is guaranteed to remove and prevent tumours. That alone causes the natural extinction of the cancer microbes and a breakdown of the cancer mechanism.

---

63 Ralph Moss PhD - Questioning Chemotherapy

I'm not claiming to be a medical expert but an expert is only someone who 'has great knowledge or skill in a particular area' and I'm doing OK in my general area which I consider broadly useful. The medical experts I meet typically only specialise in one area be that oncology, neurology, haematology, urology, cardiology, endocrinology... Like an invasion of body part snatchers! These are medical experts who we would hope to be more generally clued up on health than the rest us, but most have only a superficial understanding of the whole human, how all the parts interact or what best fuels and protects it. A prescription, a blood test or a referral to one of a large number of body part specialists just about sums up an average visit to the doctor. Not one ever mentioned nutrition to me. Within this system, knowledge of body parts is broken down into a product inventory and nutrition, the competitor, is brushed aside like a conspiracy theory. It's no wonder there's so much confusion about health and the disease process.

It's not just the cancer researchers who aren't piecing the puzzle, this is a problem with medicine and the sciences more broadly. Specialities are necessary but the system is controlled to the extreme and so the left brain has no idea what's occurring within the whole. The left brain doesn't see the whole or think it needs to look. It is the left brain that does well academically but teasing it to look outside the academic textbook is a tricky thing to achieve since rules are rules and territorial incursions will be strictly enforced by the high priests of the religion of science.

Most people think great God will come from the skies. Take away everything and make everybody feel high. But if you know what life is worth, you will look for yours on Earth. And now you see the light. Stand up for your rights.

Bob Marley (1945 – 1981)

Science When it Suits

You never change things by fighting the existing reality. To change something, build a new model that makes the existing model obsolete.
R. Buckminster Fuller (1895 -1983)

What becomes clear the more one looks is that the art of science lies in the eye of the beholder. To put it another way, it matters not what the science says more what he who pays for the science says. Science is meant to be about discovery about following the signs, the evidence - the science - to wherever that may lead. But science isn't guiding us. We guide science with the beliefs we currently hold and if we limit the input the output will be limited. We are still burning fossils fuels to move ourselves around the planet and generate heat, yet the other worldly biological entities we mock and ridicule, like the idea of healing naturally, are zipping across the universe using super high tech engineering and efficiency.

This drug thing isn't about science it's about money and restraining the science is the money. We have allowed the dirt bag with the most money, the most laboratories and the most scientists on the payroll to tell us what the science says, or doesn't say depending on what it's worth. Beliefs and bank balances pay the piper and science as we know it is not so much a science as a means to an end.

And how can any of it be settled? Orthodox science is 300 years old and is still cutting up rats for fcuk sake. Science is the new kid on the block in the human story and is just as lost. Science like horny teenager has been distracted by temptation. Or the scientists have.

The irony is that science does confirm the coolest stuff that the scientists try to pretend doesn't exist.

Science, for example, tells us or would do if we looked beyond what we believe to be true, that the legendary Bigfoot/Sasquatch is very real and living among us. Mainstream scientists and the mainstream media tell us this is an unproven myth spread by conspiracy theorists, for reasons unknown, while the gatekeepers pour their scorn. Yet DNA evidence proves that the officially registered *Homo sapiens cognatus* (Sasquatch) is as real as the countless witnesses have been testifying for as long as anyone can recall. It is a contradiction, is it not, how one witness can send a man to death or to spend the rest of his life in a prison, yet when we are confronted with too many witnesses to count who each have a story to tell that sits ill with our beliefs, we accuse them **all** of making it up! Crop formations? Aliens anyone? Sasquatch? Cancer cure? Just where is the evidence that proves every single encounter or experience of this nature is fake? Science says? The Bible perhaps needs reassessing in light of denying all these witnesses, understanding as we do it too is based on witness testimony. Old witness testimony documented hundreds of years after the Jesus event and later edited beyond recognition by men and represented as the word of God. Really? That Bible story makes perfect sense but talk of unknown species is bonkers?

ZooBank, the International Commission on Zoological Nomenclature have officially validated *Homo sapiens cognatus* as a blood relative of ours. According to the best science there is and a lot of credible scientists', Sasquatch is part human. The mitochondrial DNA is 100% human female which was crossed around 12-15,000 years ago, we may assume through a breeding interaction, with an unknown primate species: the father of our modern day Bigfoot. Leaving us today with a wild relative that blends into the remote forests and mountains of the planet so successfully that the majority of the city dwelling humans are clueless! Great Uncle Sasquatch chose to live in the wilderness! I think about that for a moment and it makes me tingle with joy. Others cringe and deny. Never! They sneer, in blasphemy of the very science they worship.

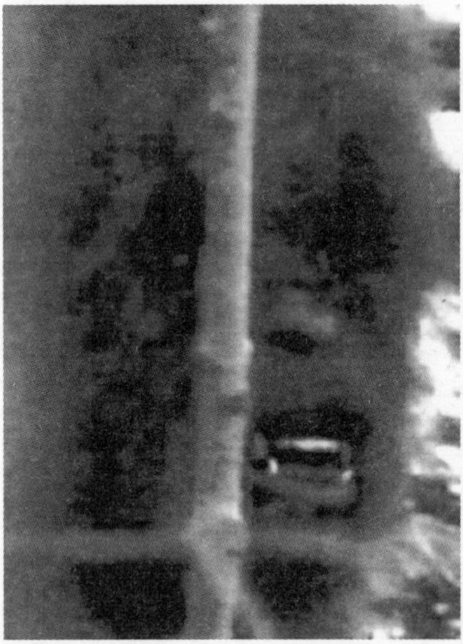

Whoever the father turns out to be this is a status that cannot be taken away, no matter what they don't say on the news and on those go nowhere 'search for Sasquatch' documentaries where we are bored to the closing titles by a left brain presenter working for the status quo and a pile of plaster casts of big foot prints, some real, some not, while ignoring the definitive DNA. Let the search continue! Sound familiar?

Keep your head down girl. Matilda, hair sample number 37 in the North American Genome Project. Filmed by the Erikson Project.

Field researchers provided samples for the Sasquatch Genome Project (SGP), including hair, tissue, blood, mucus, scratched tree bark, saliva and even a toenail. The SGP team then spent 5 years and hundreds of thousands of dollars testing 111 samples which were submitted from 34 different hominin research sites in 14 U.S. states and two Canadian provinces. Hundreds of thousands of people on all continents (except Antarctica) have testified, and some do so regularly, to the activities of this elusive human animal which vary in size and colour dependant on state, country and continent. We hear most of the Abominable Snowman/Yeti, in the Himalayas, Bigfoot/ Sasquatch in North America and the Yowie in Australia. From my research I believe we will one day learn that they can drift between dimensions and use telepathy to communicate and are acutely intelligent. A recurring theme from those having close contact on the North American continent is that the smell of this creature is nauseating and musky, quite gross. Or as one witness in Australia reported in March 2018 "like five-week old road kill" And why not!

The peer-reviewed research was conducted by this non-government team of scientific experts with specialities in genetics, forensics, imaging and pathology and was led by Dr Melba S. Ketchum of DNA Diagnostics in Texas. In all, so far, they have sequenced 20 whole and 10 partial mitochondrial genomes, as well as 3 whole nuclear genomes using double blind studies, the latest cutting edge science and the professional services of 12 independent science laboratories. MtDNA analysis, nuDNA analysis, forensic analysis, histopathology, and next-generation whole genome sequencing is a lot of tecky sounding stuff that have together proven far superior to belief systems. And isn't this more exciting than bellowing "hoax" and walking off? The science is quite clear: this mystical creature is around 15,000 years old as real as granddad and it's a hybrid.

> *Mitochondrial whole genomes were consistent with modern humans. In contrast, novel data were obtained when nuclear DNA was sequenced. Next generation whole genome sequencing was performed on three samples. Phylogeny trees generated showed homology to human chromosome 11 and to primate sequences.* ***The data indicates that the Sasquatch has human mitochondrial DNA but possesses nuclear DNA that is a structural mosaic consisting of human and novel non-human DNA.***[64]

But the scientific community is in denial. It is perhaps as well that scientists don't approve for if our cousins were accepted by the orthodox, aside the social ramifications, its leaders would only demand live specimens for research into treatments for cancer and Parkinson's and all that, because they're not real humans not like us but close enough to hold promise for cures. Like mice. Maybe some Squatch farms where organs could be harvested for humans with needs? Could save money, save lives, help the economy, generate much needed employment and pay for new hospitals for all the sick people with nowhere warm to die.

What say someone was, or is, using planet Earth as a laboratory?

Someone is certainly messing with us!

We can't simply ignore all of this and remain credible. Here's another taster, with the very same science they wholly depend upon to diagnose cancer in humans and to instigate the death delivering treatments. Here the radiation scanners confirm what is clear from physical appearance that these **reptilian humanoid beings** discovered in cave networks in Nazca, Peru in 2017 are real. And represent an orthodox scientists' worst nightmare. Can you look at the following images and in all honesty believe them to be fake?

---

64 http://www.denovojournal.com/denovo_015.htm
http://www.sasquatchgenomeproject.org/index.html

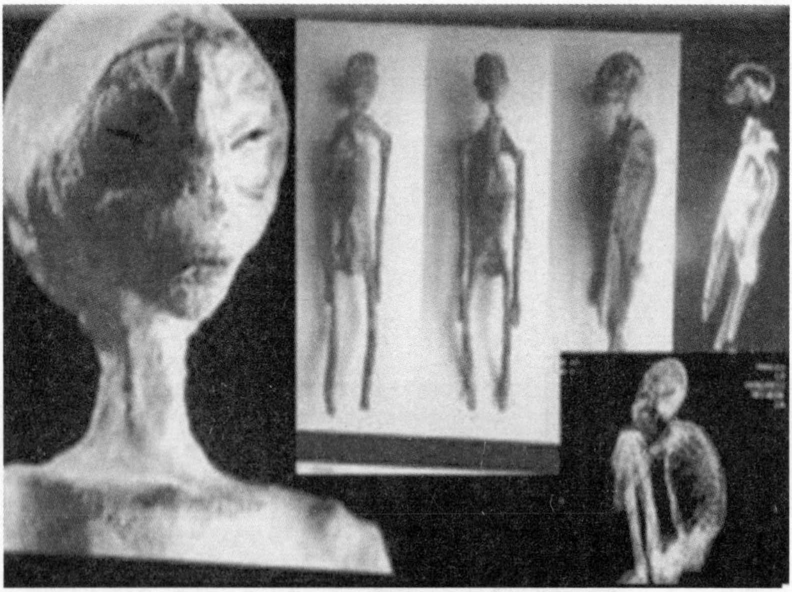

They always demand a body as proof. Here's some.

It's just one more discovery that alone changes everything and invites us to wonder what else they have missed while ridiculing stray thoughts and witnesses. There are many such anomalies to our way of thinking coming to light at this time of enlightenment, often at an archaeological pace, but this is the proverbial spaceship on the White House lawn and I think it's special. At writing a group of six three fingered beings, of more than one species, have been unearthed. One is carbon dated circa 1700 years old. They are immaculately preserved specimens of unknown origin head to toe with top quality DNA. What's unique here is that all of the internal organs are intact, something thought impossible in mummification – achieved with a simple herbal concoction and clay.

The internal organs and brain material can be seen in CT scans. One of the reptilian creatures, the smaller species of the group found as a family of three, is carrying eggs and some are fitted with devices.

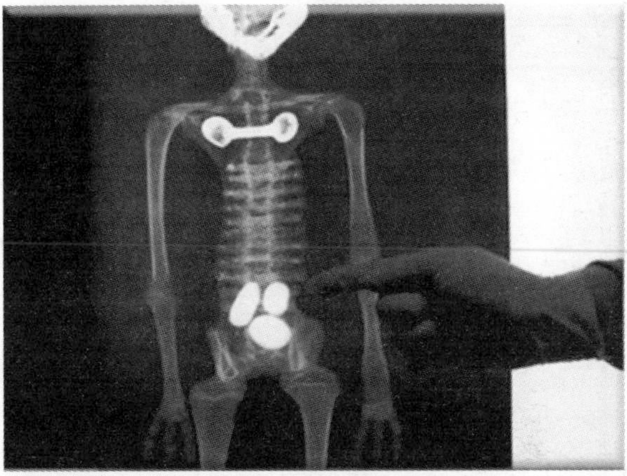

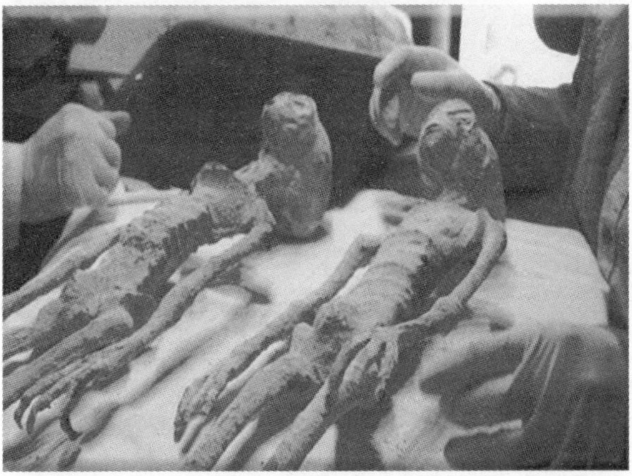

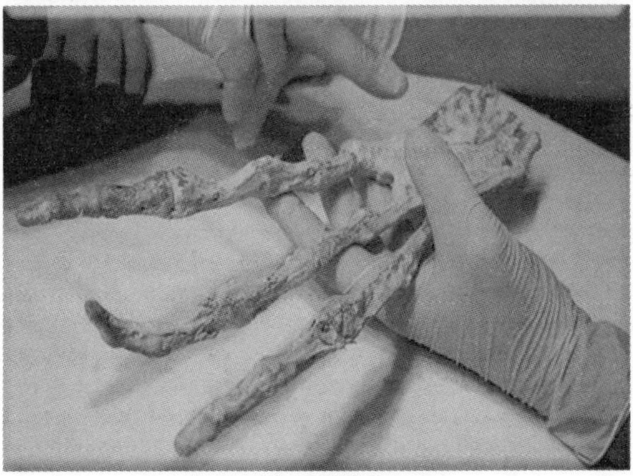

Images from Gaiatv.com

As the scientists and all the science involved in this discovery stand with me in awe, the status quo don't want us to know. We can but wonder at how many wanna-be experts will look for proof of fakery in this story, at first all expectant and then desperately so. All of those who want to find it and all those who don't can't. But it doesn't matter; their role is to maintain their fixed vision of life and death for another two thousand years and to deny any other reality; to brand all evidence illegitimate, to challenge the story as a hoax, false, fake, trickery, unbelievable, impossible, no matter what. And of course they would know all about that. The DNA to come from these creatures they will call "contaminated" or swamp gas or a hallucination. But simply denying reality to oneself doesn't change it for everyone.

When it gets really awkward like this someone sneers and blurts out something about David Icke and little green men in the hope that diverts attention, but nowadays that just makes matters worse.

The take home message is perhaps that anything is possible. We are allowed to imagine and theorise and wonder, but we don't have to! When we open our minds on our current reality we will open doors on the reality we want. A reality full of these wonders. And we might wonder, if 'science' and 'everyone' can have been so wrong about the presence of reptilian humanoids here on Earth, what else has been overlooked? Cancer cure? If we don't ask we'll stay right where we are in our own mummified state.

The 911 story may seem a little off my topic too, but it fits neatly into our study of science and the science of manipulation. And it matters.

The science tells us that the events of 911 as most people believe them simply cannot be true. It's another challenging topic for sure, but the real story has a lot to offer the inquisitive mind and evolutionary necessity of humanity. Most people believe the Twin Towers collapsed to the ground after hijacked planes slipped inside, but all the high tech ground monitoring systems record that this all important inevitability of a collapse simply did not happen. This one critical flaw alone makes the official story a conspiracy theory (it's a story entirely composed of contradiction and anyone who claims otherwise is not being honest with themselves) but we have really good science coming out of our ears on this one too!

What Dr Judy Wood B.S, M.S, PhD discovered in her exemplary forensic investigation into the events in New York on 911, is that most of those two 500,000 tonne towers were turned to dust in a few brief seconds in mid air and **did not collapse to the ground**. As unfathomable as that claim may sound it is a fact based on all the known science and stands unchallenged. One only has to observe the momentary - evaporation of skyscraper - events of that morning and study the inconsequential remnants of rubble once the thick dust carpet had settled over the city to realise that most of the material is missing. The big buildings did not fall down. According to all the available evidence this dust covering was the disintegrated debris of molecularly disassociated concrete and steel. Aluminium cladding and paper are pretty much all that remain undamaged.

Just as revealing in this exquisitely detailed and comprehensively referenced 500 page hardcover scientific study 'Where Did The Towers Go' is the evidence pointing to the use of directed energy. This is important for many reasons not just for sparking never ending war. The title of Judy Wood's investigation is the elephant in the living room. It is to the point and poignant and our answer to that question must tally with our hypothesis of what happened and with the science. As yet the only hypothesis meeting all those demands is that of directed energy turning steel to powder in seconds, as we can see occur in slow motion, leaving remains no more than 2% of the original building height, thick dust for miles and no adequate seismic impact recorded. While professional cue card readers appear all knowing when telling 'the news', of 'collapses' caused by a bearded bogeyman on dialysis in a cave half way around the world, no evidence of a skyscraper hitting the ground has been presented by anyone ever and of course there has been no presentation of evidence at any trial. Religious fanatics in flying machines is a conspiracy theory. Our modern day Sherlock Holmes family of news delivering experts, albeit reliant on a script, or blueprint, and the ever helpful experts, insiders and sources they allude to and George 'trust me' Bush were the ones who solved the crime of the century, within minutes. On telly! And that simple story has run amok.

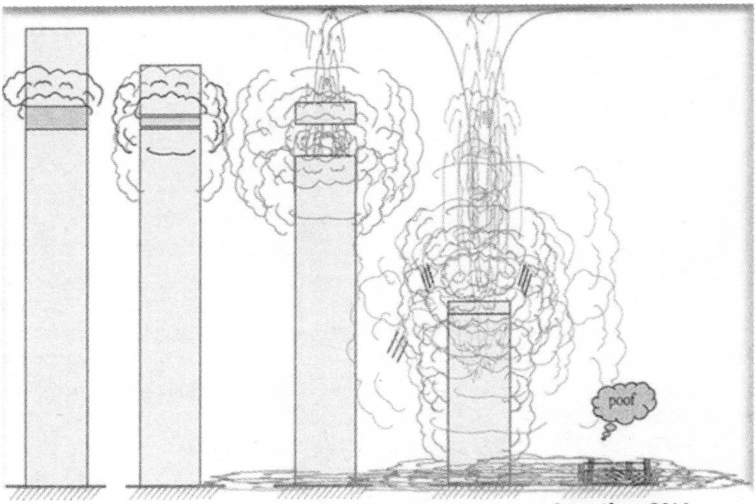

Less than 2%!

Drjudywood.com

Science is very rigid in that explosive moment when two objects meet at high speed. Seriously there is no getting away from it! The force of impact is sudden, must be equal and devastating to the weaker of the two. This bored me to death at school but I'm listening now and I try to tease the curiosity of others who are often just as uninterested! It was Isaac Newton who taught us by his Third Law of Motion, that when one body exerts a force on a second body the second body exerts a force equal in magnitude and opposite in direction on the first. So, when a fly hits your car windscreen, or you hit a fly, you win because the fly is a fly. If you were to punch a steel girder, well you'd be an idiot and of course the steel would win. When half a million tonnes of structural steel and concrete hits a 100 ton aluminium airplane, or equally the other way around, the airplane crumples like the fly.

Except on 9/11, when the science was suspended, and we were all shown on TV what for all the world appears to be a plane pass clean through the enormous heavy mass of steel and concrete as though it were butter. Leaving a silhouette of itself don't you know, like the Road Runner through a mountain! Seriously, check your windscreen. Not once did a fly pass through, at any speed. Either the laws of motion need rewriting or there is something very wrong with what we were shown on TV on 9/11/2001 and with desperate repetition ever since.

I can find no science to replicate this stunning science breakthrough, so how can we assess at what speed it becomes possible to pass aluminium clean through steel? I think it matters to discover new sciences. Science says it is not possible at present, but look...

It isn't a bird. Is it? Science says it isn't a plane passing through steel yet it casts a shadow, as might a missile.

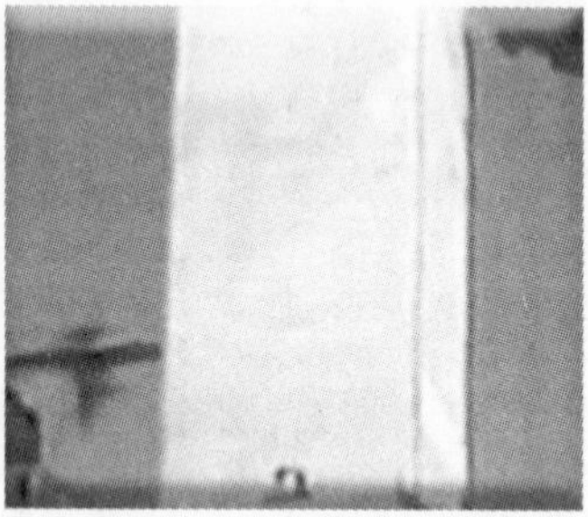

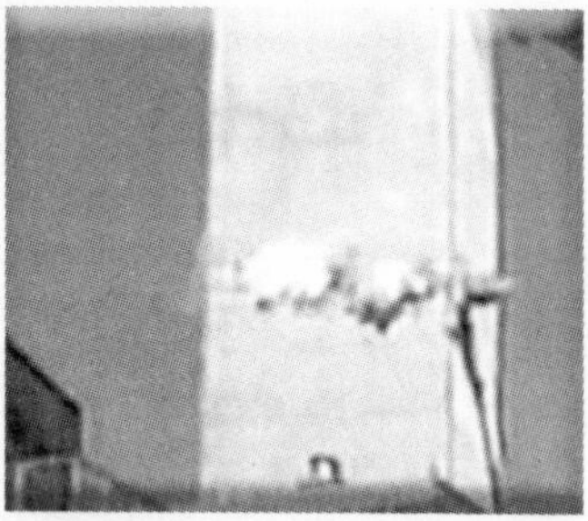

Please have the good grace to allow me to consider this questionable.

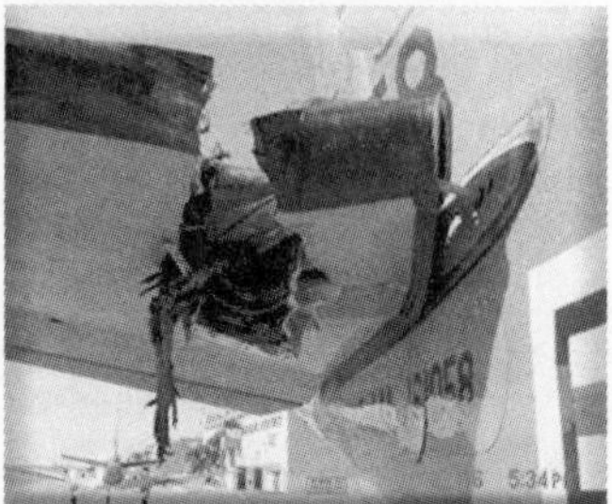

We can agree that's both a bird and a plane but at what speed does it become possible for a bird to pass clean through a plane and not be damaged?

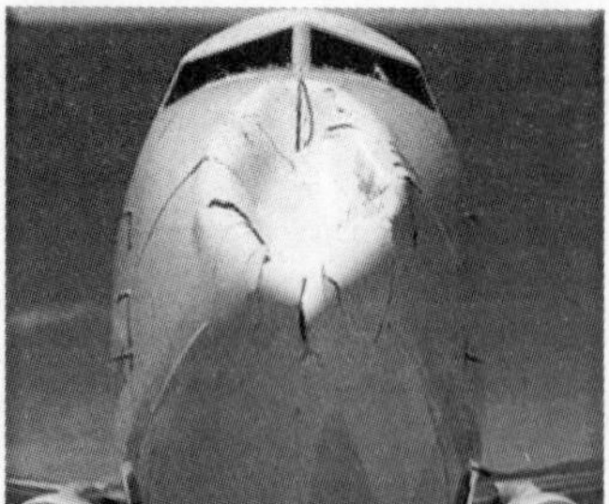

Punched on the nose by a bird! Not so tough when they aren't on stage performing for a TV audience.

Science question. How long would it take for 110 floors to pancake collapse downward one floor onto the next through the path of greatest resistance and for the entire mass to hit the ground as it must in one almighty explosion of energy?

It took around 10 seconds to disappear each tower according to the footage. But compare that to what science says should have happened...

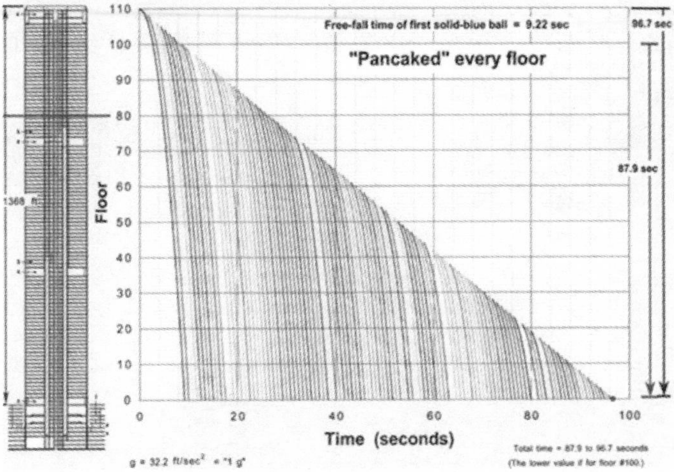

Minimum time for the collapse, if every floor collapsed like dominos.[65]

Columbia University's Seismology Group recorded seismic events of 10 seconds and 8 seconds in duration, which correspond to the collapses of WTC2 and WTC1, respectively

That says there was no pancake collapse. So the official story is a conspiracy theory. Funny that. The seismic impact was miniscule at 2.1 on the Richter scale for the demise of WTC 2 and 2.3 for WTC 1. Each significantly under-representing the impact of 500,000 tonnes of material slamming into the ground by a factor of 30! So that bit didn't happen, according to all the science.

> *Each tower's collapse should have registered nearly 3.5 on the Richter scale, given the order of magnitude... and ... potential energy and dimensions. The apparent fact that the Richter reading peaked at 2.3 and the disturbance lasted only 8 seconds is our first indicator that the* ***mechanism of destruction could not be a conventional one****. **An energy technology of some kind had to have been used to eliminate the towers,** while preserving the bathtub and surrounding structures. Conventional technology, which uses kinetic energy (bombs, gravity) cannot explain the elimination of the towers.* Judy Wood B.S, M.S, PhD

65 http://drjudywood.com/articles/BBE/BilliardBalls.html

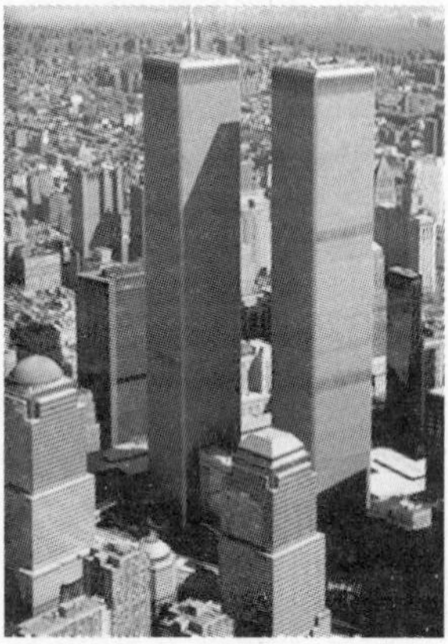

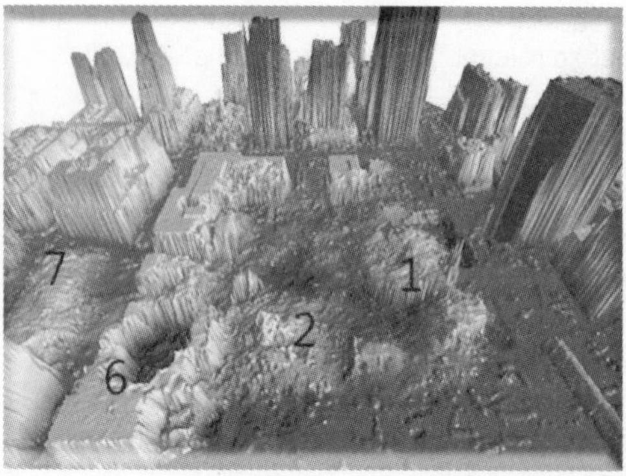

Judy Wood's investigation is extremely thorough and impressed me like nothing I've studied before or since. I'd describe this as the best way to do scientific research and for that alone her book should serve as a reference point for students of good science. It's honest and carries no bias. She followed the evidence to its conclusion; she made some mind blowing discoveries but makes no assumptions on who done it. But she has proven, and will one day be recognised for unravelling single-handedly *what* happened in New York on 911. Only this hypothesis explains the vast amount of missing debris, the sheer speed of demise and the absence of material impacting with the bedrock. Whatever our religious beliefs or prejudices are, knocked down by planes doesn't add up. But look at this infrared image from 4 days later and ask yourself if turned to dust and blew away in the wind doesn't have a bit of a feel about it.

We have come to see the cancer microbe at the centre of our cancer research in a similar way to these buildings and we found a way to influence their demise in a very similar fashion using unseen energy fields, and to much less than 2%! This resonance was described in the 1930's by Royal Raymond Rife as the Mortal Oscillatory Rate. We are of course using our knowledge of directed energy to disrupt disease and not the rise of the new human.

If we have the courage to follow the evidence in this story to its logical conclusion we can see through what we saw on 9/11 to something even more remarkable. Evidence suggests someone has access to an energy technology that could set us free of debt and our dependence on fossil fuels but has weaponised it and is using it to mesmerise and control us and keep us at war with each other.

In that, the same scientists and assorted experts tease us to "fight" the ever shifting natural elements on our planet while ignoring climate change across the universe, as they tease us to fight cancer with chemo and fight infections with injections, all based on incomplete information. I don't mind what anyone else does in their war with the weather but I'm not getting involved. Seems to me like a lost cause and too many unanswered questions like when will we know this war is won and the weather is back where it should be? Polluting the planet with outdated technology is bonkers but so is ignoring solutions staring us in the face.

The wide coverage of chemtrail clouds across continents must also be factored into any climate action calculations before anyone can talk of settled science. These ever widening man made grid patterns in the sky are not a side effect of aviation fuel, that's condensation and it evaporates. As it doesn't always evaporate like it used to, what role does it play in heating or cooling the planet as it forms the new layer of insulation? I see the sun driving the climate and no sun means no life, yet somehow not only are we encouraged to hide from it when it shines under cancer causing chemical sun block potions, but we seem to think we have more power!

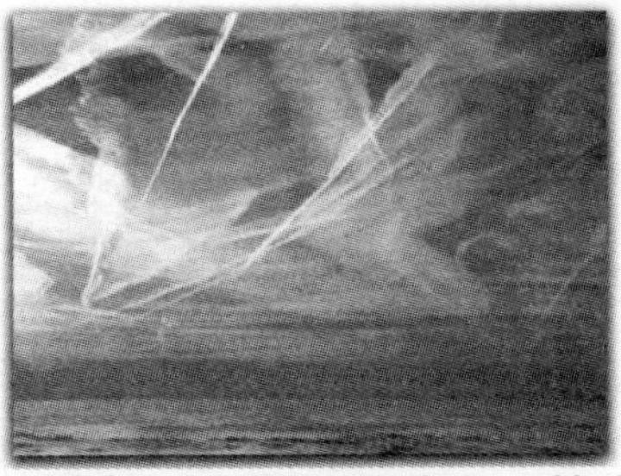

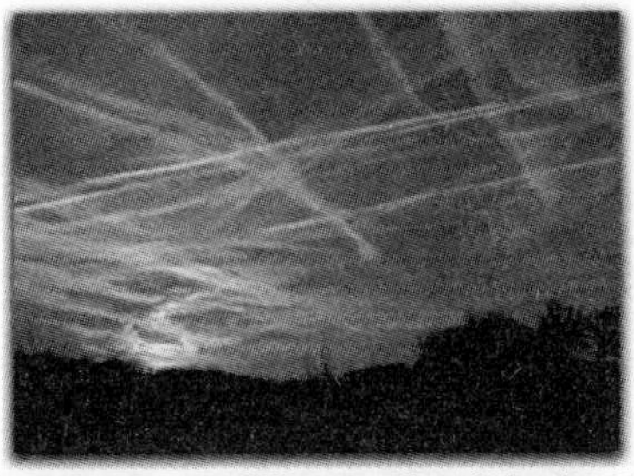

A heavy chemtrail spray day **blocking out the sun** **filling out the night sky**

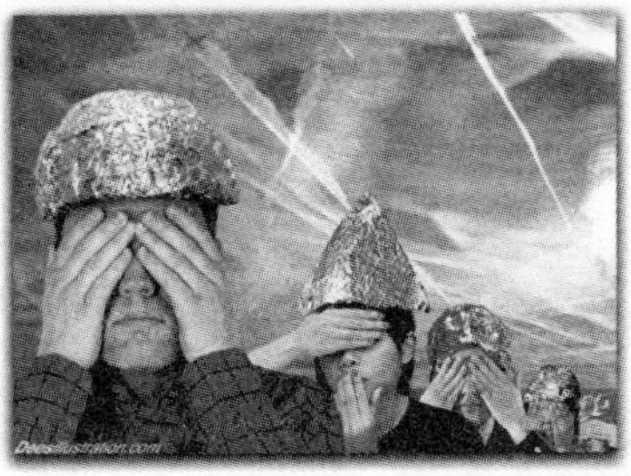

Mr. blue sky please tell us why you had to hide away for so long.

A few recent official observations from a variety of sources that just feed my crazy thoughts:

- On the **Sun**: "We are living with a very unusual sun at the moment."

  "It is quite amazing that the flaring regions continue releasing such strong flares. I think the last week will go into the history books as one of the most dramatic solar activity periods we have seen in modern times."

- **Mars** is having "Global Warming", huge storms, the formation of new clouds and the disappearance of polar icecaps. "**The long-term increase in solar**

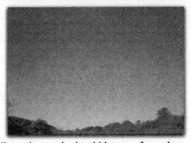

irradiance is heating both Earth and Mars. This temperature spike is so extreme it's almost unbelievable. To get a temperature change of the same scale on Earth, you'd be going from the depths of winter in Fairbanks, Alaska, to the height of summer in the Mojave Desert."

- 'Global warming on **Pluto** puzzles scientists'. Images show that Pluto is changing colour and is now 20 per cent more red than it used to be.

- **Saturn** let out an "unprecedented belch of energy," leaving scientists puzzled not only by the size of the storm but the source, which rapidly changed the temperature.

- **Jupiter** has had a 200% increase in brightness of surrounding plasma clouds. "The storm is growing in altitude. Before when they were just ovals they didn't stick out above the clouds. Now they are rising."

- Images of Jupiter's volcanic moon **Io,** taken with the Hubble telescope show the surprising appearance of a 200-mile-wide 'feature' near the center of the moon's disk. This represents a more dramatic change in 16 months than any seen over the previous 15 years, say researchers.

- **Venus** has had a 2500% increase in auroral brightness and substantive global atmospheric changes in less than 30 years.

- **Uranus** is experiencing "Really big, big changes" in brightness, and increased global cloud activity.

- **Mercury** is alive! Magnetic tornadoes, evidence of a strong magnetic field and polar ice has been discovered.

- Global warming has also been recorded on Neptune's moon **Triton**. Benny Peiser, a social anthropologist at Liverpool John Moores University said *"I think it is an intriguing coincidence that warming trends have been observed on a number of very diverse planetary bodies in our solar system. Perhaps this is just a fluke."* *

Ah, the old coincidence theory! Some view it as a shift, a renewal, an evolutionary process we should welcome. It's happening whether we like it or not and I do! [66]

It's all worth thinking about while we're going to extremes!

We shall no longer hang on to the tails of public opinion, or to a non-existent authority, on matters utterly unknown and strange. We shall gradually become experts ourselves in the mastery of the knowledge of the future.

Wilhelm Reich (1897-1957)

---

[66] https://www.gaia.com/video/planetwide-disturbances-mars?fullplayer=feature

* https://www.livescience.com/1349-sun-blamed-warming-earth-worlds.html

Laetrile is B17 is Amygdalin is an Anti-Cancer Agent
(from seeds!)

That the NCI [National Cancer Institute], with enthusiastic support from the ACS [American Cancer Society] - the tail that wags the NCI dog - has effectively blocked funding for research and clinical trials on promising non-toxic alternative cancer drugs for decades, in favor of highly toxic and largely ineffective patented drugs developed by the multibillion dollar global cancer drug industry. Additionally, the cancer establishment has systematically harassed the proponents of non-toxic alternative cancer drugs.

Samuel Epstein, The Politics of Cancer - Revisited

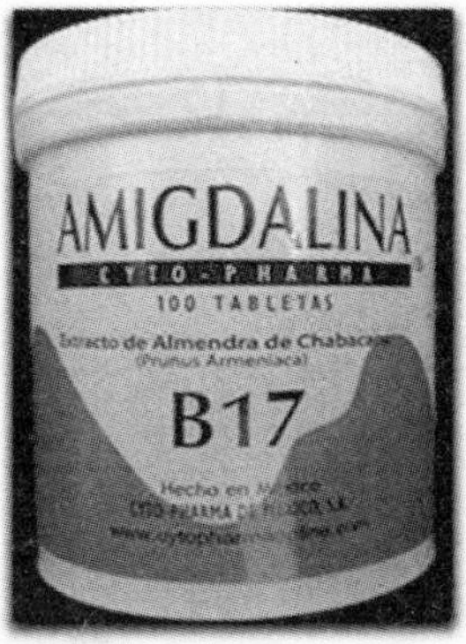

Science tells us that vitamin B17 kills cancer cells and that vitamin C kills cancer cells. Science says the Gerson Therapy cures cancer. Science tells us that chemotherapy causes cancer, radiation causes cancer, mammograms cause cancer and vaccines cause cancer. Jeez, now what do we do? Do we believe the opposite of what the science says or do we go with the science? We do neither. We keep an open mind and we question everything. Everything. And eventually the scientists will catch up with the science.

For 5 years between 1972 and 1977 amygdalin (vitamin B17), was meticulously animal tested at the prestigious Memorial Sloan-Kettering (MSK) cancer centre in Manhattan under the direction of Dr Kanematsu Sugiura, a highly respected scientist with over 60 years experience. This gentleman and his team tormenting captive animals reasserted what was already known from the human experience, that this simple extract of fruit seeds specifically apricot seeds can stop the spread of cancer, can improve health, relieve pain and prevent cancer.

> *The results clearly show that Amygdalin significantly inhibits the appearance of lung metastasis in mice bearing spontaneous growth of the primary tumors... Laetrile also seemed to prevent slightly the appearance of new tumors... the improvement of health and appearance of the treated animals in comparison to controls is always a common observation... Dr Sugiura has never observed complete regression of these tumors in all his cosmic experience with other chemotherapeutic agents.* [67]

The established order relies heavily on laboratory animals to blind us and guide them through the gold mine of human ills, and here we have more proof of the futility of it all. We can find ample testimony from cancer patients of their success with this nutrient, in spite of these suppressed findings in animals, yet all we hear

---

[67] A Summary of the Effect of Amygdalin Upon Spontaneous Mammary Tumors in Mice Sloan Kettering Report June 13, 1973 http://www4.secondopinionfilm.com/wp-content/uploads/2014/01/anatomy_of_a_coverup_so_02.pdf

from the usual suspects is denial and disapproval. They don't approve! Good. More for those of us who do. B17 didn't prove compatible with my needs, as it happens, but it clearly has a significant anti cancer role as can be seen from the behaviour of MSK bosses once the truth started to leak from within their walls. The full story of how to buy an industry and bury a cancer cure is told in G. Edward Griffin's 'World Without Cancer - The Story of Vitamin B17'.

The drug companies took over control of the medical schools and teaching institutions a long time ago and none can afford to upset he who pays the bills. Upon discovery of an unpatentable nutritional cancer therapy, such as B17, the Pharma sees competition. Who wouldn't! Seeing a risk is one thing but taking action to eliminate that risk is another and moves them from savvy investors to criminals.

> *The conspiracy to limit and eliminate competition from non-drug therapies began with the Flexner Report of 1910.*
>
> *Abraham Flexner was engaged by John D. Rockefeller to run around the country and 'evaluate' the effectiveness of therapies taught in medical schools and other institutions of the healing arts. Rockefeller wanted to dominate control over petroleum, petrochemicals, and pharmaceuticals (which are derived from 'coal tars' or crude oil). He arranged for his company, Standard Oil of New Jersey to obtain a controlling interest in a huge German drug cartel called I. G. Farben. He pulled in his stronger competitors like Andrew Carnegie and JP Morgan as partners, while making other, less powerful players, stockholders in Standard Oil. Those who would not come into the fold "were crushed" according to a Rockefeller biographer (W. Hoffman, David: Report on a Rockefeller (New York: Lyle Stuart, Inc., 1971) page 24).* [68]

Rockefeller's men politely requested a seat on the boards of the institutions they supported financially, one by one, in exchange for funding, so they could ostensibly 'monitor' how their generosity was being spent. Over time they became influential - since none of these institutions could afford to resist the men with the money - and they ultimately directed the syllabus. In due course they took over the decision making process locally, regionally, nationally and internationally and enabled the compliant to thrive and be seen as centres of excellence and leaders in their field. Those who stood their ground and stayed focussed on the old ways of healing were pushed aside and ridiculed by the men of money and might and synthetic drugs, who also in time bought out the media institutions.

Repeated experiments of B17 in animals at Memorial Sloan-Kettering over coming years showed the same anti cancer activity everyone dreams of and everyone involved knew it. While bosses tried to keep a lid on the story, the results of the second round of tests were leaked to the press by insiders at MSK unhappy with the dirty work at play. The San Francisco Examiner relayed how "100 per cent of the control mice had lung metastases, while the group given Laetrile 31 per cent had lung metastases". It's mice but this is how it goes, right, on precisely this the

---

[68] http://educate-yourself.org/fc/

medical empire is built, safely tested on animals and on it goes up the food chain to market. And this test substance just happened to be remarkably effective also, which is unusual. This was a big deal. Except it can't be controlled in the market, it's a fruit seed. MSK bosses were furious about the leak and had a choice to make.

The three most common ways people respond when facing the truth 1) they go for the messenger 2) they lie 3) with silence (or "no comment"). Less often it is with humility. Humility is rare where the big egos gather and since the Examiner had documentary proof and an outlet to share it the medical experts had to choose number 3. So they kept their heads down and refused to speak about it until the truth had blown over. Undercover of their contempt they had bought time to redesign some B17 trials: altering doses, mixing up animals, scraping, remodelling and generally juggling the science until they got the result they wanted. And then they went public to announce that scientific studies with B17 had shown no anti cancer activity after all, in the furry little scapegoats.

All this proves is that junk science is being exploited by quacks to sell products.

Quack: an ignorant, misinformed, or dishonest practitioner of medicine

B17 was duly discarded by orthodox medicine, branded a failure. And worse! So lethal had the vitamin become during these follow-up mouse experiments that in order to protect cancer patients it would have to face prohibition! I got mine from Mexico. They seem to be less irrational about healing in Mexico. This natural ingredient of fruit seeds is now on one of those fascist contraband lists with cannabis where it too must be exchanged on the healing underground by desperate people fighting for their lives. Finding no use for my supply I passed it to someone for whom it was shown to help.

The complete leaked dossier on the MSK experiments with B17 as revealed by former insider and one time Assistant Director of Public Affairs at the prestigious medical/vivisection facility Ralph Moss can be read here... [69]

Retrospectively, I think the results were arrived at because I did not follow most of the scientific literature nor the laboratory findings, as far as they did not accord with the clinical confirmations. "Der Efolg am Krankenbett ist entshcheidend," Professor Kassmaul said (The result at the sick-bed is decisive). I do not want to make the mistake Winston Churchill expressed so clearly: "Men occasionally stumble over the Truth, but most pick themselves up and hurry off as if nothing has happened."

Max Gerson - A Cancer Therapy

[69] http://www4.secondopinionfilm.com/wp-content/uploads/2014/01/anatomy_of_a_coverup_so_02.pdf

Designing a cancer protocol

I look upon cancer in the same way that I look upon heart disease, arthritis, high blood pressure, or even obesity, for that matter, in that by dramatically strengthening the body's immune system through diet, nutritional supplements, and exercise, the body can rid itself of the cancer, just as it does in other degenerative diseases. Consequently, I wouldn't have chemotherapy and radiation because I'm not interested in therapies that cripple the immune system, and, in my opinion, virtually ensure failure for the majority of cancer patients.

Dr Julian Whitaker, M.D.

The general cancer spread continued its rebirth in me for another eight months following chemo, but incredible as it sounds, and is, that was all the time we needed. We were buying in what we could and testing everything at regular VEGA readings. Amygdalin, vitamin C and Essiac tea, quercetin, Agaricus Blazei mushrooms... We needed to give our creation a name. Up popped the MannIcure. Well, you would wouldn't you!

The foundation of enema's, organic everything and juices daily is a given. An early enema and two 16oz juices are a must to start my day. A third midday and a fourth in the evening. I upped the intake of flax oil, sprouted pulses and quinoa as desired rather than the limits on my Gerson protocol. I did it steadily adding one at a time and minimally. Simple things but this suited my needs and the removal of restrictions was liberating, ever cautious of drifting back to convenience. There should be love of the food and love in the food. You get out what you put into anything. It has been every bit an experiment and the food and juicing have been the culture on which the rest grew.

VEGA was pivotal in the formulation of my new supplement protocol once we bailed from the Gerson boat and gave us a large degree of confidence when making big decisions, but ultimately my life was in our hands. Confirmation of our research and instincts from this superior artificial intelligence provided increasing intrigue and a curious rush of excitement as we increasingly got what we anticipated, and some big surprises, as we watched our model make.

We fished around and tried a few VEGA practitioners out. It's like anything you employ those who best suit you and your needs. Each has their own way. Not all are happy to design a protocol by measuring doses and there are quacks among them but we got to go the extra mile with good people, experiment and update on every fine detail as often as we needed for £50 - £80 a go with free some sessions thrown in. One practitioner we used for a while was so set in his ways he was actually a liability and missed important details others were desperate to support us however they could and did all we asked.

We tested the Gerson supplements I'd taken for 2 years and dropped them all except for potassium and CoQ10. For most of the previous 2 years my Gerson practitioner had advised 1 drop of vitamin D each day, which is 1000 iu, but VEGA said I needed 14,000 iu. This was one small but significant detail that matters greatly if we are to recreate that harmony. We had discovered a recurring theme regarding lymphomas and vitamin D deficiency and independent cancer researchers advise always maintaining high vitamin D levels. Since I begun to address vitamin D deficiency I have been in the high end of the range but the norm for me would appear to be way above the orthodox reference range. We know now that vitamin D receptors are widespread through the body and perhaps deficient cells turned cancerous have a greater requirement for support from the life-giving bringer of the light, reigning most high and regenerating all life on Earth every day.

We gelled with one elderly gentleman called Roger who was proficient in VEGA's superior non-invasive bioresonance diagnostic technology. He was once a surgeon who got arthritis and had to retire. By chance he'd discovered this sophisticated diagnostic tool and had trained to use it but he never really got going in practice. As such, Roger was excited when I told him I wanted him to tell me about the cancer in my body, as he wasn't licenced to involve himself in the exclusive cancer market and had never really discussed it with clients. Yet you can see it - as one might in a CT scan - but deeper. This thing reads cancer and pre-cancer and can be used to select remedies. He lit up at our deep interest in what he could reveal and his knowledge and at the idea he might be able to help us beat this naturally. Everything he was finding was accurate. It was like releasing the poor guy from a cage, he could see we were serious and we were getting the deepest insight imaginable on my health.

We got to see our friend half a dozen times before he died. The second visit was in December 2016 after we had fully fired up the MannIcure. He was stunned because 6 months earlier he said he thought I was brave but told me straight I would "have to work a miracle to get on top of all that cancer without God's help". We don't need God, God needs us to get our act together and make full use of that which he hath provided.

Having narrowed down our VEGA practitioners we set about building a comprehensive picture of me. We tested everything we had and could get our hands on for compatibility and identified deficiencies. With so much conflicting with my Gerson supplement protocol there was nothing left to doubt, we needed to find our own way in this, but still, what do we do with this mass of tumour I now had? Einstein alluded to a definition of insanity as repeating the same actions over and over and expecting different results, and here we were on that very treadmill.

I saw a doctor privately who could set me up for IV vitamin C should I choose to use it, approximately £4,000 for 15 x 100g injections. We knew from a specialist blood test that vitamin C was unlikely to debulk any more than chemo and we didn't have the money anyway. Didn't need it though as we discovered an even more user friendly way to debulk cancer and a more sustainable drip-feed of vitamin C. We were prioritising long-term healing over debulking and this fit neatly.

There are many ways to treat cancer and fully cure it but this process is inevitably simplified the less tumour the body has to deal with. Each 1 cm tumour contains billions of cancer cells and in them live the microbes we are going to be learning about and each microbe creates waste that is toxic so the more you have the more toxic you will be. While early on through Gerson I had experienced healing/toxic release reactions and revelled, these had stopped and over time I acquired a general malaise. The periodic castor oil enemas, which get deeper to the root of the disease, were just making me ill. VEGA wasn't happy with me having castor oil. I'm not convinced it'd be happy with anyone having castor oil! One practitioner relayed how another patient of hers had asked to test turpentine on her VEGA because she'd been told it might help with her candida. The machine agreed! For me it didn't nor did it like the rye bread I had been encouraged to eat either, due presumably to the gluten content. I had no idea I had a gluten issue until I sat the VEGA test. Same with the oatmeal I'd eaten for breakfast since the dawn of my awakening yet these were Gerson staples and it never occurred to me to get gluten tested, nor does it occur to Gerson practitioners to do so.

My staple Gerson menu had included rye bread and oatmeal both with gluten. Gluten is no good for anyone and I am intolerant, apparently. VEGA reflected displeasure with dairy too, something my mum tells me was an issue as a child. I have abstained in between times anyway.

VEGA in the right hands can help guide a treatment plan based on the questions we ask. You would only take to test supplements and medication you have identified for potential therapeutic value. We can visualise bouncing a micro sonar signal off an inflammation or 'soft' signal area in the body and placing our supplements in between. You get the message! I was amazed at how accurate this system proved to be, from finding known interference and allergies to diagnosing. Energy medicine will be the new norm and every home should have a VEGA. It is long past the time this system was incorporated into all medical centres and health clinics and into every self treatment programme. We really came into our own with this technology to work with. It sounds scary but it's actually much safer to become your own doctor, or at least make your decisions based on a fully rounded picture of your options which VEGA can provide. Science likes replication and you get that from this diagnostic system too.

Through August of 2016 in our laboratory of life we were strengthening defences and building an attack. I'll detail the reasoning behind each specific element in the MannIcure later in the book and will show you how we made sense of where we had gone wrong over the previous two years and how we joined together the missing pieces of this beautiful puzzle.

Everything here makes perfect sense and much more so if you think about it than the general cell-kill approach we're accustomed to, but it requires our attention to detail. We considered the problems such as immune deficiency and compiled a list of potential solutions from what we knew then did some research to find more. In due course the options grew. Isolating the best, we looked for synergy or contraindications with existing ingredients. Some elements may work better when timed apart, others in synergy.

We added into my protocol among other things **MSM organic sulphur**, **homemade ozone water**, **vitamin K2** and **mega dose vitamin D. Agaricus**

Blazei mushroom extract for immune support and its anti cancer activity. **NK Cell Activator** and **beta glucans** add another level of immune support and I needed that badly. Mainstream medicine hasn't completely missed these agents either, but again they are seldom utilised to potential in that setting. We scoured the internet and sourced the cleanest, most natural kidney support supplements we could find, the best ones we imported and included **Christopher's Kidney Formula and Uri Cleanse** tea both herbal mixtures. **Coffee enemas, Christopher's Liver Formula** and **homeopathy** for my liver and extra **CoQ10** and a **multi-vitamin**. Again VEGA suggested the need to increase my CoQ10 way beyond what my Gerson practitioner advised and **large dose liposomal vitamin C,** well documented as an effective cancer treatment was clearly encouraged. Vitamin C was shown in my RGCC [70] test to be as effective as the chemo and vitamin C has no side effects and no toxicity and it supports instead of suppressing immunity which when recovered leaves no opportunity for the cancer to rebound and overwhelm weakened defences.

I used a **Trojan horse** for infiltrating cancer cells. We employ a combination of elements such as **organic sulphur** for opening cancer cells and replenishing and **DMSO**, a wood solvent we drink. Don't laugh, this stuff is good! And orthodox medicine knows it. They've tested it as you'll see and it has value and we use it for gate crashing through the defective cancer cell walls to carry in our microbe killing agents, in this case we sent in home-made **colloidal silver** undercover of the DMSO. **Magnesium chloride salts + sodium bicarbonate** for bathing/foot soak, a magic formula in of itself for refreshing cells and balancing alkalinity. **Barley Power** from the Dutch Amish in the US and aluminium-free oral **bicarbonate of soda** to aid pH adjustment.

An RGCC blood test gives a better idea of the best agents for use against an individual cancer. It cost over £1,500 and it was interesting but of limited value. VEGA has served our purpose much better since it reads body systems in real time, but this for us was an evolving process and we were trying everything we could to find the clues. The RGCC tests your live blood and record the potential of cancer agents against cancer cells. This is arguably more relative than trying to make the results of crude animal experiments translate into human health but there are flaws. My blood is closer to me than a mouse is, but still, finding the best chemo agent against my cancer cells in my blood in a test tube to be cyclophosphamide, coming in with a whopping 82% kill rate, did not take me and my many idosyncratic complexities into account. Next was ifosfamide at 75% and trofosfamide at 70% and the other 19 such poisons offering me between 22 - 55% kill rate. Bendamustine came in at 30% and I'd say that's probably a reasonable estimate of what it achieved for me in 2015. None can heal a body.

These are alkylating agent, the first class of drugs made from mustard gas. They are highly toxic to all cells and destroy the genetic DNA. Cancer cells quickly develop

---

70 www.rgcc-genlab.com

resistance to this stuff hence the use of multiple drug regimes to hit the cancer from all angles and the inevitable relapse. Sounds smart but what does it achieve?

Of the selection of natural cytotoxic agents tested against my tumour stem cells, were ascorbic acid (vitamin C) which came in at 35%, artecin at 40%, amygdalin (vitamin B17) scored zero. VEGA also said no to B17. I should point out that these numbers don't mean cyclophosphomide would be better for me than vitamin C, since the latter can be used indefinitely and at high doses with no toxicity and has other health benefits, the former actually causes cancer and would kill me soon enough. At the end of the day neither is good enough on its own.

> *The test will tell us what natural substances will induce apoptosis... after the tumour cells and a single product have been in contact in a well plate for 48 hours. We have found this test to be very accurate over the past 10+ years and thousands of tests.* ***However it cannot take into account the many combinations of natural substances or the physiological dynamics of each individual required for life.***

We got this test off to the Greek RGCC lab just a few days before I was booked in for chemo, as is required. But this was utterly futile regarding the more beneficial chemo agents showing for me since my consultant didn't understand the test results anyway and was, as they all are, tied to what he was told to prescribe by NICE guidelines (the approved list of poisons for a particular cancer) so it didn't matter whether another product might kill a zillion more cancer cells in my lab tube results, rules are rules. And there's the other aspect regarding toxicity and side effects of chemo agents showing greater efficacy which the blood test doesn't take into account. An agent may be found to kill a lot of cancer cells but the patient too.

What we did learn from this test was the place in my protocol for vitamin C and Agaricus Blazei mushrooms. Thing is, both these natural agents are renowned for their role in immune support and cancer killing anyway so barring allergies and the inevitable exceptions to the rule it's fair to reason that most cancer patients would benefit from considering their inclusion and a simple VEGA test would answer that question.

I asked my cancer specialist what he thought of vitamin C in treating cancer. He didn't mind my questions but he thought of chemo and the mAbs like one might gold, frankincense and myrrh and suggested that my money would be better spent treating Alice, who promptly announced I was her treat. Vitamin C as a cancer treatment was pioneered by Linus Pauling, two times Nobel Prize winner. The award doesn't impress me particularly knowing as I do how such awards are directed but this guy was onto something and his findings have been repeatedly confirmed and advanced by others.

While doubting any benefit in vitamin therapy my cancer expert did by habit use a corkscrew to extract a bone marrow sample from the hip bone of each of his patients, under local anaesthetic in order to stage their cancer. Tick in a box. He agreed this corkscrew test was unnecessary and wouldn't affect his treatment plan either way. He acknowledged to his credit that he hadn't ever thought about these things because it's just the way things are. Believe it or not I was actually interested in how my bone marrow looked but was horrified to find out how bad it was!

We were at the final crossroads, the parting of the ways. It's a choice and I'd made mine. As we consolidated our experimental research, exposing masters of alchemy or mere dreamers, the ortho-docs were growing ever confident that I would soon be begging for more of their concoctions.

At concluding appointments with my orthodox cancer treatment experts the message was drilled home to me that delaying more of their failed intervention was foolish. Foolish I tell you! Doc Fear noted on 8 August 2016, 8 months after chemo ended:

> *On examination today there are numerous small volume lymph nodes bilaterally. Previously he had lymph nodes recorded on the left side of the neck. They are palpable in the anterior and posterior chain on the right side. He also has axilliary lymph nodes bilaterally...*

What this means is front and back, both sides of armpits and both sides of neck. In less words: more cancer. She didn't record any groin tumours in this report because she didn't examine for them but they were palpable too. I know because when I pee'd I'd feel them.

This same lady had been steadfast in her expert opinion soon after chemo that my disease status was now, as she put it, "the best you will ever be". Not what I was being told six months earlier just before I was initiated. She was equally certain that since the chemo couldn't get rid of all the visible cancer nothing would. She stressed to me her need to book me in for more failed treatment as soon as possible and warned me that waiting until I felt unwell "may" make "initiating" the next round of chemotherapy "more difficult". It wasn't going to be difficult for her it was going to be impossible! They don't watch and wait when it comes back, they aim to get in there fast to beat back the cancer before it goes nuts. She first wanted to scan me again with another full body CT to have another bloody look inside so she had a picture to compare to after the next assault on my innards. She was pretty determined, obsessive even. Do or die was the take home message.

She tried to tempt me with her "lesser of two evils" pitch. I was having none of it. She clearly found me frustrating but I don't do evil, period. Isn't evil evil for a reason? If it were sweet it would be a treat but it's evil. She accused me of burying my head in the sand and denying the seriousness of my situation. That was the crux of the matter, of course; I knew! We always came away from these appointments feeling jarred yet we knew what to expect and were under no illusions. Not so much information and advice or discussion of other ways and success stories, instead fear is the undertone in every exchange and the message was clear: chemo or die. Chemo and die more like. We called it the fear factory. Each appointment they ask of any weight loss, night sweats, fever or new lymph nodes. A drop in weight would cause one doctor to get disturbingly exited but there was no reasoning with this and if your weight is down from the last time, the computer brain calculates an opportunity to intervene. Yet they would weigh me at random times of the day and always fully clothed, there was no consistency, would never ask if I'd been eating or not or been doing a lot of exercise. In the winter, later in the day with heavier and more clothes I would weigh more than early morning in a pair of shorts in the summer.

Scientific research at its best. Innit? If these things matter do it properly.

August 2016 was pivotal in all this. A momentous month! My Gerson practitioners had long since retreated and were now incompatible with my hopes of survival, and the orthodox, led by Dr Fear were circling my wagon, wanting to see me **every four weeks** preparing the final assault on my immune system. And then as suddenly as cancer coming back everything changed. Just two days after the exchange with Doc Fear, 2 days before Alice's birthday, we hit the jackpot and everything fell into place. And I mean everything! The story could have so easily ended badly about now but here the story begins to turn into that fairy tale. In the space of a few days in the summer of 2016 we had literally found the root cause of my cancer and had begun to implement a cure for cancer and a whole mess of other stuff you might want to consider.

We had booked the VEGA Expert sitting essentially to establish a baseline of everything so we could build a picture, but it threw up so much more. We also booked an appointment to take a look at my live blood. You can do this with a darkfield microscope. This is a simple way to view a living specimen and monitor changes.

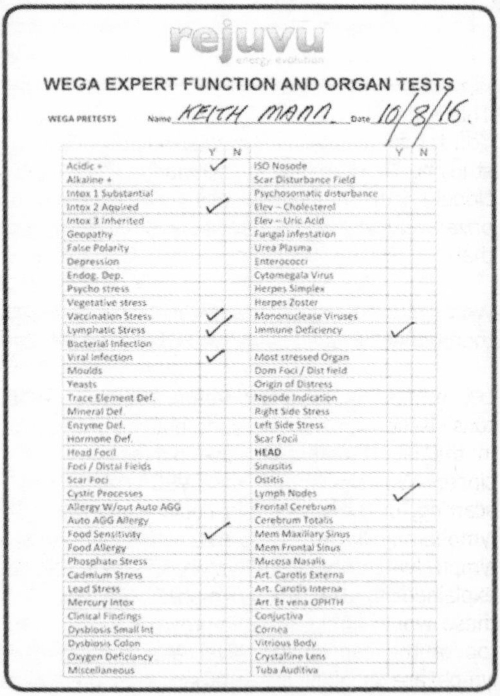

rejuvu
energy evolution

WEGA EXPERT FUNCTION AND ORGAN TESTS

WEGA PRETESTS Name KEITH MANN Date 10/8/16.

	Y	N		Y	N
Acidic +	✓		ISO Nosode		
Alkaline +			Scar Disturbance Field		
Intox 1 Substantial			Psychosomatic disturbance		
Intox 2 Aquired	✓		Elev – Cholesterol		
Intox 3 Inherited			Elev – Uric Acid		
Geopathy			Fungal infestation		
False Polarity			Urea Plasma		
Depression			Enterococci		
Endog. Dep.			Cytomegala Virus		
Psycho stress			Herpes Simplex		
Vegetative stress			Herpes Zoster		
Vaccination Stress	✓		Mononucleose Viruses		
Lymphatic Stress	✓		Immune Deficiency	✓	
Bacterial Infection					
Viral Infection	✓		Most stressed Organ		
Moulds			Dom Foci / Dist field		
Yeasts			Origin of Distress		
Trace Element Def.			Nosode Indication		
Mineral Def.			Right Side Stress		
Enzyme Def.			Left Side Stress		
Hormone Def.			Scar Focii		
Head Focii			**HEAD**		
Foci / Distal Fields			Sinusitis		
Scar Foci			Ostitis		
Cystic Processes			Lymph Nodes	✓	
Allergy W/out Auto AGG			Frontal Cerebrum		
Auto AGG Allergy			Cerebrum Totalis		
Food Sensitivity	✓		Mem Maxillary Sinus		
Food Allergy			Mem Frontal Sinus		
Phosphate Stress			Mucosa Nasalis		
Cadmium Stress			Art. Carotis Externa		
Lead Stress			Art. Carotis Interna		
Mercury Intox			Art. Et vena OPHTH		
Clinical Findings			Conjuctiva		
Dysbiosis Small Int			Cornea		
Dysbiosis Colon			Vitrious Body		
Oxygen Deficiancy			Crystalline Lens		
Miscellaneous			Tuba Auditiva		

Whatever the quacks, theorists and sceptics say about unapproved diagnostics and treatments, all they know is what they know. They have not a single positive thought about anything else. Chemo is only good for businessmen. And here's why they want us locked in their world of ignorance. This VEGA test took an hour, cost £70 and saved my life. WEGA is the European spelling.

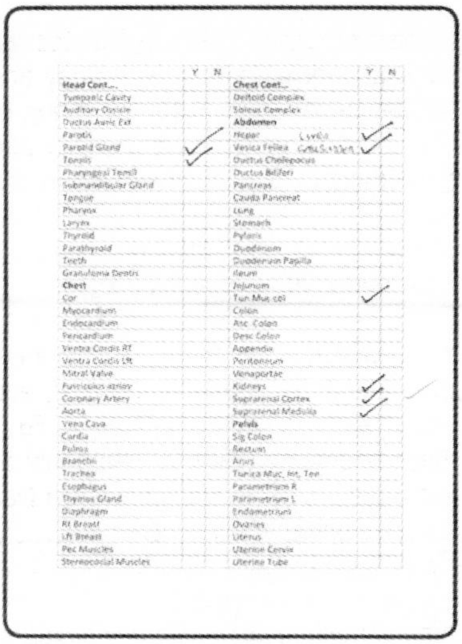

	Y	N		Y	N
Head Cont...			**Chest Cont...**		
Tympanic Cavity			Deltoid Complex		
Auditory Ossicle			Soleus Complex		
Ductus Auric Ext			**Abdomen**		
Parotis			Hepar Liver	✓	
Parotid Gland	✓		Vesica Fellea Gallbladder	✓	
Tonsils	✓		Ductus Choledocus		
Pharyngeal Tonsil			Ductus Biliferi		
Submandibular Gland			Pancreas		
Tongue			Cauda Pancreat		
Pharynx			Lung		
Larynx			Stomach		
Thyroid			Pylorus		
Parathyroid			Duodenum		
Teeth			Duodenum Papilla		
Granuloma Dentri			Ileum		
Chest			Jejunum		
Cor			Tun Muc col	✓	
Myocardium			Colon		
Endocardium			Asc Colon		
Pericardium			Desc Colon		
Ventra Cordis RT			Appendix		
Ventra Cordis Lft			Peritoneum		
Mitral Valve			Venaportae		
Fasciculus atrior			Kidneys	✓	
Coronary Artery			Suprarenal Cortex	✓	
Aorta			Suprarenal Medulla	✓	
Vena Cava			**Pelvis**		
Cardia			Sig Colon		
Pulmo			Rectum		
Bronchi			Anus		
Trachea			Tunica Muc, Int, Ten		
Esophagus			Parametrium R		
Thymus Gland			Parametrium L		
Diaphragm			Endometrium		
Rt Breast			Ovaries		
Lft Breast			Uterus		
Pec Muscles			Uterine Cervix		
Sternocostal Muscles			Uterine Tube		

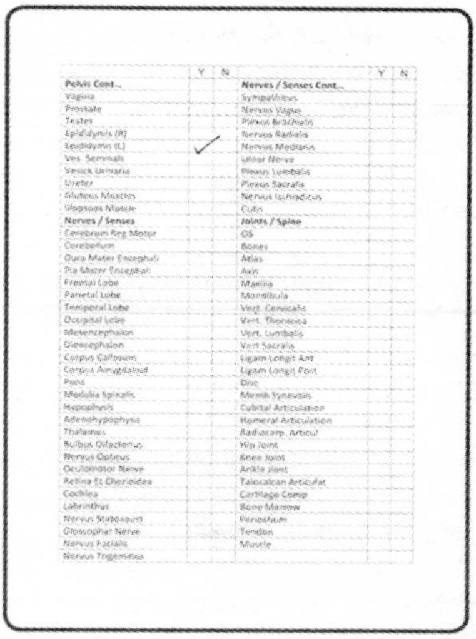

	Y	N		Y	N
Pelvis Cont...			**Nerves / Senses Cont...**		
Vagina			Sympathicus		
Prostate			Nervus Vagus		
Testes			Plexus Brachialis		
Epididymis (R)			Nervus Radialis		
Epididymis (L)	✓		Nervus Medianus		
Ves. Seminalis			Ulnar Nerve		
Vesica Urinaria			Plexus Lumbalis		
Ureter			Plexus Sacralis		
Gluteus Muscles			Nervus Ischiadicus		
Iliopsoas Muscle			Cutis		
Nerves / Senses			**Joints / Spine**		
Cerebrum Reg Motor			OS		
Cerebellum			Bones		
Dura Mater Encephali			Atlas		
Pia Mater Encephal			Axis		
Frontal Lobe			Maxilla		
Parietal Lobe			Mandibula		
Temporal Lobe			Vert. Cervicalis		
Occipital Lobe			Vert. Thoracica		
Mesencephalon			Vert. Lumbalis		
Diencephalon			Vert Sacralis		
Corpus Callosum			Ligam Longit Ant		
Corpus Amygdaloid			Ligam Longit Post		
Pons			Disc		
Medulla Spinalis			Membr Synovialis		
Hypophysis			Cubital Articulation		
Adenohypophysis			Humeral Articulation		
Thalamus			Radiocarp. Articul		
Bulbus Olfactorius			Hip Joint		
Nervus Opticus			Knee Joint		
Oculomotor Nerve			Ankle Joint		
Retina Et Chorioidea			Talocalcan Articulat		
Cochlea			Cartilage Comp		
Labrinthus			Bone Marrow		
Nervus Statoacust			Periostium		
Glossophar Nerve			Tendon		
Nervus Facialis			Muscle		
Nervus Trigeminus					

This is the kind of breakthrough every medical researcher in the world is hoping for. You see them peering into their microscopes in their shiny billion pound laboratories, studying Petri dishes, poisoning beagles, hacking at rats, looking for something. Nobel Prize? They don't really know what they are looking for in that search for the prize because the knee-jerk says nothing else exists and everyone is afraid to correct that!

We didn't really know what we were looking for but blow me did we find it! We were thoroughly intrigued by this document and couldn't wait to get home.

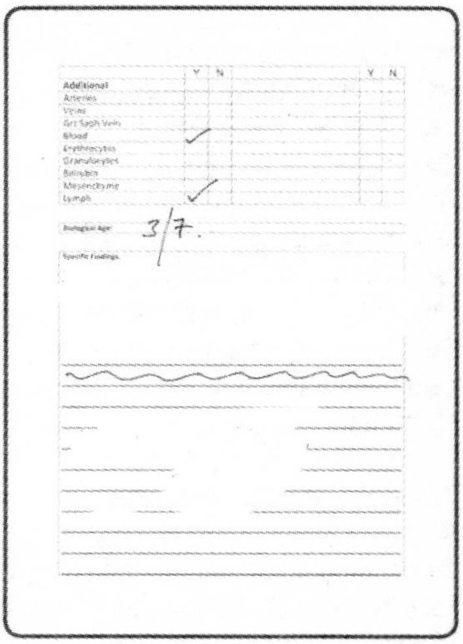

	Y	N		Y	N
Additional					
Arteries					
Veins					
Grt Saph Vein					
Blood	✓				
Erythrocytes					
Granulocytes					
Basophils					
Mesenchyme					
Lymph	✓				

Biological Age: 3/7.

Specific Findings:

Let me first isolate a few items. I had repeated tonsil issues in early childhood but these stopped in the late 1970's and have not bothered me since. We suspected the VEGA echo was scarring, or a memory, but could equally be the lymphoma, likewise the glands. Of course blood, lymph, lymph nodes and lymphatic stress can be explained by the blood/lymphatic cancer and these would all begin to improve as we got on top of the cancer. The liver and kidneys and lymph are the key detox organs and they had been under pressure for some time. Tun Muc col is the gut and the place most of our diseases originate hence the focus on simple nutrition. I knew I had swine flu at this time as a previous VEGA test picked that up, in fact the whole of 2016 was a wipe out with viruses and infection since the chemo hit took out my immune system at the end of 2015. Food sensitivity was no news either. I also had a cyst in my left testicle. The acquired toxicity is a lifetime of accumulation. No nutritional deficiencies.

Which leaves the more interesting findings.

Acidity is top of this VEGA chart and high on our priority list. PH imbalance is viewed by many as key to the cause of cancer or certainly a significant factor in its proliferation. Cancer thrives in an acidic environment and the focus of nutritional therapies is to return the environment to one of alkalinity, or balance. We must make the environment inhospitable to germs and we had been working hard at that.

So this was odd. For the previous two years I had done everything to load my body with alkaline foods and lots of green juices, as advised by many. But loading up on alkaline foods and water does not guarantee alkalinity. That was big news. What we would learn from this tick-in-a-box through our research is that a significant cause of acidity is the cancer itself. This is the lactic acid cycle, a self-perpetuating process fed by the cancer microbes within the cancer cells. The cells become weakened by our lifestyle and rather than respirate oxygen to survive they begin to ferment glucose. It is a process that will continue until the death of the host if the process isn't intercepted.

I found that the more alkalizing supplements I was loading into my body, as the cancer was growing, the more acidic I was becoming. Like using a water pistol on a house fire! As with constantly loading the gut with probiotics as opposed to fixing the cause of the depleted bacteria, we would do well to consider the viability of loading the body with high pH nutrition while ignoring the underlying cause of the acidity.

We looked into this acidic question and factored it into my new protocol. Testing my pH with saliva dip strips every morning had revealed it was actually dropping. Ideally at a green looking 7.0 - 7.4, I was now at a pale 6.2 - 6.0 and drifting down, because as the cancer was spreading and feeding itself as it grew. Patients failing on natural therapies need to consider this crucial detail. Without this little tick we may never have figured out the problem. Being immune deficient was another critical finding.

Reading 'Vaccination Stress' hit me like a truck then gave me a rush of adrenaline and I knew in that moment this was waiting for me. I was well aware that vaccines were a serious health risk for kids in particular and for OAP's, the weakest and most vulnerable, and the animals but not for me age 50 and all anti-vaccine. I latched onto that like a dog with bone and asked what more I could learn from the magic box. And there it was in all its glory - the saviour of humankind here now lighting up my twisted little mind like the key to the treasure trove – "it's the polio vaccine", he tells me. The polio vaccine! Of course it is! I only had one early on in life, that one and I knew that held a dark secret, involving monkey viruses and here it was, in its glory, the monkey virus SV40. SV40, what's that? You might well ask. You should!

We quickly went for a second opinion using an EAV diagnostic system similar to VEGA. Same finding. The orthodox will inject suspect material into a mouse to generate SV40 antibodies to tick this kind of box. We are more advanced. It's typed on the vial. You can see it - little glass bottle of liquid containing the virus fingerprint, sat on the machine in front of you squealing the sound she makes when she's found something. SV40 in me? Monkeys into Mann! Perversely I was so excited with the direction of the day and dug further, as a mole might the mud, for all I could. There was a choice of two, the Salk or Sabin vaccines both stored in the VEGA data vials. The Salk had been introduced first via needle and was soon replaced by the sugar cube delivery system we all identify with a miracle of modern medicine. But the polio virus in both products came from the same seed stock and there was no clear distinction to be drawn in this database, more leaning toward Salk when I pressed. I said it can't be. I was assured it probably was. That small detail fuelled my interest as Salk was supposedly out of circulation by 1962 and I was injected in 1966.

But that was the least important matter and my mind was racing.

Vaccines contain many ingredients that can do harm, such as metals and chemicals and these can be isolated in an investigation such as this. Vaccine stress recorded on VEGA on the other hand represents DNA damage caused by the viral components and other unknown micro-organisms in the vaccines and as you will see this tick in my box has ramifications for us all.

How awesome that we have access to the kind of forensic technology that can unravel a many decades-old crime! I knew I'd had this vaccine but 1966 was a long time ago. It's the kids of today I feel for. They don't have a hope. Vaccines in general fire me up but I had no idea how close to home this thing was. It was 1966/7 and I reacted so badly so my mum says I dodged any more. I know they got me with a tetanus jab once at Accident & Emergency as a teenager. I was a busy teenager, in and out of A&E with injuries, but I was invincible so I would always tell them 'yes' when I was asked if I was "up to date" because I didn't need injecting to protect me! I asked of VEGA where the vaccine stress was located in my body. Guess what? In my lymphatic system! Well that floored me! I'm not sure how to make a coincidence out of all of that and I have tried. It should give citizen stupid a hard time so they will simply refer back to the technology being unacceptable to the orthodox, but that doesn't matter to the rest of us. This all suggested to me that the origin of my cancer was the polio vaccine, but that's just crazy talk right because vaccines save lives; it been on the news and everything. Everyone says so, so it must be true.

You wish!

This was like an information overload. We knew right away from the picture this test had painted that we had pieced together the missing pieces of me and the cancer puzzle and we immediately factored all this into what became the MannIcure. But over the next few months so much more poured out of the can of worms we had opened up. While we did our own version of watch and wait to see what impact our radical ideas might have on my cancer, we quickly got the feedback everyone wants when treating cancer, I was free to do what I wanted with my life so I healed as I honed in on that polio vaccine. You are going to have to join me on that journey before I can talk you through my rebirth. This is how 2016 panned out. This is stunning information and I appreciate it may not be what you were expecting to find in a story about curing cancer, but I urge you to pay attention.

The rest of this story I have abbreviated as best I can. Vaccines are like an open wound, an area you don't touch. Accept and be silent is the pervasive message. Ask no questions and they'll tell you no lies.

I asked. Of course I asked! I had in my hands a treasure trove of information and a clue to something so big you have to tell everyone. I'm one of those geeks that want to know all about crop formations and alien abductions of course I want to know all about me! And this was it in droves. I hadn't realised it at the time but this was what I had always been looking for. I knew from the rush I felt when I heard "polio vaccine". Like you might feel on matching all the numbers on your lottery ticket. You have to read them again and again but you know. I knew, but I asked to hear it again. I'd been rooting around the vivisection/vaccine subject for as long as I was conscious and knew that it didn't add up, always hoping for a chink in the armour of the deception and denial that would show everyone I was right. You might think that an animal rights activist with a long criminal record and a well established role in calling out the vivisectors making outrageous unpopular claims about vaccines causing cancer would be a hard sell, but you might be surprised.

And how is this vaccine damage affecting my ability to heal? And how can it be repaired?

The next day I applied through my doctor for my old medical records to see what they held. And then I went on the internet and asked some questions and ordered some books. I quickly found that claims of vaccine damage are actually common and that there are 'vaccine courts' similar to kangaroo courts used as the official clearing house to reverse engineer the public perception of the damage and trickle some compensation to the lucky victims granted the long-term care they can't live without, but this typically relates to a sudden or recent self-evident vaccine injury. Vaccine damage is generally unspoken of in official circles and culpability is publicly denied with long-term damage said to be impossible. But record keeping lacks desire and credibility and they could of course only deny my 50-year-old discovery. Of the VEGA practitioners I contacted vaccination stress shows up in between 25 and 45% of clients with a higher probability in the kids. That's just the DNA damage that leads to cancer which of course can take time to manifest. Others acquire a mercury or aluminium burden or perhaps some life-threatening allergies and there are no safeguards.

Buckle up for a bumpy ride.

Belief in myths allows the comfort of opinion without the discomfort of thought.
John F. Kennedy (1917 – 1963)

It's in the Vaccine.
The Monkey Cancer Virus is in the Vaccine.

The chief, if not the sole, cause of the monstrous increase in cancer has been vaccination

Dr Robert Bell, former Vice President of the International Society for Cancer Research at the British Cancer Hospital

Maurice Hilleman was lauded as the worlds leading vaccine expert who was head of Merck's vaccine programmes in the 1950's. A hero to some who went on to develop dozens of vaccines. Working on a dream to eradicate polio (poliomyelitis), Hilleman along with other jolly chaps such as Sabin and Salk, manufactured some unprecedented mayhem upon the human race. And I exaggerate not one word. I'd told this story in the past, funny enough, on various internet forums and my website and to anyone who would listen, not really knowing it was about me. I had no intention of covering vaccines in this book but what do you do when the truth pokes you in the eye?

According to the testimony of Hilleman himself, 50 years earlier little Keith, "Monkey Mann" to the envious, along with hundreds of millions of other little humans ever since, were injected with a cancer causing monkey virus known as SV40 hidden in the polio vaccine. If you think that's way out there, well I've got loads of it so prepare yourself because this is going to get really weird. Also quite fun! And if you are hungry for the truth this is delicious.

Hilleman would later postulate with telling insight that "vaccines have to be considered the bargain basement technology for Twentieth Century". And he should know. He was the king of the vaccine experts, right? He had been messing around with wild caught monkeys in the 1950's and growing this polio vaccine in their kidneys, like you do. Oh, by the way, they do precisely this as the norm in all vaccine production and they use all manner of unlikely live organ and tissue cell cultures to grow the vaccine bacteria and viruses, each containing its own universal community of microorganisms and viral particles and who knows what.

Hilleman, Mr. Vaccine, wasn't always happy in his work. He complained a lot about a problem they were having with what he describes with suitable disdain as his "lousy monkeys". These were terrified wild caught beings trapped in cages in shiny laboratories surrounded by psychopaths, and the monkeys were not playing science with the scientists. In the 1950's, drug companies were beginning the drive to persuade everyone from pensioners to puppies to be injected with a new, improved range of disease prevention potions being heavily invested in to prevent all future suffering. And central to this are the lab animals. They suffer terribly of course, or they wouldn't be needed, but they are only put through this so we can all be free of disease. There is no other way. That's science according to scientists.

In an unreleased 1986 National Institute of Health film interview, recorded by Harvard Medical Historian Edward Shorter, Hilleman vents his frustration at these monkeys. Not just uncooperative stressed out and a long way from home, these were living breathing biological weapons of mass destruction, set to be unleashed on humanity. These experiments have always been immoral, unscientific and more than a little bit dangerous. And as we may deduce from the story unfolding before us, messing with Mother Nature is a big mistake. [71]

Hilleman radiates clinical with not a care for the world. His biggest gripe was that the monkeys were diseased and their damn viruses were putting obstacles in his path to greatness. But never mind needs must. And a vaccine was needed, apparently, and the Three Stooges were going to deliver - monkey virus or no monkey virus into human babies the vaccine will go. Does this sound like a good idea to you? I think it's time to decide.

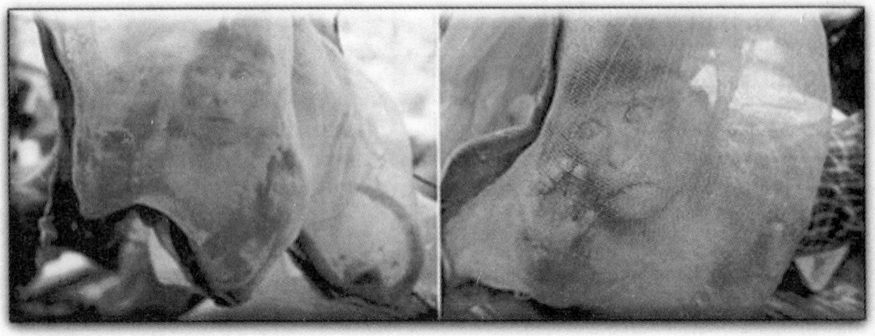

When one claims a necessary evil but cannot sustain necessity all one is left with is evil.

What we dug up in trying to understand Vaccination Stress in me is only a sniff of this particular swamp. I've cut it back to its core so not to overwhelm, so there can be no doubt, but the essence for me was in just those two words. They very quickly became three words: Vaccines cause cancer. And then a book full!

We have free will to choose, to ignore or to embrace the tricky subjects. Free will is a gift. But with that treasure comes a deep responsibility to those in our care on whom we impose our will, believing as we do that we are doing the best thing. It is important for all concerned that we get it right when we are talking about something so serious as a vaccine or a cancer treatment, but we can only get it right when we know what's right and what's not right. So, we need to know both sides, and when we have all the information we will then make the right decision and the best decision. Only then! Until that point we have not given our informed consent we have been coerced, manipulated or deceived. Informed is to ***be in possession of all relevant facts.***

> *The giving and obtaining of consent is viewed as a process, not a one-off event. Consent obtained before the occasion upon which a child is brought for immunisation is only an agreement for the child to be included in the*

[71] https://www.youtube.com/watch?v=2MpHKPZLaqw

> *immunisation programme and does not mean that consent is in place for each future immunisation. Consent should still be sought on the occasion of each immunisation visit.* ***The individual must be informed about the*** *process,* ***benefits and risks of immunisation*** *and be able to communicate their decision.* ***Information given should be*** *relevant to the individual patient,* ***properly explained and questions should be answered fully.*** [72]

We've had over 200 years being told how great vaccines are and we see increasingly as the human spiritual awakening gathers its insatiable momentum that any hint of doubt or distrust is crushed. Well this is some of the information they denied you when asking for your informed consent. What you do with it is up to you. I'm going to tell the world.

I'm sorry.

From PubMed, 2003:

> *Association Between SV40 and Non-Hodgkin's Lymphoma*
>
> ***Millions of people worldwide were inadvertently exposed to live simian virus 40 (SV40) between 1955 and 1963 through immunization with SV40-contaminated polio vaccines. Although the prevalence of SV40 infections in humans is not known, numerous studies suggest that SV40 is a pathogen resident in the human population today. SV40 is a potent DNA tumor virus*** *that is known to induce primary brain cancers, bone cancers, mesotheliomas, and lymphomas in laboratory animals. SV40 oncogenesis is mediated by the viral large tumor antigen (T-ag), which inactivates the tumor suppressor proteins p53 and pRb.* ***During the last decade, independent studies using different molecular biology techniques have shown the presence of SV40 DNA, T-ag, or other viral markers in primary human brain and bone cancers and malignant mesotheliomas.***
>
> *Evidence suggests that there may be geographic differences in the frequency of these virus-positive tumors. Recent large independent controlled studies have shown that* ***SV40 T-ag DNA is significantly associated with human non-Hodgkin's lymphoma (NHL).*** *In our study, we analyzed systemic NHL from 76 HIV-1-positive and 78 HIV-1-negative patients, and nonmalignant lymphoid samples from 79 HIV-1-positive and 107 HIV-1-negative patients without tumors; 54 colon and breast carcinoma samples served as cancer controls.* ***SV40-specific DNA sequences were detected in 64 (42%) of 154 NHL, none of 186 nonmalignant lymphoid***

[72] https://www.gov.uk/government/uploads/system/uploads/attachment_data/file/144250/Green-Book-Chapter-2-Consent-PDF-77K.pdf

> ***samples,*** *and none of 54 control cancers. For NHL from HIV-1-positive patients, 33% contained SV40 DNA and 39% Epstein Barr virus (EBV) DNA, whereas NHLs from HIV-1-negative patients were 50% positive for SV40 and 15% positive for EBV. Few tumors were positive for both SV40 and EBV.*
>
> ***SV40 sequences were found most frequently in diffuse large B cell and follicular-type lymphomas. We conclude that SV40 is significantly associated with some types of NHL and that lymphomas should be added to the types of human cancers*** **associated with SV40.** [73]

How is this possible, I hear you ask. A cancer causing monkey virus showing up in human cancer - must be some kind of freak one off unforeseen accident, discovered and repaired with haste and remorse? You'd hope! Let's see how long we can cling on to that theory.

The Creation and Production of the Polio Vaccines

> *In the 1950s, scientists like Doctors Jonas Salk and Albert Sabin had isolated the poliovirus strains to make vaccines. Dr Salk's strains would be inactivated with formaldehyde and injected into children. Dr Sabin's strains would be attenuated or weakened by transferring or passaging the live viruses through different host cells and then fed to children orally.*
>
> *Because his goal was to create a live attenuated vaccine, Dr Sabin had to isolate the poliovirus strains and then passage the strains through a myriad of host cells in order to attain the right virulence - strong enough to illicit an immune response, but weak enough so as to not cause polio in the recipient. Sabin's oral polio vaccine (OPV) is a trivalent vaccine and was, therefore, comprised of three types – Type I, II, and III. For example, Type I has the following lineage: In 1941, Drs. Francis and Mack isolated the Mahoney poliovirus **"from the pooled feces of three healthy children** in Cleveland." **Dr Salk then subjected the strain to passages through fourteen living monkeys and two cultures of monkey testicular cultures.** In 1954, the strain (now called Monk14 T2) was given to Drs. Li and Schaeffer who **subjected the virus to nine more passages through monkey testicular cultures**. Next, the strain (now called Monk14 T11) **underwent fifteen more passages in monkey testicular cultures, eighteen passages in monkey kidney cells, two passages through the skin of living rhesus monkeys, and additional passages through African Green monkey skin and monkey kidney cell cultures... In 1956, Dr Sabin took this virus and passaged it through seven cultures of African Green Monkey kidney cells.** That same year, the pharmaceutical company, Merck, Sharp & Dohme, **passed the strain... through a rhesus monkey kidney cell culture.** The resulting material was called Sabin Original Merck (SOM) and was provided to Lederle in 1960*

[73] https://www.ncbi.nlm.nih.gov/pubmed/15202523

> *as the seed material to manufacture its polio vaccine. Types II and III were created in a similar fashion.* [74]

What could possibly go wrong? Well just about everything did go wrong. This is what some call science. Doesn't it give you that warm feeling, like our destiny is in safe hands?

Seriously, filter through kidneys? Which organ would be more prone to contamination? You could filter it through the anus and get a cleaner sample. Imagine the hysteria if ISIS or whoever we are meant to fear just now was cooking up biological time bombs in some basement laboratory and spreading disease. The mainstream media would be going crazy whipping up hysteria for war, to save lives! And this wasn't just one kidney in the pot, this was a big old cocktail of so many thousands of wild monkey kidneys all mixed in and mashed up in a blender and made into some kind of nutty scientist seed stock broth. They use fancy words to flavour their behaviour but crazy, kidneys, blenders and broths neatly sum it up. Not so comforting but easier to understand. And to complete the circle of tragic - the waste disposal organs of these wretched souls are a vivisectors favourite because they're easy to access. Get that! No major surgery or breaking open the rib cages all they had to do was to anaesthetise the monkey shove it face down on the table, stick a knife up the side of the spine and bingo - got yourself a kidney and not much mess.

We are talking about a shopping list for full scale vaccine production using upwards of 5,000 mostly Indian rhesus macaques alone every day in the US, many more dying en route. Every last one of these abductions is sickening enough but to add insult to injury large amounts of the resulting brew from these animals was so visibly contaminated with exotic simian viruses that it was discarded like the rest of the animal. But the hidden viruses in the final concoction were not so readily disposed of and were left to fester for some time in the future. Around about now for some of us!

Cancerous bird embryos, dog kidneys and extracts of cow's blood have all led to serious contamination of human vaccines. Those they concoct for use on animals are just as messy with more of the same and maybe some suckling mouse brain or sheep brain-derived proteins, goat nerve tissue or cats' kidneys as the seed stock. Oh yes they do and the DNA damage is spreading. Hard to image what kind of mind devises such a scheme, but on our level we can easily see the potential for harm from injecting a living pathogen grown in cat brains into someone we love. I imagine it and it makes me sick but this is what some people do for a living. We don't need to image because the evidence is widespread, way beyond SV40. Polio was just the launch pad, the testing ground.[75]

Viruses are tricky things to grow and cancers can be caused by viruses. Once a home-grown target colony of virus or bacteria is established in the lab the same

---

74 http://www.sv40foundation.org/

75 https://www.frontiersin.org/articles/10.3389/fmicb.2010.00147/full

seed stock will be maintained way into the future. There are non-animal origin alternatives available for growing some vaccine viruses and have been since the early 1960's. Frying pan and fire come to my mind, but which would you choose? One goes by the code name WI-38 and is made from aborted human foetal material. That's right. Female. Abortion. 12 weeks old. Into the blender. We'll come back to this. These vaccines are so enticing it's really hard to choose.

In 1936, Albert Sabin and Peter Olitsky at the Rockefeller Institute had managed to grow the polio virus in a culture of brain tissue from a human embryo. In spite of the success they achieved in this Sabin and Olitsky were concerned about using brain cells as a vaccine medium, **fearing nervous system damage in vaccine recipients,** so it was shelved. These people do crazy for a living and isolating these viruses has been a challenge so this kind of voluntary abstinence is a big statement. They clearly understood the potential problems of growing vaccine viruses in live pieces of people, yet the practice persists.[76]

The polio vaccine is our canary in the coal mine. It was a disaster from its inception when the seed stock was found to be uncontrollably contaminated with rouge monkey viruses. The formation of the actual idea of a polio vaccine was arguably the pinnacle of this entire saga, because from then on one vaccine disaster has led into the next.

In early experiments on the human population in the US in the 1950's, in what became known as the Cutter incident (after the company who manufactured it), 260 people contracted polio from the Salk vaccine and there were 200 cases of what was called "paralysis" and several deaths recorded. Polio/Paralysis, Greed/Need - depends who you ask, if you ask me. This brought about the downfall of the Salk polio vaccine. According to millionaire vaccine inventor and mandate fanatic Paul Offit MD "The disease caused by Cutter's vaccine was worse than the disease caused by natural polio virus". This is a not unusual side effect of vaccines but vaccine-induced polio isn't half the story.

The official line today, albeit quietly stated, is that the problem with Salk's polio vaccine was solved after it was discovered and by 1963 all was rosy again in the vaccine lab. But when we delve deeper we find weeds in their garden of roses. In fact the roses are long gone. Poisoned! And on that contaminated plot a vast invasive vaccine schedule has taken root, sucking the life.

For anyone closely following this polio thread and battling that unfortunate human instinct to feel some small comfort for being born after the purge of the first poisoned vaccine in 1963, when the safe Sabin brew was dripped into the sugar cube as the replacement, I have some more news. The dates that the early vaccine was infected with SV40, as quietly confessed to in the medical literature here, there and everywhere are not entirely accurate. And we shouldn't be in any way surprised at this trickle feed of the truth because this is standard operating procedure. Put simply virus in vaccine yes, virus out no. The monkey virus and the polio vaccine are

[76] https://www.historyofvaccines.org/content/articles/early-tissue-and-cell-culture-vaccine-development

inseparable. The Salk vaccine was unleashed in 1955 and soon after Cutter happened, officially because of an isolated manufacturing mishap and consequently the SV infection was discovered. This was hushed up and wasn't revisited for at least four decades.

All this time the same rhesus kidney seed stock has been used in polio vaccine production. In some parts of the world around 1999 as a kind of April Fools prank, they shifted polio production from the Three Stooges monkey kidney stock (with SV40's) to a different monkey kidney stock and associated disease matter. This disaster in the making they call Vero who we are also going to come back to.

In 1960, the pharmaceutical company Merck & Co. wrote to the U.S. Surgeon General:

> *Our scientific staff have emphasized to us that there are a number of serious scientific and technical problems that must be solved before we could engage in large-scale production of live poliovirus vaccine.* ***Most important among these is the problem of extraneous contaminating simian viruses that may be extremely difficult to eliminate and which may be difficult if not impossible to detect at the present stage of the technology.*** [77]

This was known to just about everyone in the field, but the mad scientists and assorted vivisectors in this polio vaccine programme still reckoned they were smart enough that they could deactivate the viruses with their dumb ass meddling. Whatever you think of vivisection and vaccines, when you see how thoroughly they cocked this up you will probably feel a sense of unease at the crude stupidity of the entire methodology.

SV40 by the way represents the 40th family of simian virus that these buffoons actually found swimming in the monkey kidneys they were extracting and grinding up into their potions. There are more than 40 known, there may be hundreds or thousands in any given vaccine but it only takes one family member to cause cancer.

When children had begun dying (and contracting polio) from the original Salk injectable polio vaccine (circa 1955 – 1963) and the SV40 contamination was discovered, it was withdrawn and a new improved sweeter version was produced and fed to the people from 1963 onwards with the SV40 virus allegedly "destroyed" with formaldehyde. This was as impossible for them to achieve then as it is now, but that remains the official line. And it isn't just one vaccine with this kind of contamination, it's all of them, as you will see. Diseases emerge within us when the conditions suit their needs. SV40 likes the conditions we humans make of ourselves.

Unbeknown to the polio vaccine scientists through these decades, there was a second form of the SV40 virus asleep in the original polio vaccine seed stock that

---

[77] http://www.sv40foundation.org/How-OPV-produced.html

would take longer to 'wake up' when tested for than the known SV40, so no one knew it was there and no one found it. We'll call this SV40. I'm not sure why they don't, perhaps because they know they never killed it, because they can't. Alternatively it would be SV41, but they see another 'form' of SV40. Anyway, the monkey virus would wake up when it was good and ready and not when a textbook says it should. We are all unique and don't fit the rules. So SV40 the sleeper cell broke a rule the scientists made without even getting up, creating confusion for the scientists and cause for a decades' long cover up. It's a lie that grew so big the consequences so grave no one dares to break ranks. But I'm not in the club.

Remember the story of Vlad The Impaler? Check out Simian Sabin.

By 1963 we were being groomed on the sweet tasting Sabin polio vaccine, complete with the sleeper SV virus that hadn't come to life yet and is not affected by any agent used to kill them. But even if it had been discovered then what? There are many hidden viruses in these vaccines mixing into the human genome as we speak.

There has been an awful lot of testing done on the polio vaccine over the years but still the truth has remained under the control of the scientific community until very recently when those of us with the real power to take science out of the dark ages have begun to do so. That's you and me. This is all about you and me.

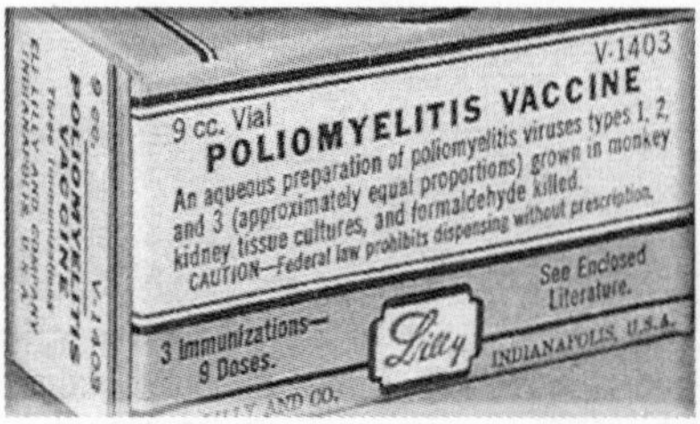

Much more recent testing of batch samples of the sweet vaccine used after this 1963 cut-off date, proved that the vaccine used until at least 1999, when SV40 was finally rediscovered, had been grown from the **exact same live virus seed strains** as the 1950's Salk injectable vaccine so were inevitably contaminated. In the earlier tests, according to the laws of scientists, the virus was supposed to take 14 days to mature in culture but it didn't, did it. So some bright sparks decided the virus wasn't there. And that has been the science ever since on which we entrust everything we love. But the virus was there, it was just a little bit late, sometimes dependant on the amount of virus in the test sample, up to five weeks late. By which time the vaccine safety box 'No Sign of Rouge Viruses' has been ticked and everyone has gone home.

This is not my idea of science, but never mind. At least with no *sign* of any rouge monkey viruses in the polio vaccine seed stock, for the time being there was piece of mind and a safe polio vaccine for everyone to enjoy. Yeah, of course the children would be safe in the hands of the drug companies! To be blinded by science in the 1960's is understandable but not with 60 years of experience. They give us cancer and they make children commit suicide and homicide with their antidepressants!

The better information on this incredible story is found in the independent media but it's not hard to piece it together from the trickle feed of the truth filtering into the mainstream medical literature.

Conspiracy theorists writing for the National Institute of Health:

Simian virus 40 in humans

> ***SV40 footprints in humans have been found associated at high prevalence with specific tumor types such as brain and bone tumors, mesotheliomas and lymphomas and with kidney diseases, and*** *at lower prevalence* ***in blood samples from healthy donors.*** [78]

And the Lancet Journal:

Association between simian virus 40 and non-Hodgkin lymphoma

> *We saw no significant differences in the mean age of patients with SV40-positive and SV40-negative non-Hodgkin lymphoma within the HIV-1-infected group...* ***Five of the patients with SV40-positive non-Hodgkin lymphoma were born after 1963****, the last year that SV40-contaminated poliovirus vaccine was used in the USA.*
>
> *Seroepidemiological studies have shown the presence of SV40 neutralising antibodies in 16% of HIV-1-infected patients and 11% of HIV-1-uninfected individuals,* ***some of whom were born after 1963*** *and could not have been exposed to SV40-contaminated poliovaccines.* ***Our study found that five patients with SV40-positive non-Hodgkin lymphoma were born after 1963—a finding similar to previous studies involving brain and bone cancers in which some patients with SV40-positive tumours had been born in recent decades. These observations suggest that polyomavirus SV40 might be causing infections in human beings long after the use of the contaminated vaccines.*** *However, how SV40 is transmitted among humans, and the prevalence of infection, remain to be established.* [79]

I can think of one possibility why we have a monkey virus sweeping through the species, of which there aren't really that many to choose from. That the contamination of the vaccine continued ad infinitum? There is another scenario that could equally explain some of the disease manifestation we are experiencing. We do of course inherit damaged DNA. That could see it go on long after the vaccines are finally rejected by the majority but wouldn't necessarily be detected in the same way this direct contamination is. Either way...

In 1986 paediatric oncologist Daniel J. Bergasel found that **10 of 20 early childhood choroid plexus tumors and 10 of 11 ependymomas tested positive for SV40 gene sequences**. This is an awful lot of doctor-induced cancer to be sloshing around in young children.

---

78 https://www.ncbi.nlm.nih.gov/pmc/articles/PMC1941725/

79 http://www.thelancetnorway.com/journals/lancet/article/PIIS0140-6736(02)07950-3/fulltext

> *I was in shock when I discovered that - because you don't find monkey viruses in humans.* ***Monkey virus should not be present in human brain tumor.*** [80]

Indeed not.

If you think about it there must be a really good reason why we haven't heard this crazy cancer-vaccine story discussed on the talk shows and on 'the news' and in a crowded house of representatives or two because this is as big as it gets. And it can not reasonably be buried as conspiracy theory since it's documented officially as a fact. Perhaps the reason it hasn't been publicised all over the world where the vaccine is used is because it was so long ago now and because *now* they fixed the problem? I'm afraid that isn't going to wash, and even if it were the case under the current medical treatment approach cancers continue to spread and thrive. What might have something to do with limiting what we see and hear are the half dozen billionaires who control most of the media in the mainstream and Big Pharma's dependence on vaccines. Best explanation I can see.

Whatever, we have cancer being injected into people on a vast scale and there can be no excuse.

Here we can reaffirm those wacky conspiracy theorist conspiracy theories claiming not only that SV40 survived the clumsy formaldehyde deactivation process, but that SV40 was no lone ranger. We say there are loads of them in all the vaccines, officially there are now more than 40 and counting. We might consider them as sleeper cells. How many more we may never know but it hardly matters how many there are when any one of them is showing up in the brain cancers in human infants.

> *To confirm the presence of SV40 T antigen sequences, we further analysed samples of non-Hodgkin lymphoma in which SV40 DNA was detected. Sequence analysis of amplified products obtained from ten samples of non-Hodgkin lymphoma... showed the DNA sequences to be identical to those of the SV40 T antigen gene... Sequence analysis of PCR products from five samples of non-Hodgkin lymphoma (three from HIV-1-infected and two from HIV-1-uninfected patients) confirmed that* ***their origin was SV40****. We then compared these five lymphoma-associated T antigen C sequences with a catalogue of SV40 sequences (GenBank).* ***One*** *C sequence* ***was similar to that of SV40 strain*** *CPC/MEN,* ***previously detected in several primary human brain cancers, one was different from any previously reported SV40 sequence, and three*** *(one from an HIV-1-infected patient and two from HIV-1-uninfected patients)* ***were similar to that of SV40 strain*** *MC-028846B -* ***a virus first detected in a sample from a contaminated polio vaccine from 1955****. These results substantiate our belief that the T antigen gene of* ***SV40 was present in the non-Hodgkin***

[80] https://www.nejm.org/doi/pdf/10.1056/NEJM199204093261504

> ***lymphoma specimens tested****, and that detection of SV40 sequences was not the result of laboratory contamination.* [81]

This is insane! I'm not great at mathematics but I can count. We are only seeing the tip of this iceberg here but already we are swimming in this stuff. That was in the Lancet in 2002. Here's more:

The National Institute of Health:

> *These results suggest that* ***SV40 or a closely related virus may have an etiologic role in the development of these neoplasms during childhood****, as in animal models.* [82]

Close relative? SV41? 42? Secret Agent 007? I suspect if they start numbering all their injectable cancer causing viruses it'll be too much too soon, so the scientists are settling with "similar" for now. Trickle feed the truth to the plebs.

In July 2002, the National Academy of Science Institute of Medicine (IOM) Immunization Safety Committee convened a study into the link between SV40 and human cancer which culminated in a report published three months later:

SV40 Contamination of Polio Vaccine and Cancer.

> ***The committee's scientific assessment concludes that moderate to strong lines of biological evidence support the theory that SV40 contamination of polio vaccine could contribute to human cancers. Specifically, the evidence is strong that SV40 has transforming properties in several experimental systems. The committee concludes that concerns about exposure to SV40 through inadvertent contamination of polio vaccines are significant because of the seriousness of cancers as the possible adverse health outcomes and because of the continuing need to ensure and protect public trust in the nation's immunization program.*** [83]

Trust the program! It's undeniable there is a serious problem here but a mind made up is a mind made up and these animal sacrifice extremists at understandinganimalresearch carry on beating their drums of war no matter what mess their idiotic theories stir up. On the cancer causing monkey kidney grown polio vaccine they have long encouraged all human children to consume, they insist:

> ***This advance alone has saved millions of lives****, and the World Health Organisation is close to eradicating polio completely through its worldwide*

[81] http://www.sciencedirect.com/science/article/pii/S0140673602079503

[82] http://jvi.asm.org/content/77/9/5039

[83] https://www.ncbi.nlm.nih.gov/books/NBK221112/

> *vaccination programme.* ***Forty years of research using monkeys and mice led to the introduction of the vaccine in the 1950s.*** [84]

SV40 is lethal; it is highly oncogenic and is routinely used to inflict cancer in lab animals, it readily transforms rodent and human cells in culture, it causes cancer in humans and it is the main side effect of the polio vaccine now showing up in the brain tumours of our children. Go vivisectors! Go chop up some rats; see if you can't find a cure for stupidity.

The discovery of our stealth SV40 originally came from injecting samples of the failed polio vaccine directly into the brains of hamsters of a few hours old. [85] These most vulnerable beings have no immune system to protect themselves from the prowess of these scientists, and in due course the suspect SV40 virus reappeared within the vivisector-induced baby hamster brain tumours. Hamsters infested with SV40 typically develop lymphomas, brain tumours, osteosarcomas, and mesotheliomas. This was all coming to light in 1960 and a tidal wave of research only confirms the impact of this the most intensively studied animal virus. And what did they do with the findings of this animal research, the finest of human endeavours; of scientific research at its best? *Shhhh! Keep it in-house and do more research. Look for more stuff to investigate further, keep the research grants flowing.* There's no stopping these people when they discover a way to maintain or make a disease.

What we were left with was business as usual and the pure art of scientific research gone to waste!

Hilleman & Sweet said in 1960:

> *The discovery of this new virus vacuolating (SV40) represents the detection for the first time of a hitherto "non detectable" simian virus of monkey renal cultures and raises the important question of the existence of other such viruses…* ***all 3 types of Sabin's live poliovirus vaccine, now fed to millions of persons of all ages, were contaminated with vacuolating virus.*** [86]

It's not looking good for the king of the vaccines.

One university student of something or other told me in a condescending email about how "the exaggerated cancer risk to a minority is worth it for saving the world from the scourge of polio". "Fill your boots", I replied. Loyalists should be vaccinated to their hearts content, as long it's first proven to pose no infection risk to innocent bystanders, of course.

---

[84] http://www.understandinganimalresearch.org.uk/why/human-health/polio-vaccine/

[85] Eddy et al, 1961. https://www.sciencedirect.com/science/article/pii/004268226290082X

[86] http://www.sv40foundation.org/cpv-link.html

But just what are we afraid of anyway that we go to such bizarre lengths to protect ourselves? According to the independent vaccine researchers such as Dr Sherri Tenpenny:

> *Polioviruses are transient inhabitants of the gastrointestinal tract. Up to 95% of all polio infections are completely asymptomatic. Approximately 5% of polio infections consist of a minor, nonspecific illness consisting of an upper respiratory tract infection (sore throat and fever) and gastrointestinal disturbances (nausea, vomiting, abdominal pain, and diarrhea). This influenza-like illness, clinically indistinguishable from the myriad of other viral illnesses, is characterized by complete recovery in less than a week with resultant life time immunity. Less than 1% of all polio infections result in paralysis. Most importantly, the vast majority of individuals who contract paralytic poliomyelitis recover with complete—or near complete—return of muscle function. Any weakness that is still present 12 months after onset of paralysis is usually considered permanent.* [87]

According to the UK government:

1997: *Polio Eradication: Surveillance Implications for the United Kingdom*

> *Poliovirus infection may be inapparent. For each clinically recognized poliovirus paralytic case, there may be between 60 and 1000 inapparent infections. In a review of UK polio cases, Joce et al... found that not all clinically suspected cases were being notified, and even some confirmed cases had not been notified.* [88]

Vaccine advocates hone in on the iron lung as an argument for vaccinating everyone, but what was this horrific medical torture chamber for? A coffin for life?

---

87 https://www.newswithviews.com/Tenpenny/sherri3.htm

88 https://academic.oup.com/jid/article/175/Supplement_1/S156/878681

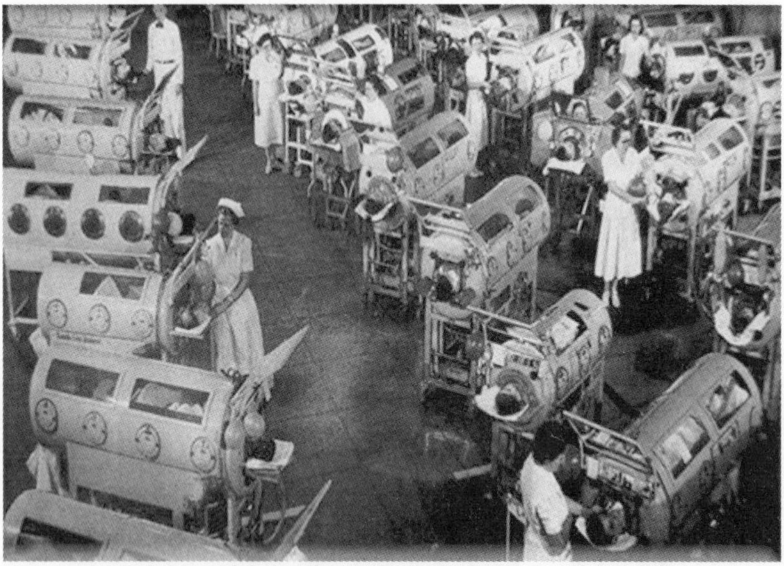

Iron lung ward during the 1940s, then prevalent in U.S. hospitals.

Nah! A bit cumbersome maybe, like the early computers and mobile phones, but as the ventilator of the day it was a useful piece of life-saving medical equipment to aid breathing in severe cases. As the patient recovers the aid can usually be removed.

Ventilators are much safer and less bothersome than the monkey vaccines, trust me!

But what a ridiculous choice! Is that it? What about those repetitive claims of necessity?

In the UK polio infection numbers bounced up and down erratically from one year to the next until 1951 when this uneven infection rate begun plummeting naturally and purposefully toward extinction. In 1950 the recorded incidence peaked at 7760 with 755 deaths. In 1955 there were 6331 reported infections, 270 reported dead. By 1960 there were 378 notifications and 46 dead. A whopping 95% decline in ten years to 1960. Yet only one year earlier, in a population in excess of 51 million and with the vaccine agenda in utter disarray after the disaster of the polio-causing Salk polio vaccine, and with that product undergoing recall, only a mere 12% were subject to vaccination. So 88% didn't get it. Get it? 95% decline, 88% unvaccinated. No need to be a mathematician to figure this one out either! [89] [90]

[89] http://www.post-polio.org/ir-eng.html

[90] https://www.ncbi.nlm.nih.gov/pmc/articles/PMC1592614/

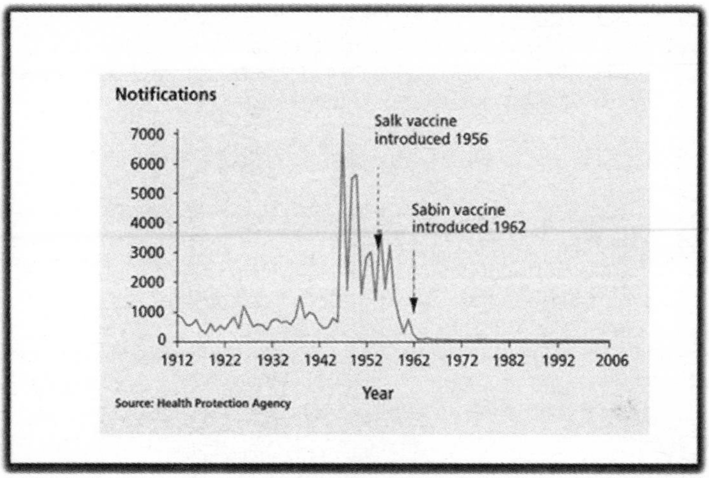

A picture paints [91]

This natural decline of the polio virus and its virulence would continue unhindered, in spite of the vaccine-induced infections and idiotic vaccine efficacy claims. This fell in line with improved medical care, a revolution in social hygiene and a phase out of the pesticide DDT, which is a key suspect in aggravating the polio-like phenomenon and is well known for its impact on the nervous system and for causing muscle weakness and respiratory dysfunction. Death from DDT poisoning is usually the result of respiratory arrest, as it happens.

The pesticide stood accused of damaging nerves and allowing the entry of normally-harmless enteroviruses, such as polio. In hearings before a US Select Committee in the early 1950's to investigate the use of chemicals on food, we find early clues:

> *The introduction... of DDT... and the series of even more deadly poisons that followed, has no previous counterpart in history. Beyond question no other substance was ever before developed so rapidly and spread indiscriminately over so large a portion of the earth in so short a time.* [92]

Toxicity testing on many animal species had foretold of the all too obvious danger of these destructive chemical cocktails, but animal experiments have no place in human health and well being and so they are ignored:

> *Somehow a fantastic myth of human invulnerability has grown up with reference to the use of these substances. Because their affects are cumulative and may be insidious and because* ***they resemble those of so many other conditions****, physicians for the most part have been unaware of their danger.*

---

[91] https://www.gov.uk/government/uploads/system/uploads/attachment_data/file/148141/Green-Book-Chapter-26-Polio-updated-18-January-2013.pdf

[92] Hearings before the house select committee to investigate the use of chemicals in food production, 81st Congress 2nd Session. https://www.archives.gov/legislative/guide/house/chapter-22-select-food-and-cosmetics.html

> *Since shortly after the last war a large number of cases had been observed all over the country in which a group of symptoms occurred the most prominent feature of which was* ***gastroenteritis, persistently recurrent nervous symptoms and extreme muscle weakness.*** [92]

Ah those fantastic human myths! Do these symptoms sound strikingly familiar?

Gerson quotes two British authors in 1958 in '50 Cases' describing their experience of DDT poisoning in humans:

> *A running nose, cough, and persistent* ***sore throat*** *are common, often followed by a persistent or recurrent feeling of constriction or a lump in the throat. Pain in the joints,* ***general muscle weakness****, and exhausting fatigue are usual; the latter are often so severe in the acute stage as to be described by some patients as* ***paralysis.*** *Most striking about the syndrome is the persistence of some of the symptoms, the tendency to* ***repeated recurrence*** *of others over a period of many months... even after a year.*

Post polio syndrome (PPS) is a label given to the repeated recurrence of symptoms in polio survivors. Remember...

> *Polio is a non-specific illness consisting of an upper respiratory tract infection (****sore throat*** *and fever) and gastrointestinal disturbances (nausea, vomiting, abdominal pain, and diarrhoea)...* ***clinically indistinguishable from the myriad of other viral illnesses...*** *less than 1% of all polio infections result in paralysis... vast majority recover with complete or near complete return of muscle function...*

I wonder...

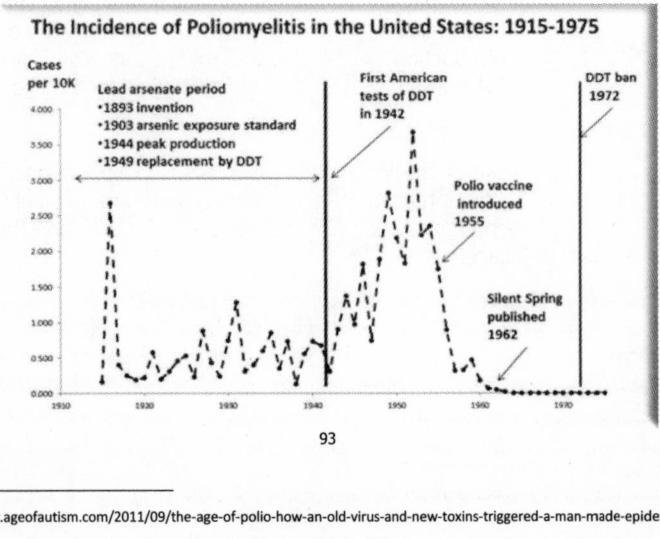

[93]

93 http://www.ageofautism.com/2011/09/the-age-of-polio-how-an-old-virus-and-new-toxins-triggered-a-man-made-epidemic-1.html

This pattern of polio passing in spite of any vaccine was replicated in various countries. According to Stetten and Carrigan in 'NIH [National Institute of Health]: An account of Research in its Laboratories and Clinics'.

> *By about 1960, three different attenuated live virus vaccines... Sabin... Cox... Koprowski... were ready for large scale clinical trials. Evidence of waning immunity in persons who had received the Salk vaccine several years earlier made the prospect of live virus vaccines most attractive. The extensive clinical trials conducted in South America... Africa... Poland... and in Russia led, in 1962, after much agonising analysis of data, to approval by NIH of only the Sabin... Poliovirus Vaccine.* [94]

The replacement oral polio vaccine was introduced into the UK in due course and then very slowly taken in through the 1960's by an untrusting population, who can now begin to see the error of our ways and are spitting it out again. However they spin it polio was no longer a threat by time the rebranded monkey-cancer-vaccine was let loose.

Even if this could be blamed on a natural viral invasion of our species and not something self-inflicted, against a mostly "inapparent" transient viral infection they have pillaged the jungles of the higher life and replaced the possibility of that with the risk of cancer or something else you can't readily get rid of.

Further diluting the polio horror story, we find that around the time the polio vaccine was adding cancer material to the human gene pool the definition of polio was adjusted. So, one might now be found to have Acute Flaccid Paralysis instead, which is "clinically indistinguishable from polio paralysis but twice as deadly" [95] and can be caused by any exposure to toxins.

The new definition of polio requires a patient to exhibit paralytic symptoms for weeks, and residual paralysis has to be confirmed twice during the course of the disease. Prior to the introduction of the vaccine the patient only had to exhibit paralytic symptoms for 24 hours, but with the advance of science these are flexible details. [96]

And what are we to make of the increase in diagnosis of aseptic meningitis and of the Coxsackie viral infections that may mimic mild or non-paralytic polio and were once categorised as such? It's all very uncertain and unscientific, and there's more, in fact it's all over the place!

---

94 (ISBN: 978-0-12-667980-9) https://www.elsevier.com/books/nih-an-account-of-research-in-its-laboratories-and-clinics/stetten/978-0-12-667980-9

95 https://www.ncbi.nlm.nih.gov/pubmed/22591873

96 http://www.vaccinationcouncil.org/2011/11/17/smoke-mirrors-and-the-disappearance-of-polio/

There are 6 Group B Coxsackie viruses (and 24 Group A). In the category of pathogenic enteroviruses. They can cause spastic paralysis and are associated with pancreatitis, juvenile diabetes, aseptic meningitis, herpangina, pleurodynia, myocarditis, pericarditis, meningoencephalitis, heart arrhythmia and hepatitis. But there is no vaccine for the Coxsackie and for most of us the virus apparently passes through undiagnosed.

On coxsackie:

> *In the UK outbreaks occur regularly in nurseries, schools and childcare centres. Most adults have developed immunity.* [97]

Coxsackie is named after the small US town where it was found. 'Atypical polio' reflects the symptoms this virus causes, the polio-like symptoms. Atypical Polio has since been reclassified as Chronic Fatigue Syndrome, or ME. In 'What Doctors Don't Tell You' Jan 2014 we get a taste of how some cases of Chronic Fatigue Syndrome may be 'polio by another name'.

> *Research into Post-Polio syndrome and chronic fatigue has made the astounding discovery that the virus that most often triggers CFS is closely related to the one that causes polio. But a body of evidence is growing linking Chronic Fatigue Syndrome (CFS), also called myalgic encephalomyelitis (ME), to this terrible disease, largely caused by attempts to eradicate polio. Other researchers demonstrate that CFS is just another form of polio, which has increased with the advent of polio vaccination. As one type of gut virus has been eradicated, so other forms have had the space to proliferate.* [98]

There are far too many questions for this to be settled science or even science for that matter and perhaps this explains why we are not meant to talk about it. So let's look at some more pictures! This slight of hand plotted in the following graphs from the vaccinationcouncil.org shows the potential for this 'alternative' polio diagnosis to present for the world a vaccine-induced polio cure.

---

97 https://patient.info/doctor/coxsackievirus-infection

98 volume 6 issue 9 http://www.anapsid.org/cnd/diffdx/polio1.html

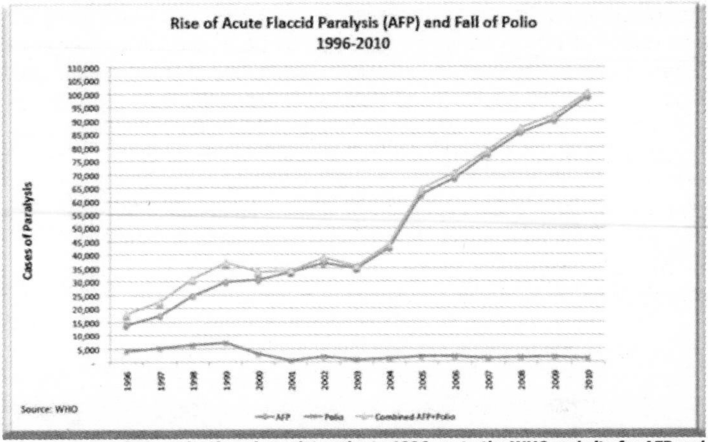

If you are wondering why there is no data prior to 1996, go to the WHO website for AFP and you will see that there is no data prior to 1996, and note that AFP continues to rise in 2011.

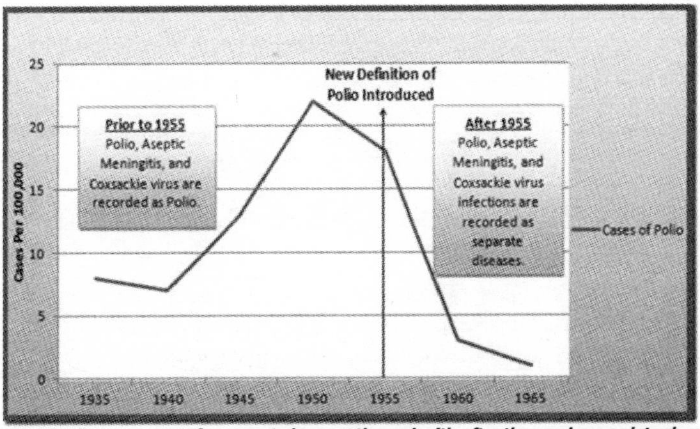

Cases of polio were more often reported as aseptic meningitis after the vaccine was introduced, skewing efficacy rates.

Source: The Los Angeles County Health Index: Morbidity and Mortality, Reportable Diseases.[99]

It was hoped that following polio eradication, immunisation could be stopped. However the synthesis of polio virus in 2002, made eradication impossible. It is argued that getting poor countries to expend their scarce resources on an impossible dream over the last 10 years was unethical. Furthermore, while India has been polio-free for a year, there has been a huge increase in non-polio acute flaccid paralysis (NPAFP). ***In 2011, there were an extra 47,500 new cases of NPAFP. Clinically indistinguishable from polio paralysis but twice as deadly, the incidence of NPAFP was directly proportional to doses of oral polio received.*** *Though this data was*

[99] http://www.vaccinationcouncil.org/2011/11/17/smoke-mirrors-and-the-disappearance-of-polio/

> *collected within the polio surveillance system, it was not investigated. The principle of primum-non-nocere was violated. The authors suggest that the huge bill of US $8 billion spent on the programme, is a small sum to pay if the world learns to be wary of such vertical programmes in the future.* [100]

Referring again the UK government polio eradication report we discover a **considerable failure of reporting.**

> *The rate of reporting of AFP in the UK study was lower than that from any country... undertaking such surveillance. The low UK AFP rates, along with the progressive decline of reporting through the study period, suggest that there has been considerable failure of reporting.* [101]

OK one or two silly mistakes can happen when you are trying to save the world and it was all a long time ago and things have now improved, obviously! Science makes things better, right? Otherwise it makes things worse because nothing stays the same and so there would be no point in having scientists.

Remember it's the fake horror story about millions dying of polio that they use to sell the entire vaccine programme on the back of. Since the polio vaccine was a disaster from the start nothing good could ever come from it.

Outbreaks of polio caused by cVDPVs (vaccine-derived polio viruses) have been reported across the world and are known to be able to mutate into deadlier entities. MSN News reported in 2009 that genetic analysis has proven such mutated viruses have caused at least seven separate outbreaks in Nigeria paralysing 124 children, and counting. [102]

- ***Most cVDPVs were recombinants of mutated poliovaccine strains and other unidentified enteroviruses. The co-circulation in children and genetic recombination of viruses... can lead to the generation of pathogenic recombinants, thus constituting an interesting model of viral evolution and emergence.*** [103]

- ***In Pakistan many non-polio enteroviruses have been isolated from AFP (Acute Flaccid Paralysis) cases but unfortunately, these cases were never being explored further either by the polio eradication programme or the country health care system****. As a result, no clear and detailed information about the epidemiology of NPEVs in the country is available except few reports.* ***Acute flaccid paralysis is a heterogeneous neurologic condition defined by the sudden onset of***

---

100 https://www.ncbi.nlm.nih.gov/pubmed/22591873

101 https://academic.oup.com/jid/article/175/Supplement_1/S156/878681

102 http://www.nbcnews.com/id/32418446/ns/health-infectious_diseases#.WlHhrLp2vlU

103 http://journals.plos.org/plospathogens/article?id=10.1371/journal.ppat.1000412

> ***weakness and floppiness in any part of the body in a child <15 years of age or paralysis in a person of any age in whom poliomyelitis is suspected. The predominant cause of AFP is infection with poliovirus.*** [104]

This is a recurring theme and may one day swamp us. Polio never needed this kind of pseudo-scientific meddling to start with yet it was all based on "good science", of the time according to the celebrated hero of vaccine intervention, Maurice Hilleman. It wasn't good science then and it hasn't evolved. Hilleman goes further in his Edward Shorter interview, even making a claim of responsibility for "importing AIDS". He reveals that "the Yellow Fever vaccine had leukaemia virus in it" and that all Merck's vaccines were contaminated. On AIDS, which is related to the SIV (Simian Immunodeficiency Virus), he says that was an accident. Phew!

This is all delivered very matter of fact and might sound like the ramblings of a madman, but only because that is how the truth is usually wrapped up. This dude is blowing a whistle. We just have to listen.

It wasn't until I actually had experience with a group of children who were totally unvaccinated that I started to see. I had never seen such healthy children. They did get whooping cough, they did get chicken pox, they had the normal childhood illnesses but they never required antibiotics, they were never sick for longer than 24 – 48 hours. They were brighter, smarter... ***It was like talking to aliens.*** *That was one of the things that got me to really start investigating further.*

Dr Suzanne Humphries

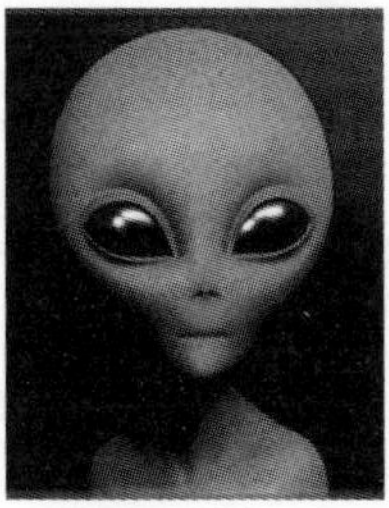

104 https://www.nature.com/articles/srep17456

You couldn't make it up

By altering the population's resistance to a particular organism, we alter the balance of infectious agents in the environment. The circulation of wild polio viruses 1-3 has declined through vaccination. However, this has left us open to the other 69 polio related viruses, which have thrived.

Dr William Campbell Douglas - Chronic Fatigue Syndrome: The Hidden Polio Epidemic

Monkey cancer in vaccines should be as far out there as it gets but what about that human foetal material? This is where the same scientific method has reached by 2017. Remember, when someone says "it's just a conspiracy theory" they either know all this and are covering it up or they are ignorant.

Varicella chickenpox has always been a mild irritation but has nevertheless been a target for the vaxers. And quite a success too, apparently. Should we celebrate? We no longer need to worry about a dose of the pox and the lifelong immunity associated with it. Instead, the quelling of this irritant has created a new problem in the form of shingles, which is caused by the same varicella virus. The older generations are no longer being naturally exposed to and therefore boosted safely and naturally by the suppressed chickenpox virus once common among us, so we are now more susceptible to shingles, which is a much more unpleasant experience. You'd think wouldn't you that the realisation of a disease made worse by vaccination would cause pause for thought, at least. And it did. And in that time they thought of an opportunity to sell another vaccine. The upgraded chickenpox vaccine that saved the kids from the pox is the zostavax shingles vaccine, to help the aged.

> *The Oka strain of the varicella-zoster virus (VZV) was isolated from fluid taken from the vesicles of a 3-year-old boy with a case of chicken pox.* ***The virus was isolated in primary human, embryonic lung cells (HEL) and was passaged 11 times. The strain was further passaged 12 times in guinea pig embryo fibroblasts (GPE) to attenuate the strain and once in human diploid cells (WI-38)*** *to passage 24.*

So far this vaccine virus (the bit you want) was brought to life through the remains of a 14 week old aborted male foetus (HEL - MRC-5) and passaged eleven times, then it went through guinea pig material twelve times, then through the extract of an aborted female foetus (WI-38) and was finally filtered through minced baby cow. It doesn't really matter why, does it? This of course sounds crazy but in the world of crazy this is actually for your benefit as they are trying in their naïve way to clean the bit you want in your vaccines and remove stuff you don't. It doesn't sound anything like a good idea to me and this scientific discussion paper on ema.europa.eu suggests as much:

> *Process-related impurities arising from the VZV vaccine bulk manufacturing processes are classified as cell-substrate or cell-culture derived.* ***Cell-substrate-derived impurities may include proteins derived from the host cell line; cell-culture-derived impurities may include antibiotics (e.g., neomycin), serum, or other media components.*** *VZV process*

> *uses cell growth medium containing bovine calf serum. Serum protein clearance is provided by rinsing the cell layers to* ***remove as much serum as possible*** *prior to virus harvest.* [105]

Alerting us to "other media components" in the vaccines, such as the SV range of cancer causing agents, is another big red flag.

When they talk of harvesting or isolating these viruses what they fail to mention is that the virus colony in question cannot be isolated from the medium in which it grew. You want the croutons you get the soup.

Once this is all blended with an assembly of equally unlikely ingredients such as hydrolysed pig gelatine and MSG (monosodium glutamate), it is then injected into test subjects and with an "immune response to vaccination demonstrated", the vaccine is good to go to market. This doesn't feel like good enough research. Surely if our immune system didn't respond to these unnatural invasions we would be dead? And the funny thing is, the vaccine manufacturers admit that in spite of all this **"there is no established correlation with vaccine efficacy"** and an immune reaction. Put another way, we don't go from vaccine to immune as a matter of course. Besides, efficacy is created against a set of rules in a controlled test whereas the vaccines are a real world experiment.

This funny business with the aborted human foetus in vaccines has to be a relative of cannibalism, has it not? Is there even a word to describe it? It certainly isn't vegan. Is this secret cousin of the Cannibal family something religious people are happy to associate with? Do vegetarians want it in their children? Calling all humans... Who is happy about this? Attorney Marc J. Bern, of Marc J. Bern & Partners LLP, says he has been inundated with "thousands of complaints" from the over 60's, who are central to the shingles vaccine campaign and have been feeling the early effects. The vaccine victims are reporting those post-vaccine 'events' we are hearing so much about and they want action. Don't we all! In a statement to FiercePharma.com, Bern said that the injuries

> *... run the gamut from* ***contracting shingles as a result of the vaccine*** *all the way to serious personal injuries such as blindness in one eye, individuals who have serious paralysis in their extremities, brain damage, all the way to death. Merck has failed terribly... to warn about the very serious side effects and the failure of the vaccine to do what they claim it does.*

No shit! But even that almost pales to insignificance when you dig a little deeper so let's do that. **The WI-38 cell line is "*a diploid human cell culture line composed of fibroblasts derived from lung tissue of an aborted white (Caucasian) female fetus*".** [106]

This female child-like product was 12 weeks.

---

105 http://www.ema.europa.eu/docs/en_GB/document_library/EPAR_-_Scientific_Discussion/human/000674/WC500053460.pdf

106 https://en.wikipedia.org/wiki/WI-38

The Coriell Institute for Medical Research tell us that the

> ***MRC-5 cell line was developed in September 1966 from lung tissue taken from a 14 week fetus aborted for psychiatric reason from a 27 year old physically healthy woman. The cell morphology is fibroblast-like.*** *The karyotype is 46, XY; normal diploid male.* [107]

See, delicious.

This means that every child injected with the chicken pox vaccine is also getting cellular material originally harvested from an aborted human foetus which was surgically removed from a mother who was a psychiatric patient. Added to which is the neurotoxin MSG and various animal DNA and blood by-products. But they won't get chicken pox. Well, that's not strictly true. They do.

The WI-38 / MRC-5 cell lines are used in all the following human vaccines:

Adenovirus/DTaP, IPV (polio) (Vero monkey kidney cells in the UK, also used to grow BoostrixIPV), Hib/Hep A, Hep A/Hep B, MMR (MMR-II), MMRV, Rabies, Varicella (chicken pox) and Zoster.

For more murk take a look into the murky world of the Vaccines and Related Biological Products Advisory Committee (VRBPAC). This is from their September 2012 meeting where we find them exploring this rather unlikely topic of

> *Cell Lines Derived from Human Tumors for Vaccine Manufacture*
>
> ***All of the new mammalian cell lines being considered are immortal, having been transformed by various oncogenes or are spontaneously immortalized, and some are derived from human tumors****. Over the last 20 years, it has been recognized that* ***cell lines derived from tumors may be the optimal and in some cases the only cell substrate that can be used to propagate certain vaccine viruses.***
>
> ***The CEM T-cell line established from cells from an individual with leukaemia... The A549 cell line established from cells excised from the lung of an individual with adenocarcinoma of the lung... The HeLa cell line was established from cells of a cervical carcinoma in 1952.*** *These cells contain approximately 50 copies of the HPV-18 genome. The HeLa cell line is permissive to many human viruses. HeLa cells have been engineered to be producer lines for adeno-associated virus... AAV has been used to produce investigational gene-therapy products and investigational vaccines.*

---

107 https://catalog.coriell.org/0/Sections/Search/Sample_Detail.aspx?Ref=AG05965-C&PgId=166

> ***Although the possibility of unknown oncogenic factors remains as a theoretical concern with cells derived from human tissues, current knowledge related to the mechanisms of oncogenesis supports the notion that it is highly improbable that any whole cell or complex of cellular factors from a tumor-derived cell will be present in sufficient quantities and lead to the development of tumors in the vaccine recipient.*** [108]

Supporting a notion is the same as agreeing with what someone else says. A notion is not a science, it's a belief. And just how many "oncogenic factors" does it take before cancer is diagnosed in this vague science? Isn't it a precious moment in the career of the oncologist, the day the patient dreams to hear the expert announce they "got it all"? The same cancer experts who carve out margins of flesh and take off limbs and warn of more cancer to come if **any** cancer cells remain? I jolly well think it is.

> *Current recommendations for testing of mammalian cell substrates and vaccines are generally based on three main safety concerns: the presence of residual, potentially tumorigenic, live cells in the vaccine; the presence of residual DNA from the cell substrate; and the potential presence of adventitious agents.*
>
> ***Furthermore, many tumor-derived cell lines*** *support infection and replication of a wide variety of viruses and therefore* ***may be more susceptible to infectious viruses present in the host... or through contaminated human or animal-derived reagents used during cell-line derivation and passage history. There may be additional concerns in the case of virus-like particles (VLPs) such as co-packaging of "unwanted" oncogenic RNAs or DNAs that may be transferred to the recipient by vaccination.***
>
> ***Emerging technologies that can detect both known and novel viruses have generated great interest and extensive discussions regarding the application of these methods for the evaluation of biological products. Although the advantages of these methods are recognized, currently they have not been recommended for use due to technical challenges that are being addressed. These challenges include standardization and validation, data analysis, interpretation, and storage, and development of follow-up strategies for investigation of a positive result.*** [108]

What we can take from this is that they have talked about it extensively at meetings like this and cannot overcome the fact there is not a hope in hell of protecting the population from these needle delivered death viruses. They failed to kill the simian viruses in the 1950's and they are using the same methods today!

---

[108] http://whale.to/v/FDA%20Briefing%20Document%20Sept%2019,2012.pdf

> ***Small amounts of residual cell substrate DNA unavoidably occur in all viral vaccines as well as other biologics produced using cell substrates. There are several potential ways DNA could be a risk factor. DNA can be oncogenic*** *or infectious; in addition,* ***it can cause insertion mutagenesis through integration into the host genome. A major concern about residual cell-substrate DNA has been the potential for the induction of cancer, particularly if the DNA was from a tumorigenic cell or from a cell line established from a human cancer.***
>
> ***Although there were no standardized assays to test for oncogenic activity of DNA, the Committee agreed that cell DNA and lysates should be evaluated in three newborn rodent species. The species were newborn nude mice, newborn hamsters, and newborn rats.*** [108]

This is standard operating procedure: carry on regardless, design some animal studies to fudge and then at least reality can be shrouded in repetition of how rigorously the product has been tested on animals. That's always reassuring for the public, somehow comforting to know. And for the scientists to feel proud that science can test stuff and can generate data. You can do an awful lot with data.

> *These species were selected based on their broad sensitivity to oncogenic viruses. The recommendations were to administer by the subcutaneous route in the three newborn species... Animals should be monitored for more than four months, and any tumors would need to be assessed for their species of origin to determine whether they arose spontaneously or were induced by the test article.*

This is good science! And then what happens?

> *The oncogenic and infectious risk of residual DNA in vaccines can be* ***reduced*** *by the implementation of manufacturing steps designed to* ***lower the amount of DNA, decrease*** *the size of the DNA,* ***and/or*** *to* ***reduce the activity of residual DNA by chemical treatment or gamma irradiation.*** [108]

Feel safe yet? And, just in case all those risk 'reductions' make them look soft, we find the piece de resistance of this committee's work as almost a footnote. Referring to the deliberations of a 1997 World Health Organisation Study Group they conclude:

> *The value of 100 pg of host cell DNA vaccine dose remained the* ***recommended standard*** *for a decade. However, the issue was revisited in 1997 for several reasons.* ***First, vaccine manufacturers could not always meet this level of residual cell-substrate DNA for some viral vaccines****, such as with certain enveloped viruses.* ***Second, more information was available as to the oncogenic events in human cancers****, where it has been established that multiple events, both genetic and epigenetic, are required. And third, for continuous non-tumorigenic cell*

> *lines such as Vero, the major cell substrate that was being considered at the time, the presence of activated dominant oncogenes in these cells was* ***unlikely****. The outcome of the 1997 WHO meeting was that* ***the amount of residual cell-substrate DNA allowed per dose in a vaccine produced in a continuous cell line and administered by [needle] was raised from 100 pg to 10 ng****.* [108]

That's a massive hike up from 100pg to 10,000pg.

Is "unlikely" similar to possible or more like maybe? It's settled then: no risk in using human cancer cells in human vaccines! Good old science. We may observe also how all this new information regarding a greater understanding of "oncogenic events in human cancers" (how cancer develops), has not led to less cancer or better treatment but instead benefits the drug companies who are excused yet another bothersome safety study! With that, and the kids left to mop up the mess with a **9900% increase** in cancer causing viruses left swilling around in their vaccines, this is everything a breakthrough in cancer is not meant to be!

You want to laugh but it doesn't feel right because it isn't really that funny.

Continuous cell lines are also known as immortalised. They are seed stock from a long time ago from which the same standardized viruses can be grown in theory for ever thus ensuring some stability in the vaccine batches. The thing about cancer cells is that they immortalise and continue to replicate in the same way. So what is the difference between continuous, cancerous and immortal cells? Probably more than we will ever understand but not enough to make any of them safe to be injected into OAP's and puppies. So the bit we want in the vaccines is not just brewed in a manner we may find a little bit creepy, but it also causes cancer. These supercharged growth mediums help to keep manufacturing costs down. In their ideal world the vaccine pharma will be able to shift from needing tens of millions of birds' eggs each flu season (each flu vaccine requiring between one and two chicken embryos) or large isolation tanks bursting with kidneys, to a Petri dish of hyperactive cancer cells reproducing themselves like crazy. [109]

Flu vaccines, measles and the new improved polio vaccine among others are created in these ancient animal cell lines, such as the Vero from African green monkeys harvested in 1962 and MDCK line which is what became of a Cocker Spaniel in 1958.

At an earlier murky meeting of the vaccine fanatics, they discussed the cancer causing nature of animal cell lines in human vaccines.

> *It has been important to note that this cell line* ***[MDCK] is a neoplastic cell line or a continuous cell line and we do not currently understand how these cell lines become neoplastic. There is a concern that***

108 http://whale.to/v/FDA%20Briefing%20Document%20Sept%2019,2012.pdf

109 https://www.google.co.uk/patents/US5753489

> ***intact cells may find their way into the final product and lead to tumor formation. The presence of residual cellular DNA is also a concern due to the potential presence of oncogenes****, which could confer the transformed phenotype or the possibility of infectious genomes also being present.* ***Our regulatory approach for addressing such concerns has been to limit the amount of DNA in the final product and to reduce its biological activity... or... to reduce the size the DNA fragments.*** [110]

According to Dr Kemble who presented at the same meeting on behalf of his employers at MedImmune (AstraZeneca) the makers of Flumist, one dose of their vaccine contains "less than a nanogram of MDCK DNA". He goes on to assure the meeting that this is OK since WHO guidance allows for 10 times that amount. Or so...

> *The* ***median*** *size of that DNA is* ***approximately*** *450 base pairs and we really* ***cannot detect much*** *above that but* ***when we try and quantitate*** *these gels* ***what we can claim*** *is that 90 per cent of the DNA is* ***less than*** *1000 base pairs.*

That sounds like much more doggy DNA than should be inside anyone but the sacrificial dog!

Dr Peden closes the meeting with an honest acknowledgement: **"I think in conclusion... we can say the DNA appears to be more of an oncogenic risk than we reported or even realised"**. [111]

I happen to agree! But David Mott, president and CEO at MedImmune was unmoved by the trivia, he described Flumist as "the product of choice, particularly for children", but then he would, wouldn't he.

It's a constant fight when you have a vaccine-injured child. It's not just the disability, it's the ignorance. The hatred from the medical community towards families like ours is intense.

Jillian Moller mother of induced autistic Emily. One of the 'lucky' ones, finally awarded compensation for damage done. [112]

---

110 Biological Product Advisory Committee. Transcript of Meeting, Sept 25 2008. Timothy Nelle: http://wayback.archive-it.org/7993/20170404043202/https://www.fda.gov/ohrms/dockets/ac/08/transcripts/2008-4384T1_1.htm

111 Dr Peden: http://wayback.archive-it.org/7993/20170404043209/https://www.fda.gov/ohrms/dockets/ac/08/transcripts/2008-4384T1_2.htm

112 https://www.huffingtonpost.com/david-kirby/post2468343_b_2468343.html

Eye of newt, and toe of frog, wool of bat, and tongue of dog

Beyond containing polysorbate 80 and cancer and other viruses, and likely mycoplasma, the Gardasil vaccines are contaminated in an additional way. It and all the new vaccines are contaminated with genetically engineered DNA. It can contaminate people's DNA, just as genetically engineered crops can contaminate normal crops. Gardasil itself is contaminated with a man-made version of the HPV DNA, the very virus it was supposed to protect against, which now it threatens not only altering kids' healthy DNA with synthetic DNA (!) but with a diseased version. [113]

In addition to the cancer viruses and foetal DNA there are other ingredients we are invited to consent to in this medical contract and so should bring a few into our investigation.

1969 medium supplemented with calf serum

Aluminium hydroxide/phosphate - highly neurotoxic. This ingredient is added with a view to forcing an immune reaction. Aluminium has an affinity for phosphorous which is found in abundance in the myelin sheath of the brain and cell membranes. Bonding to and dislodging this protective coating causes inflammation and irritation and allows the aluminium to accumulate and is a suspect in neurological illness such as Alzheimer's.
Amorphous aluminium

Amino glycoside
Ammonium sulfate
Amphotericin B – antifungal.
Baculovirus and Spodoptera frugiperda cell proteins
Beta-propiolactone

Bovine foetal/calf serum/albumin - Here we can reflect upon the rise of Bovine Spongiform Encephalopathy or 'mad cow disease' as they dubbed it to deflect some attention, more like mad scientist disease if you ask me. Feed dead cows back to their brethren, chop them up cook them and feed them to the children! Safe as houses they told us against all our instincts and then came the human variant Creutzfeldt-Jakob disease (vCJD). Another creation of the medical experts! These institutional inmates and their MrDrPhD straightjackets are chasing shadows of their own creation and bouncing into their own limitations with this meddling. As such it later dawned on the boffins that they hadn't just messed up with the meat science, but by brewing up vaccines in dead cows the vaccine science might have some holes in it too. At just such a gathering in 2001, this time of the Joint Committee Vaccination and Immunisation (JCVI), they talked about another highly unlikely topic:

---

113 http://salem-news.com/articles/november292011/vaccines-contaminated-se.php

Ruminant and Human Materials in Vaccine Manufacture.

> ***The Committee asked by which date the vaccines already distributed would no longer include any whose production process may have involved the use of potentially BSE infected Category 1 or 2 material.*** *The Committee was told that a* ***Category 1 material was only used at the master seed/working seed stage of the manufacture of a very few vaccines****, not in routine vaccine production itself. Master seed material* ***often*** *antedates the BSE epidemic in the UK, and was diluted many fold to the extent that any* ***exposure to infected material****, if ever present,* ***would be remote.*** [114]

Chicken fibroblasts - the potential for inter-species activation of unknown retroviruses is multiplied significantly with each foreign protein added.

CTAB (cetyltrimethylammonium bromide)

Betapropiolactone

DL-alpha-tocopherol (vitamin E) derived from soya bean oil. Like every other ingredient DL - alpha-tocopherol is experimental in human vaccines. There is no safety data and minimum toxic dose has not been established either orally or directly into the blood. This is a man made dietary supplement used as an antioxidant in fats and oils and in animal feed, it is also used as experimental medication. It is in the top 3 most frequent allergens in sunscreens. The processes of making vitamin E artificially uses a chemical called trimethylhydroquinone.

> *This is one of the biggest problems that the Cosmetics Database has with... vitamin E, because the finished products can contain traces of hydroquinone. Hydroquinone is in a class of chemicals called aromatic organic compounds. This means not just that it's aromatic in the sense of it being fragrant, but it contains a benzene ring. I view most compounds with simple benzene rings with caution for their possible xenoestrogenic effects. Animal studies have found hydroquinone to alter immune function and to increase the incidence of renal tubule cell tumors and leukemia in F344 rats.* [115]

And in the test tube too.

> *But the relevance to humans is uncertain. Quantitatively, however, the use of hydroquinone in cosmetics is unlikely to result in renal neoplasia through this mode of action. Thus,* ***hydroquinone is safe*** *at concentrations of ≤1%* ***in hair dyes and is safe for use in nail adhesives.*** *Hydroquinone should not be used in other leave-on cosmetics.* [116] Or vaccines?

The same element spelt D-alpha tocopherol is the natural original vitamin E.

---

114 http://parentsandcarersagainstinjustice.weebly.com/uploads/2/5/2/8/25284293/04_jcvi_meeting_04th_may_2001.pdf

115 http://chemicaloftheday.squarespace.com/qa/2011/4/26/tocopherol-vs-tocopheryl-acetate.html

116 https://www.ncbi.nlm.nih.gov/pubmed/21164074

Formaldehyde/formalin - preserves dead bodies. Supposed to neutralise those unwanted viruses in the vaccine growth medium, such as SV40, but it doesn't. It is suggested that formaldehyde in fact locks in the viruses by temporarily hardening the outer protein layer. Formaldehyde is listed by the US National Toxicology Program as a known human carcinogen.

Gelatine - is a mixture of peptides and proteins and who knows what produced by partial hydrolysis of collagen extracted from the skin, tendons, ligaments and bones of meat animals. Known to cause anaphylaxis via vaccines.

Glutaraldehyde - is toxic, is a powerful sterilant and irritant. It is used for the inactivation of bacterial toxins to create toxoid vaccines such as pertussis toxoid component in the Boostrix DTap vaccine and ProteqFlu used on horses. Glutaraldehyde is sometimes used for the tanning of leather and for embalming. [117]

Human diploid cells - originating from aborted human foetal tissue.

Hydrolysed porcine gelatine

Madin Darby Canine Kidney (**MDCK**) - a continuous kidney cell line from a female Cocker Spaniel.

Modified Mueller's growth medium
Modified Mueller and Miller medium -

> *Involves the use of a variant and somewhat unstable strain of Clostridium Tetani and a culture medium containing a pancreatic digest of casein, cystine and tyrosine, beef heart infusion, glucose and inorganic salts and a high concentration of iron. Casein is a milk protein. "Pancreatic digest" means that enzymes from the pancreas of an animal are used to break down the soup so the tetanus bacterium can eat it.* [118]

Monosodium glutamate (MSG) - this ingredient when eaten causes neurons to become over excited and burn out. So unwanted as a food item that they have to sneak it into us as a 'flavour enhancer' and a heap of other cover names, but maybe it's safe in vaccines?

MRC-5 - is a continuous cell line from lung tissue taken from a 14-week aborted white male human foetus.

Octoxynol-10 (TRITON X-100) - is a detergent. Mutagenic and carcinogenic.

Peanut oil (emulsified) – aka Adjuvant 65, patented by Merck & Co., Inc. in 1964. If the point of the vaccine mixture is to force the immune system to respond with

---

117 https://en.wikipedia.org/wiki/Glutaraldehyde

118 http://pamfa.org/index.php/modified-mueller/

antibodies to the enclosed antigen, is it not conceivable that a similar immune reaction could occur each time the immune system is rechallenged with peanut and therefore cause peanut allergies?

PER C6 - is another human cell line. This foetus made 18 weeks before being put to work. The vaccine virus grows in the retinas of the deceased. Dr Alex Van Der, the scientist who developed this product observed of the Frankenstein technology:

> *In all the cases, it is quite clear aborted babies might have been healthy, with no life-threatening condition or other medically indicated reasons to abort them. But is the abortion morally right or the use of the tissue cell lines?*

Phenol red indicator
Phenoxyethanol - antifreeze.
Potassium diphosphate
Potassium monophosphate

Polymyxin B antibiotic, side effects include neurotoxicity.

Polysorbate 20
Polysorbate 80 (Tween 80) - best known for its use alongside chemotherapy for brain cancer treatment due to its ability to cross through the blood/brain barrier. Its purpose in vaccines, anyone's guess! To take viruses and aluminium and mercury to the brain and to the foetus? Why not!

Porcine (pig) pancreatic hydrolysate of casein

Poultry embryo/eggs/proteins -

> *Fertilised chicken eggs are susceptible to a wide variety of viruses.* ***All the egg based vaccines are contaminated****... influenza measles mumps yellow fever and smallpox vaccines. As well as the vaccine for horses against encephalomyelitis virus.* [119]

Recombinant human albumin

Semi synthetic media
Sodium phosphate-buffered isotonic sodium chloride
Sorbitol

Soy peptone broth - soy allergies anyone?

---

119 Dr Andrew Lewis head of DNA Virus laboratory in the Division of Viral Products, to the Vaccine and Related Biological Products Committee. Transcript of meeting 19 Nov 1988 (Page 19: The Vaccine Papers, Janine Roberts)

Squalene - an oil based adjuvant believed to be linked to the widespread devastation caused to military personnel by the Gulf War Syndrome group of doctor induced diseases.

Sucrose

Thimerosal/Thiomersal - (is the brand name, mercury is around 50% by weight of the product) gets a lot of attention as the mutagenic mercury based vaccine preservative/adjuvant made of the most neurotoxic element on earth after radiation and it causes alterations in DNA. Keep well out of reach of small children and animals if you ask me. And I'm not alone and our concerns are well understood and well founded. But check this out. According to nhs.uk in August 2017:

> *Thiomersal is no longer used in any of the vaccines **routinely** given to **babies and young children** in the NHS childhood immunisation programme.*

Sounds good, like some kind of progress. They clearly understand that mercury shouldn't be given in a needle, but what's always the first priority once a product or idea has been sold to the public and is profitable? Not safety, that's the bottom of the list. The illusion is most important and this is classic. When all else fails they fall back on there being only 'trace amounts' found in the vaccines, which they define as 1mcg, as if a little is somehow OK!

But if we trace this story back a little we find the full story has not been told. You know when someone over-talks to cover up for something or make it sound plausible? Well for me there were a few too many words in that NHS statement and we will shortly see why it matters. Anyway, why is it important to announce that mercury is no longer in some vaccines? Was it not thoroughly tested in a whole battery of ever complex science experiments and found to be absolutely essential, safe and beneficial for babies? If not, why was it injected into them in the first place? Why is the developing world being flooded with hundreds of millions of mercury laced vaccines that the UK establishment want to pretend they are protecting our children from? We are going to investigate.

Tri(n)butylphosphate - is a kidney and nerve poison

Urea

Vero cells - are a continuous line of kidney cells from an African green monkey harvested in 1962. This is a replacement or alternative polio vaccine virus growth medium. Replacing SV40 with what?

Washed sheep red blood cells

WI-38 - continuous lung fibroblast cell line from an aborted human female.

Yeast protein - yeast, wheat, gluten allergies?

- *Saccharomyces cerevisiae is best known as the baker's and brewer's yeast, but its residual traces are also frequent excipients in some vaccines. Although anti-S. cerevisiae autoantibodies (ASCAs) are considered specific for Crohn's disease, a growing number of studies have detected high levels of ASCAs in patients affected with autoimmune diseases as compared with healthy controls, including antiphospholipid syndrome, systemic lupus erythematosus, type 1 diabetes mellitus, and rheumatoid arthritis.* [120]

We hear it said that dairy allergies may be common because the human body hasn't adapted to digest the breast milk of another animal, and there may be something in that as it is rather an unnatural behaviour. But allergies go way beyond dairy and now increasingly even include fruit. Fruit! What if the human body is generating defences toward food ingredients increasingly the cause of allergic reactions because of their presence in vaccines? There is no evidence to the contrary. Sensitivity follows injection into the blood of intact foreign protein, a well known trigger for an allergic reaction in all species. Follow it later by eating the same molecules in a food and you have the perfect ingredients for a reaction that may be fatal or subtle, or both.

Delayed-type hypersensitivity (DTH) is an immune response to an invader also known as a cell-mediated immune response, produced when sensitised T cells attack foreign antigens and secrete lymphokines that initiate a secondary humoral immune response. Also called cellular hypersensitivity reaction or a delayed hypersensitivity reaction. It's good or not so good largely depending on whether there's a vaccine involved in the raid.

The vaccines contain ingredients such as aluminium that force an immune attack on the antigen, if peanut oil is embedded in the mix any time during manufacture the body will consider that an enemy combatant too and attack it. Literally **any** variety of oils may be present in **any** vaccine or **any** other food proteins and in **any** combination. There are no rules. The oils they use may be any vegetable, nut, seed, fish or animal or synthetic and do not have to appear on the package insert, yet allergies can kill. So reckless and inconsiderate are these people that peanut oil is a common ingredient in vaccine adjuvants. Allergies don't sound like much but are a life changing side effects and for those affected every meal carries a serious danger. Vaccines are very unstable with batches and even vials varying in potency and values and inducing varying effects. Barbara Feick Gregory has compiled a list of all the known vaccine ingredients including life giving essentials such as mussels, emu oil, chicken fat oil, bananas, kiwi, lard oil… [121]

---

120 https://www.ncbi.nlm.nih.gov/pubmed/23292495

121 http://barbfeick.com/vaccinations/allergy/951-vaccine_allergy.htm

Aside from soya and milk casein and pork gelatine, calf serum causes beef allergy, chick embryo cell culture has been known to cause egg allergy, Chinese Restaurant Syndrome is a monosodium glutamate allergy and neomycin also causes allergies.

Latex is a natural rubber that some have become allergic to since the rise of latex stoppered vaccines. Latex (NRL) is in the vial stoppers of many vaccines and sometimes the tiny particles can be seen floating in multi-dose vaccine liquid.

> *We hypothesize that **immune reactions triggered by close contact with NRL** might influence the functions of B lymphocytes by altering expression of certain proteins identified in our experiments **thus contributing to the occurrence of autism**.* [122]

Overlapping with a latex allergy we can find tropical fruit allergies such as avocado, banana, kiwi, papaya, peach or nectarine. Alice was found have all these and more and since she was weak, premature and jaundice and fully vaccinated as a child with multiple doses of MMR, DTP and polio etc before she was one year old this is no surprise. In fact when you go through some of the vaccine patent applications, it soon becomes clear that every recorded allergy could be traced to vaccines.

This vaccine adjuvant patent for example claims a method for increasing antibody production in response to vaccine administration:

> *Suitable pharmaceutically acceptable carriers include, but are not limited to, water, salt solutions, alcohols, gum arabic, **vegetable oils** (e.g., corn oil, cottonseed oil, peanut oil, olive oil, coconut oil), fish liver oils, oily esters such as Polysorbate 80, polyethylene glycols, gelatine, **carbohydrates** (e.g., lactose, amylose or starch), **foods**, magnesium stearate, talc, silicic acid, viscous paraffin, fatty acid monoglycerides and diglycerides, pentaerythritol fatty acid esters, hydroxy methylcellulose, polyvinyl pyrrolidone, **etc**.* [123]

Anything goes - into the blood - and no safety studies! Of course the vaxer's solution to all this is not to say *Whoa hos! This has gone far enough,* and stop. Rather, as is quite normal, they instead see an opportunity to open up the market some more.

> *A team led by a researcher at the Stanford University School of Medicine has developed vaccines that vastly reduce or eliminate dogs' allergic reactions to three major **food** allergens: peanuts, milk and wheat. The vaccines' benefits lasted at least three months.* [124]

This is progress, for some. None of the previous range of vaccines has required 4 doses per year! And this vaccine is just for three of the allergies they have created and there are loads more of them to chase, increasing with every new vaccine!

---

[122] https://www.ncbi.nlm.nih.gov/pubmed/20957522

[123] http://www.freepatentsonline.com/5569457.pdf

[124] https://news.stanford.edu/news/2004/november17/med-vaccine-1117.html

The vaccines will apparently provide new hope for the millions of us who now suffer from food allergies.

> *"Food allergy is* ***an important problem*** *for which there is no good treatment", said some PhD.* ***"Developing a cure for this growing problem will help millions of people and save lives"****.*

Helping people and saving lives, now there's an idea.

In this poser on sciencedirect, 'Food allergy: Past, present and future' they tell us,

> *Severe food-allergic reactions were rare 35 years ago, but now represent the single leading cause of anaphylaxis treated in American emergency departments, and data from the USA and Australia indicate that there has been a marked increase in hospitalizations due to food allergy in the past two decades. The reason for this rapid rise in food allergy among industrialized countries around the world* ***remains an open question.*** [125]

Of course it does. In trying to answer this puzzler the quacks have come up with a cracking theory! In this not only are the victims inevitably to blame, but so desperate to point the finger even the vaccines come under friendly fire!

> *According to one study these* ***allergies' prevalence in children doubled from 1997 to 2001. The so-called "hygiene hypothesis" attributed this escalation to too much cleanliness in modern life****.* ***Under this theory, infections are critical to help protect people from allergies.*** [126]

Infections are critical to strengthen us but the purpose of all these vaccines is to prevent infections!

I need to lie down.

Rare in 1980... doubling in 1997... Hmmm... what was going on around then? Can't think of anything. Although washing machine sales did go up, so did shampoo so maybe they're right. We are too clean! I know, what's needed is a vaccine so we don't need to wash. A daily injection! Boom! That's what they're working towards next! Then maybe 'the multi-vit multi-hit nutrient special' - *all you need for you and your family to live for as long as you may live. Save time eating, food shopping and cooking: let us inject you once a day to set you free, to work more.*

No error is fully confuted until you have seen not only that it is an error, but also how it became one.
Thomas Carlyle (1795 -1881)

---

[125] https://www.sciencedirect.com/science/article/pii/S1323893016301137

[126] https://news.stanford.edu/news/2004/november17/med-vaccine-1117.html

Atchoose not to

Doctors put drugs of which they know little into bodies of which they know less for diseases of which they know nothing at all.
Voltaire (1694 – 1778)

Given how shoddy the safety testing of vaccines are generally, is it any wonder that the notion that anyone really understands the potential impact of theses pick and mix potions sounds complete and utter bonkers? It's hard to know where to start. And stop. Let's do the mercury. This has attracted some attention but clearly not enough. Enough to keep it low key but not enough to deter them.

For those who still trust in the integrity of the medical profession and understand the danger of mercury in any form in the human body then that medical reassurance via the NHS about no mercury in the kiddie's needles may offer some comfort, but being suspicious of character I decided to pull up some vaccine data and see for myself. And I didn't have to go far to confirm my suspicions. On the European Medicines Agency website we can find the product information for the latest flu vaccine, Adjupanrix. This is the upgraded Pandemrix H5N1. It's a similar product with a slightly different viral antigen and it will be unleashed on the unsuspecting public as soon as the WHO gives the go ahead. The viral antigen they use will not be the same as the wild version circulating through communities in the coming flu season since the flu virus doesn't send its DNA profile ahead of arrival for a colony to be brewed up ready for the vaccine. The ortho-docs are chasing a virus around with no hope of keeping up with its evolution, but that almost becomes funny when you consider the rest of the story.

The flu vaccine is brewed up in contaminated birds' eggs and it contains 5 micrograms of thiomersal. So the UK establishment isn't really lying just not disclosing the full truth. And unfortunately, that really matters. In this NHS statement there is much more under the surface than on it. On the face of it this removal of thiomersal from vaccines "routinely" given to babies and young children is a tacit acknowledgement of a grave wrong done that must be addressed. But without announcing it what the ortho-docs were covertly doing by 2017 was experimenting on two humans at once by injecting mercury via pregnant mothers **directly into the unborn child**.

It's worth noting that if you are pregnant and you timed it wrong you could be talked into two winter season flu shots, plus the Boostrix-IPV (DTaP(polio) with its aluminium hydroxide and aluminium phosphate and propagated in Vero monkey kidney cells, which all taken together makes for a heady mix of stuff building up in your baby. And remember they are targeting this flu vaccine at expectant mothers from 16 weeks intending them to pass immunity to their baby in the womb, because mums do that, which is why we try to do the right things when pregnant and when breastfeeding. I say we.

Most important of all to remember in all of this is that "**Individuals for whom no valid consent has been received" cannot be vaccinated**. So, those who want them say "yes please" and those who don't say no. Or nothing at all. The beauty of free choice!

> *The scientific evidence that... thimerosal cause(s) reproductive toxicity is clear and voluminous. Thimerosal dissociates in the body to ethyl mercury. The evidence for its reproductive toxicity includes severe mental retardation or malformations in human offspring who were poisoned when their mothers were exposed to ethyl mercury or thimerosal while pregnant.* [127]

Bear in mind also that research on mercury toxicity usually relates to oral ingestion of methylmercury, in seafood for example, and not intramuscular uptake of the ethylmercury that bypasses the majority of our natural gut-based defences. And as no safe "reference dose" (RfD) has been established for the mercury they inject through the skin in vaccines we may conclude this to be a reckless venture.

So if a doctor or nurse or chemist fails to **fully** inform the patient of the real disease risk of not vaccinating, **and** the risk of injecting known poisons, **and** of the alternatives to this illegitimate medical intervention, then there is no informed consent. This is even more serious than an incorrect diagnosis or wrong prescription. Informed consent is a critical factor in the contract between health practitioner and patient and forms the foundation of civilisation. They got quite agitated about this kind of thing at Nuremberg and set out to instil an ethical code back into humanity. But whatever others might say and think it is our responsibility to enforce boundaries around ourselves and our children from which all predators are repelled.

On 12 March 2015, the London Supreme Court delivered arguably the most significant decision in the field of medical negligence for a generation, ruling that:

> *The doctor is... under a duty to take reasonable care to ensure that the patient is aware of any material risks involved in any recommended treatment, and of any reasonable alternative or variant treatments. The test of materiality is whether, in the circumstances of the particular case, a reasonable person in the patient's position would be likely to attach significance to the risk, or the doctor is or should reasonably be aware that the particular patient would be likely to attach significance to it.* [128]

By allowing the appeal in this case, rather than adjudicate retrospectively on a legal point the Supreme Court is reaffirming the General Medical Council (GMC) existing guidance on consent to medical treatment. Doctors must fully advise patients of the options for treatment, the risks of each option and the benefits. It is then for the patient, not the doctor, to decide whether to participate or not.

---

127 https://oehha.ca.gov/media/downloads/crnr/hgbayer1.pdf

128 https://www.supremecourt.uk/cases/docs/uksc-2013-0136-judgment.pdf

The patient-focused test, as it has been called, corrects the notion of a relationship between the patient and the doctor as one of medical paternalism. This is not about them and us, this is about us and them. What we have is a relationship where the patient is treated as an adult capable of deciphering the facts, all the facts, before making a decision the patient may pay a heavy price for.

Fully informed means you should be aware that the flu vaccine also contains the AS03 adjuvant which is composed of squalene, dl-α-tocopherol and polysorbate 80. Aside the contaminated poultry proteins, cancer causing formaldehyde, mercury and the mutagenic carcinogen octoxynol 10, there's a whole mess of other crap in there I won't list but you can see for yourself in the data. Meanwhile we probably have enough to be getting on with. [129]

This snippet from the Adjupanrix vaccine safety data gives a hint of how they've streamlined the testing criteria:

> *Epidemiological* ***studies relating to another AS03-adjuvanted vaccine (Pandemrix H1N1****, also manufactured in the same facility as Adjupanrix), in several European countries* ***have indicated an increased risk of narcolepsy*** *with or without cataplexy* ***in vaccinated*** *as compared with unvaccinated* ***individuals****... These data suggest that the excess risk tends to decline with increasing age at vaccination.* ***There is currently no evidence to indicate that Adjupanrix may be associated with a risk of narcolepsy.***

Well isn't that odd! Are we referring to Adjupanrix or are we not? I don't like it when science is all unscientific. Pick and mix data for pick and mix potions! There can't be any epidemiological date on Adjupanrix because they haven't exposed people to it yet! So we don't know then if the vaccine they want us to have in the next flu season increases some risk of a neurological condition or not. Eek! So that means it isn't safe, right? But is it dangerous?

> *Caution is needed when administering this vaccine to persons with a known hypersensitivity (other than anaphylactic reaction) to the active substance, to any of the excipients listed... to thiomersal and to residues (egg and chicken protein, ovalbumin, formaldehyde, gentamicin sulphate and sodium deoxycholate).*
>
> *However, in a pandemic situation, it may be appropriate to give the vaccine, provided that facilities for resuscitation are immediately available in case of need.*

You might want to revisit that list of ingredients before agreeing to this one! They often enquire about our allergies, but have you had squalene injected before? What about the unborn children of pregnant victims of these concoctions? How is it

---

129 http://www.americanpharmaceuticalreview.com/Featured-Articles/117498-Potential-Mycoplasma-Contaminants-Inactivation-during-Production-of-Inactivated-Egg-Based-Viral-Vaccines/

rational to curse expectant mothers for one glass of wine **and** for questioning vaccines? I say we, I am not judging anyone, I don't think either is a good idea but in my minds eye I see the wine as the safer of the two.

Very common effects according to the vaccine maker include: headache, fever, fatigue, arthralgia, myalgia, induration, swelling, pain and redness at the injection site. Common effects include: lymphadenopathy, ecchymosis at the injection site, sweating, increased shivering and "***influenza like illness***".

Is that like the flu?

And lest we forget that the car we just bought with three wheels, no gears and the wrong fuel, might not work:

> ***As with all vaccines, Adjupanrix may not fully protect all persons who are vaccinated***.

Even that isn't the whole truth. After analysing 116 studies involving several millions of people comparing the flu vaccine to placebo (whatever that might be) or no intervention at all, the Cochrane Library revealed over 70% vaccine failure rate. Taking into account the widespread use of fake placebo trials this is an extremely generous calculation.[130]

So, according to the official data recipients are test subjects who may be given a flu-like illness or something much worse and most likely won't be protected from the flu. Not looking like a bargain at any cost! But what of the original guinea pigs, the ever present essentials of this bargain basement technology, did we gain anything from their sacrifice?

> *The ability to induce protection against... [some flu] vaccine strains was assessed non-clinically using ferret challenge models. In each experiment, four groups of six ferrets were immunised intramuscularly with an AS03 adjuvanted vaccine...*
>
> *Control groups included ferrets immunized with adjuvant alone, non-adjuvanted vaccine or phosphate buffered saline solution. Ferrets were vaccinated on days 0 and 21 and challenged by the intra-tracheal route on day 49 with a lethal dose of [the viruses].*
>
> *Of the animals receiving adjuvanted vaccine... [between] 87% and 96% were protected against the lethal challenge... Viral shedding into the upper respiratory tract was also* ***reduced*** *in vaccinated animals relative to controls,* ***suggesting a reduced risk of viral transmission.***
>
> *In the unadjuvanted control group, as well as in the adjuvant control group, all animals died or had to be euthanized as they were moribund, three to four days after the start of challenge.*

---

130 http://www.cochrane.org/CD001269/ARI_vaccines-to-prevent-influenza-in-healthy-adults

> *This medicinal product has been authorised under 'exceptional circumstances'. This means that for scientific reasons it has not been possible to obtain complete information on this medicinal product.* [131]

The mind boggles. It worked in the lab animals that were vaccinated with the relevant virus but this is not how it works in the real world in humans since no one knows what the virus will be!

Maybe squalene is the life saving ingredient that brings all the nasties together in a kind of vaccine Happy Meal that's good for everyone? Let's see.

The 'Final Report on the Safety Assessment of Squalane and Squalene' in the International Journal of Toxicology in 2014:

> *It is concluded that both Squalane and Squalene are safe **as cosmetic ingredients** in the present practices of use and concentration.* [132]

Hmmm. You find that a lot. There's no mention of vaccines anywhere in this settled science; no reference to the safety of injecting it **into** pregnant ladies, fluffy kittens, children or the elderly.

This oil adjuvant many believe is the culprit in the physical demise of hundreds of thousands of healthy military personnel who were forced under threat of court martial to take experimental vaccines during the 1991 Gulf War. Batches were made with squalene at the time when it was still officially classified deadly and unapproved for use in humans or animals. But times have changed. Remember the hypothesis about a toxic substance best not injected? This is a classic case of not paying attention! Is it at all conceivable that this hypothesis about once a toxin always a toxin could be disproven in the space of so few years with squalene now detoxified and rendered safe to be added in to vaccines? Unlikely, I know, but it's the kind of claim they make.

Many experiments with animals show that squalene and aluminium in vaccines cause autoimmune disease and kill brain cells. Investigative journalist Gary Matsumoto writes in 'Vaccine A -The Covert Government Experiment That's Killing our Soldiers and Why GI's are Only the First Victims'

> ... ***when an oil is injected, the immune system responds to it not only specifically, but with heightened intensity because the oil adjuvant resembles so closely the natural oils found in the body.*** *A 'cross reaction' then happens, sending the immune system into chaos destroying any oils found anywhere in the body that resemble the adjuvant oil. Demyelinating diseases like multiple sclerosis are an example of this destructive autoimmune process.*

---

[131] http://www.ema.europa.eu/docs/en_GB/document_library/EPAR_-_Product_Information/human/001206/WC500049544.pdf

[132] http://www.beauty-review.nl/wp-content/uploads/2014/08/Final-Report-on-the-Safety-Assessment-of-Squalane-and-Squalene.pdf

Wow! Matsumoto cites more than two dozen peer-reviewed scientific papers from 10 laboratories located in far flung countries documenting how squalene-based adjuvants can trigger autoimmune diseases such as lupus, rheumatoid arthritis and MS in rats, mice, guinea pigs and rabbits. The same animals we treat like trash yet claim some dependence for our survival. So, if we are 'into' animal experiments or are pro-vaccine we need to choose between what the animals tell us and what the vaccine makers say. Being a supporter of both could make this a real puzzler.

Don't ask your doctor.

Aluminum Adjuvant Linked to Gulf War Syndrome Induces Motor Neuron Death in Mice

> *In addition, **the continued use of such adjuvants in various vaccines** (i.e., Hepatitis A and B, Diphtheria, Pertussis, and Tetanus) **for the general public may have widespread health implications.** Until vaccine safety can be comprehensively demonstrated by controlled long-term studies that examine the impact on the nervous system in detail, **many of those vaccinated may be at future risk for neurological complications, while those currently receiving injections may develop similar problems in the future.*** [133]

This represented the official line from the US government in 2005:

> *Squalene in the form of an emulsion (emulsified squalene, such as an adjuvant called MF59) has been added as an adjuvant to some investigational vaccines in the U.S (**Burdin et al., 2004**). There is no squalene adjuvant in any US-licensed vaccine. Whatever the arguments for or against squalene as a vaccine adjuvant, the fact is that none of the anthrax vaccine administered to U.S. troops contained squalene as an adjuvant. Based on manufacturing records, FDA can verify that no squalene was added to any vaccine formulation used during the Gulf War. This includes the anthrax vaccine. To date, the FDA has licensed, and US manufacturers have used, only aluminum salts for example, aluminum hydroxide, aluminum phosphate, aluminum potassium sulfate) as adjuvants.* [134]

They have since been forced to admit there was squalene in some of these vaccines tested on their military personnel, but fall back on the old coincidence theory of accidental cross contamination.

> *Because of the difficulty of removing squalene-containing fingerprint oils from laboratory glassware, it is hard to know whether the squalene is truly present in some lots of the vaccine or is introduced by the testing process itself. DOD,*

133 www.whale.to/vaccines/shaw.pdf

134 https://medvetenskap.files.wordpress.com/2009/09/squalen.pdf

FDA, and several civilian advisory committees agree that squalene at such low levels has no adverse health consequences. [135]

The monsters who experiment on their own loyal servants first pointed the finger at their troops, blaming psychological trauma: not as tough as they thought they were! That theory didn't fit with the symptoms or the fact many of the victims hadn't been on frontline duties, so then they picked on lab technicians claiming they must have touched the inside of the Petri dishes or some such with their sticky fingers when testing for the presence of squalene, thus leaving signs of the squalene our body naturally produces, which thus became mixed with the nice clean pure life saving – squalene free - anthrax vaccine all those bone idle soldiers claim made them ill.

Statement of Congressman Jack Metcalf to the Subcommittee on National Security, Veterans Affairs, and International Relations September 27, 2000:

Mr. Chairman, I want to thank you for the opportunity to once again be a small part of your courageous effort to answer questions regarding Gulf War Illnesses and vaccines used by our military personnel. Your determination to move forward and find answers has provided vital leadership for this Congress on this critically important issue.

Indeed, ***we have an obligation to pursue the truth, wherever it may lead us.*** *To do less would be to act dishonorably toward the dedicated men and women who stand between us and a still dangerous world.*

For that reason, I have issued a report culminating a three year investigation into the conduct of the DOD (Department of Defense) with regard to the possibility that squalene, a substance in vaccine adjuvant formulations not approved by the FDA, was used in inoculations given to Gulf War era service personnel. ***According to the GAO (General Accounting Office), scientists have expressed safety concerns regarding the use of novel adjuvant formulations in vaccines, including squalene.***

The report reveals that the FDA has found trace amounts of squalene in the anthrax vaccine. The amounts recorded are enough to "boost immune response," *according to immunology professor Dr Dorothy Lewis of Baylor University. Therefore, my report concludes that, Mr. Chairman, you are absolutely correct in demanding an immediate halt to the current AVIP (Anthrax Vaccination Immunization Program).*

My report further states that an aggressive investigation must be undertaken to determine the source of the squalene, and the potential health

---

[135] Anthrax Vaccination Program Questions and Answers: https://www.hsdl.org/?view&did=18410

consequences to those who have been vaccinated, both during and after the Gulf War. [136]

According to Dr Viera Scheibner, a former principal research scientist for the government of Australia:

This adjuvant contributed to the cascade of reactions called "Gulf War Syndrome," documented in the soldiers involved in the Gulf War. The symptoms they developed included arthritis, fibromyalgia, lymphadenopathy, rashes, photosensitive rashes, malar rashes, chronic fatigue, chronic headaches, abnormal body hair loss, non-healing skin lesions, aphthous ulcers, dizziness, weakness, memory loss, seizures, mood changes, neuropsychiatric problems, anti-thyroid effects, anemia, elevated ESR (erythrocyte sedimentation rate), systemic lupus erythematosus, multiple sclerosis, ALS (amyotrophic lateral sclerosis), Raynaud's phenomenon, Sjogren's syndrome, chronic diarrhea, night sweats and low-grade fevers. [137]

What's flu like again?

Any intelligent fool can make things bigger and more complex... It takes a touch of genius – and a lot of courage – to move in the opposite direction.
Albert Einstein (1897 -1955)

136 http://www.autoimmune.com/SqualeneInVaccine.html

137 Adverse effects of adjuvants in vaccines. Nexus. Dec 2000;8(1)–Feb 2001;8(2). http://www.whale.to/vaccine/adjuvants.html

Blowing the Whistle on the MMR

ProQuad... is a combined, attenuated, live virus vaccine containing measles, mumps, rubella, and varicella viruses. ProQuad is a sterile lyophilized preparation of... ***M-M-R II... propagated in chick embryo cell culture... rubella virus propagated in WI-38 human diploid lung fibroblasts****... Oka/Merck strain of* ***varicella-zoster virus propagated in MRC-5 cells. The cells, virus pools, bovine serum, and human albumin*** *used in manufacturing are all tested to provide assurance that the final product is free of potential adventitious agents.*[138]

Some whistleblowers are more of a threat to the established financial order of things than others and not all are provided a prominent media platform to reveal what they know. None are more dangerous than those who expose vaccines. Dr Andrew Wakefield springs to my mind. He was a consultant gastroenterologist in the right place at the right time, depending on your perspective, but he was not meant to get a platform to reveal his findings before they could be 'reviewed' and that's why they stole his career from him. Vaccines and cancer treatments represent the ultimate in power and control and exposure makes the emperor edgy. But we don't need all these whistleblowers anyway it's not like the truth about vaccines and cancer treatment is hidden. Although there is one coming up whom we really must hear from as he designed the study that says MMR is safe but proved otherwise.

Do we even know what the MMR fuss was all about? It could have been about a lot of things but it ended up being about Dr Andrew Wakefield, which was perhaps the least important factor. But that's how it works. So just what were they hiding behind the good doctor's reputation?

Measles **M**umps **R**ubella vaccine - as safe in kids as radiation! Side effects, they warn, may include "seizures, a severe headache, **a change in behaviour or consciousness**, or difficulty walking". I remember measles and it wasn't that bad! We are bred to fear missing an injection that can like a kick in the head lead to a change in behaviour and consciousness.

Here is a sniff of how measles was described in 1959, nine years before a measles vaccine was launched in the UK. From the British Medical Journal Feb 7 1959, page 354:

> *These writers agree that measles is nowadays normally a mild infection, and they rarely have occasion to give prophylactic gamma globulin.*

BMJ February 7 1959

> Page 380: *Bed rest, for seven days for moderate and severe cases and of five to six days in mild cases, seems to cut down the incidence of such complications as secondary bacterial otitis media and bronchopneumonia.*

---

138 https://www.fda.gov/downloads/BiologicsBloodVaccines/Vaccines/ApprovedProducts/UCM123793.pdf

Despite their initial alarming severity, they tend to resolve spontaneously, and treatment apart from first principles seems useless.

In the majority of children the whole thing has been well and truly over in a week... and many mothers have remarked "how much good the attack has done their children", as they seem so much better after the measles.

Page 381: *The follow-up of all epidemics reveal that patients have not suffered any permanent disabilities. This could be due to the treatment given being satisfactory or to the excellent recuperation powers of a sturdy population.* [139]

My mum assures me this is how it was and measles has been nothing to fear since we cleaned up our living conditions. A dose provides natural lifelong immunity and viral challenges give strength to the system. If you don't use it you'll lose it, right? I had it once. Challenges are necessary for growth and it is typically those who have been through difficult experiences that come out better for it. Ill-health is a reminder of its worth and makes us more humble. And don't all these infectious diseases dilute in severity over time the more they pass through the population in spite of artificial intervention? By Jove I think they might!

According to the NHS in 2017:

Measles is a highly infectious viral illness that can be very unpleasant and sometimes lead to serious complications. It's now uncommon in the UK because of the effectiveness of vaccination. ***Anyone can get measles if*** *they haven't been vaccinated or* ***they haven't had it before****, although it's most common in young children. The infection usually clears in around 7 to 10 days.*

Well everything from taking a train journey to taking a vaccine can lead to serious complications but a week to clear an infection is pretty impressive! And anyway, anyone can get measles vaccinated or not, *unless* you have had it before!

Today's US MMR 'jab' includes: chick embryo cell culture, those WI-38 human diploid lung fibroblasts, has vitamins, amino acids, fetal bovine serum, sucrose, glutamate, recombinant human albumin, neomycin, sorbitol, hydrolysed gelatin, sodium phosphate, sodium chloride.

UK jab: may contain traces of recombinant human albumin, is produced in chick embryo cells, and in WI-38 human diploid lung fibroblasts, has sorbitol, sodium phosphate, potassium phosphate, sucrose, hydrolysed gelatin, medium 199 with Hanks' salts, MEM, monosodium L-glutamate, neomycin, phenol red, sodium bicarbonate, hydrochloric acid and sodium hydroxide.

---

[139] http://www.informedparent.co.uk/mmr

The NHS in March 2017 claimed that the frequency of severe life changing reactions to the MMR is "Not known" and "cannot be estimated from the available data."

Andrew Wakefield has a different view; simple but startling. One which seems far more credible based on my observations and includes further studies of children similar to his and confirmation from the CDC itself. He reckons: "If autism does not affect your family now, it will. If something does not change - and change soon - this is almost a mathematical certainty."

That's it! That's what the fuss **should** have been about. So of course they changed the subject!

Wakefield was branded a quack for publishing a peer reviewed paper in the Lancet describing the clinical history and findings in a group of a dozen children who had been referred with autistic regression and gastrointestinal symptoms and were found to also have intestinal inflammation. A common factor raised by most of the parents and properly noted by Wakefield et al was the onset of this novel set of symptoms occurred following the MMR vaccine. I think that a reasonable line of inquiry as did the courageous Dr Wakefield and his team. But the world we live in is odd at times, and as that simple naïve observation shook the very foundations of the status quo, Dr Andrew Wakefield committed professional suicide.

By publicly inviting further investigation into this early research, our friend manifested the high shepherds of quackery who rounded on their stray sheep accusing him of actions they deemed "inappropriate, not in the best interests of the patients, not in accordance with professional ethical obligations, likely to bring the profession into disrepute. Actions that fell seriously below the standard of conduct expected" of a good little slave boy. Again we see the accuser accurately reflecting self. Other slaves promptly slipped into 'slave rage', jostling and calling the good doctor a quack and forcing him and his family into exile in another country. But Wakefield was right, not just to ask questions but in his hypothesis, as reaffirmed over and over by the most reliable expert witnesses of them all. It's the mums who notice when an eyelash curls on their baby. They know. They thrill at every small developmental milestone, rejoicing in their own achievement as much as that of their most precious possession. They know when all that stops. And when evolution is reversed by the nice nurse with the needle. They know.

In our topsy turvy world attacking the messenger has been perfectly normal for long enough and as such most have tended to keep their mouths shut. But times have changed.

Other effects of the MMR jab according to the product information data:

> *Bruising or bleeding more easily than normal, severe allergic reaction that may include difficulty in breathing, facial swelling, localised swelling, and swelling of the limbs, irritability, seizures (fits) without fever; seizures (fits) with fever in children walking unsteadily; dizziness;* ***illnesses involving inflammation of the nervous system (brain and/or spinal cord) were***

> ***reported*** *with the use of M-M-RVAXPRO or with the measles, mumps, and rubella vaccine manufactured by Merck & Co., Inc., or with its monovalent (single) components, during post-marketing use and/or during clinical studies.*

Autism - Autism Spectrum Disorders – ASD is now an epidemic in our children and this clinical use of any words to tell of the imposition of brain damage on a child is not fitting. Children in whom it cannot be denied are often found with mercury poisoning which is off the scale and which they are unable to detox. The word autism represents a few of the effects listed in the package information leaflet which warns the vaccine can also increase our chances of "an illness consisting of muscle weakness, abnormal sensations, Guillain-Barré syndrome, headache; fainting; nerve disorders" or a whole load of other disorders which only ever get worse. In exchange for what again, possible protection against an age-old immune boosting week off school?

These side effects are seldom disclosed to parents who only hear how safe the vaccines are. How about we drain this sea of words and just say 'Side effects may include: a living nightmare'. That's how parents describe their lives post vaccine and not only that but they also know roughly how many other kids have been damaged this way too. Most of us don't have a clue. I know a great deal more about vaccines, what they contain and what they do than the average doctor. I'm not boasting by the way, in fact I'm pretty pissed off about that. These parents know better than anyone, they network and share their stories and these are not happy endings. The gravity of this is well known but of course those with the power to inform the masses aren't going to start confessing their crimes against humanity any time soon because if they did the masses would rise up and that power and all that lovely money would be taken off them.

On the face of it we are in a bit of a pickle but in reality, if we think all this through to its logical conclusion, we have all the power. I'm keeping mine. I think together we can build a future where we sacrifice fewer children and fewer animals on any alter and we can do ourselves a favour too.

In just a few years the growth in numbers of vaccine victims has been exponential. It's in the public record and a large number of research papers prove the link. Better still, there are millions of witnesses who testify with heartbreaking clarity to the steady, sometimes dramatic deterioration of their babies following a vaccination. The symptoms often creep on and pile up, and they talk of them "fading away"; losing their ability to speak and make eye contact, toilet themselves and to walk. They regress into autism, to that lonely world of their own. And they don't come back. "A change in consciousness". Think about that for a moment. This is not just about fainting for a bit from the shock of the needle; this is about the contents of the child deteriorating.

Imagine, if at the time humanity begins to recognise its collective unconscious state and sees its long predicted conscious evolution unfolding, the predatory parasites that dictate this planet had gathered with genetically engineered viruses in vaccines to sabotage the new humans, our star children, so things stay just the way they are. And they got us to pay for it!

Ah, the audacity of evil. An evil that would if it could use its genius to degrade the species, subtly, by screwing with the gene pool so it dies out, slowly, because maybe just maybe it isn't smart enough to figure all this out. That's what they hope, but the thing is I figured it out and I'm no genius and I figured it out because a load of other people figured it and I figure if it carries on like this then millions of years of evolution can't possibly come to an end so abruptly in our lifetime. But the race is on.

These poisons are eating the brains of our children and it's being covered up. And that's official. For the record, I must stress that I of course include animals when I refer to children and babies. Everyone's an individual, everyone's unique. The animals however, get it twice. First they experiment on lab animals in cages and fail to achieve either safety or efficacy, then they persuade us to tootle along with our animals to buy from them repeat prescriptions of those animal-tested toxic vaccines, in the hope we might keep our loved ones healthy and happy for as long as possible. Perhaps the ultimate irony is that even an animal rights activist, who may be especially loyal to the notion of doing the right thing by their animals according to their animal doctor's expert advice, will boast of full vaccine compliance. Yet all the vaccines contain animal parts, are tested on animals and cause cancer in animals. But they won't be branded crazy for questioning this absurdity. Happy days!

They keep you in prison if you don't repent and you ain't getting into heaven apparently, yet the medical mafia gets away with murder again and again and again at our invite. There will always be those who take advantage of our kindness, loyalty and trust, seeing it as a weakness from which they can feed their greed. Big business, particularly the Big Pharma did not get big by being nice; status such as this in the passing world comes from being utterly ruthless.

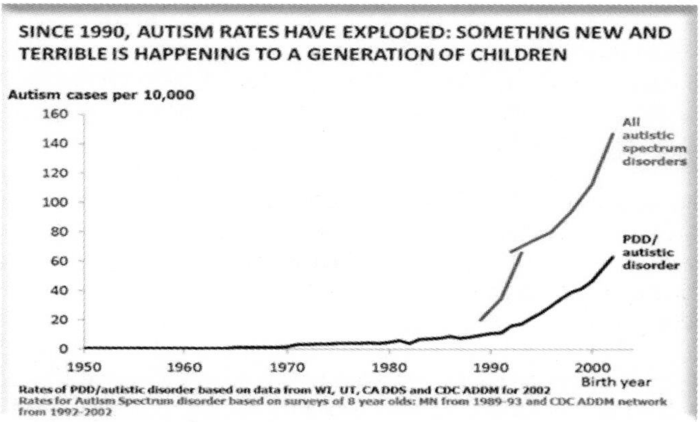

[140]

---

140 http://www.ageofautism.com/2014/03/

Since it was first diagnosed in the 1930's and for the next five decades the prevalence of autism in the US was around 1 in 10,000. In the years between 1980 and 1998 something caused 1 in 500 children to suffer this pattern of brain damage. In just two more years that had doubled to 1 in 250. This cannot be dismissed as a condition now better diagnosed because it isn't and we don't have a generation of autistic adults flapping their arms and screaming in pain.

At present there are between 1 in 25 and 1 in 50 vaccinated children struggling with this condition, depending on who you believe. If the trend continues at the current alarming rate, and why wouldn't it, the numbers predict that by 2032 every other human child will have had their consciousness modified. That's 1 in 2 and 80% of the boys with an autistic disorder, which is pretty serious. And what will the parents be doing with the rest of their lives? And when they're gone who looks after the 8 year old adults they leave behind?

The first school for autistic children opened in the UK in 1980 funded by volunteers, parents. By 2013 the BBC was reporting on a "new breed of free schools" being set up in England "to fill a local need" for society's vaccine victims.

This is an epidemic of evil whoever does the adding up and it's a pretty poor trade off for our fear of infection.

And not that it matters much but this isn't just a coincidence or an accident.

Enter Dr William Thompson PhD. An establishment Mr Big who for 17 years was glorified as a senior research scientist and statistician at the US government Big Pharma clearing house: the Centres for Disease Control and Prevention (CDC). Prior to this he worked for Merck. That's evil piled on evil and he's the frontman. But he's OK. He wasn't, but he is now. I fell for him the moment he blew the whistle on arguably the gravest crime of modern times perpetrated by the medical establishment, and that's saying something! Andrew Wakefield touched on this one and see what happened to him, but Thompson has gone one step further. Whereas Wakefield simply suggested further investigation of the possibility it was the MMR vaccine screwing with the kids, what Thompson did was open up the filing cabinets at this prestigious institution and channel the contents onto the internet. Now we have all we need to prove beyond any shadow of doubt that yes indeed the MMR vaccine does cause autism and in a big way. The results shocked everyone!

In light of Wakefield's stirring of pubic consciousness, the CDC ran a series of scientific trials with a view to generating some new data for the purpose of bringing the drifters back under the vaccine spell and to further enchant and reward those who'd stayed loyal. Equally, this official 'proof' would undermine all those litigants who claimed their children had been harmed by the vaccine and would show up the conspiracy theorists and quack lovers for what they really are. These final super science trials would show that the vaccine is super safe and more effective than ever and that the naïve uneducated parents had been duped. The vaccine agenda would be full steam ahead; with the triple dose vaccine proven, now everyone could tuck in.

So esteemed was Thompson he designed the trials. He was at the head of the most important vaccine study ever, managed by the most respected health agency in the world, sewing the seeds of deception on behalf of the Big Pharma, the most powerful commercial concern in the world. Thompson was the go-to-guy for proof the MMR was cool for kids. This study when complete would become the jewel in the crown for the loyalists, the untouchable scientific study that everyone uses to prove vaccines are indeed the magic formula humanity needs to save the children. The entire vaccine agenda rests on the findings of Thompson's work and for that alone this was **the** big deal for the status quo. Except the whole thing was a fully fledged scientific fraud. An inside job! What it all actually revealed was the opposite of a safe vaccine. As Thompson now confesses:

> *I've waited a long time to tell my story and I want to tell it truthfully.*

And then he lets it all out. Ten thousand documents online for you to read for yourself that prove the MMR vaccine study was sabotaged to suit the vaccine narrative and to cover up the damage being done to millions of children by the MMR vaccine. Charts were altered, numbers were changed, paperwork was binned and plies and piles of contradictory electronic data were deleted forever from the public record. But for our expert witness, whose conscience broke through and told him he must preserve the evidence, we would never know of the scale of this atrocity.

> ***I was involved in deceiving millions of taxpayers regarding the potential negative side effects of vaccines.*** *I have great shame now, when I meet families with kids with autism, because I have been part of the problem.*

This was more than just a federal offence, more than serious scientific fraud, more than a criminal conspiracy involving the heads of the CDC, an agency tasked with protecting the public from this very thing. It's more than a mainstream media cover up.

This is a crime against humanity.

> *We lied about the scientific findings*, admits Thompson.

The 2001 CDC study began looking at whether the age of the child figured in developing autism as proposed by Wakefield, Walker-Smith and co in London, and sure enough the numbers proved conclusively that the younger the child the more significant the risk, particularly if vaccinated between 12 & 18 months, the precise age they are scheduled by the CDC and the Department of Health to be vaccinated! Up to this age children are best protected by a healthy, informed mother and her milk and not by wealthy strangers.

This was only the beginning of the nightmare the data was exposing. The numbers then revealed a "highly significant" elevated risk of disease onset in vaccinated African American boys, up 300% compared to other ethnic groups. According to researcher Dr Brian Hooker, there have been over 100,000 African American males diagnosed with autism since the CDC discovered the extent and buried the truth about MMR. Hooker knows all about the MMR, he is a well published Assistant Professor of Biology at Simpson University, California, specialising in chemistry and biology and the father of a vaccine damaged child himself, a child who had lost his ability to speak and lost all eye contact in the days following his 15 month vaccines.

So do we have a racist vaccine? It appears it doesn't really care who it hurts. Curiously, by accident or design ethnicity is relevant in the determination of safety and efficacy of some drugs and vaccines.

'Isolated Autism' formed the next part of the study and it isn't what it sounds. You'd think wouldn't you that this had something to do with a few isolated cases of autism, but of course it's the exact opposite! It's much closer to 'all encompassing autism' and it makes using their description really awkward. They asked the question: "If early MMR causes autism what group of children is most likely to be affected?" They isolated the kids with autism from all other pre-existing injury or illnesses and found this group to be the most significant. That is, those with no developmental concerns in the year of life pre-vaccine - the healthiest children - are at the greatest risk of developing autism following MMR! The conclusion therefore is that the risk is 'isolated' to the largest possible group. Just about everyone if we take into account, as they must, that anyone unhealthy should not be vaccinated anyway!

This is explosive material proving the observable effects of the MMR. What remains to be seen is what latent or subtle injury is being done to those kids not outwardly impacted by these vaccines. Given what we do know it would be foolish to assume it's all or nothing. Boys are affected in greater numbers than the girls and this appears due to the elevated presence of testosterone in males which creates a more immediate and often explosive reaction when meeting mercury, whereas girls are more protected by oestrogen, at least in the short-term. Is it a coincidence that boys don't do so well as girls in schools?

The revelations screaming out of this CDC investigation were proving so significant that they had to be covered up. The problem for the conspirators on the inside was that the numbers were so extreme that nothing could be done to cover it up. Efforts were made to first change the analysis plan and to exclude a large number of problem kids (data) from the study, and when that failed to add up they were forced to spend the next two years cooking the books in other ways to make the numbers fit the narrative. And still they failed. The truth was not going to be buried in the data no matter how many expert scientists and genius doctors tackled the tricky task. And so, with disaster looming the whole problem simply had to be binned. Literally binned.

As affirmed via an affidavit given by Dr Thompson to Republican Congressman Bill Posey in September, 2014, [141] the ring leaders of this despicable plot held a secret "shredding party" at their workplace during August or September of 2002 where they disposed of their documents in order to cover up what the vaccine was doing to

---

141 https://www.globalresearch.ca/congressman-bill-posey-calls-for-investigation-of-cdc-whistleblower-william-thompson/5469103

children. In the history of conspiracies this ranks right up there at the top of the evil pile and these are the main conspirators: Colleen Boyle PhD CDC Division Director; Marshalyn Yeargin-Allsop M.D, CDC Branch Chief; Frank Destefano M.D CDC Director Immunization Safety and Tanya Bhasin, Research Associate. Thick as thieves, stealing the lives of families. Dr Julie Gerberding, the head of the CDC at this time of great cover up was fully implicated in a 2004 letter confirming her agency's awareness and suppression of these findings. Thompson had pleaded with his boss to come clean on this Merck MMR mess but she had herself in mind and he was brushed off and told to keep his mouth shut. Gerberding later committed perjury before she went on to grab a salary hike just one year later by accepting an invite to become Executive Vice President at the head of the Merck's Vaccine Division. Come to Daddy!

This contemptuous act represents the active industry revolving door through which many civil servants pass as they slip from regulatory government oversight, meant to protect the public, into the business of exploiting the public and back again. These people care only for themselves and have fallen into the dark side of evil and will be remembered like we remember Nuremburg.

Thompson himself a drifter through the revolving door but our exception to the rule. He had been party to this crime for 14 years and was the only dissenting voice in the CDC management conspiracy to bury the truth. You can feel his regret and the overwhelming need he has to get the truth out. He is begging the world to listen to why he could no longer take part in one of the most heinous crimes in medical history. His boss off to pastures new, his comrades committing federal offences all over the place, Thompson was forced into a corner. What he did next was smart. He broke ranks so he could get the truth out but rather than send it into the mainstream media truth filter he secretly called Dr Hooker.

Hooker wasn't just qualified and wanting the truth out about the vaccines, Hooker had been hounding the CDC for years via Freedom of Information requests to get the real data on MMR and its potential role in causing neuro-developmental disorders including autism. This data when finally released would heavily implicate the MMR in a trail of destruction. Hooker had become tired after years of being given the run around by the CDC, even prank called and threatened by people at the CDC and had always been denied requests, usually by Thompson himself. Such was the desperation to stop the truth emerging if Hooker got access to the facts that the CDC had obtained legal injunction to limit his probing!

Hooker was thoroughly frustrated but hungry as a bear just out of hibernation when he suddenly got that phone call from Thompson right out of the blue. They both desperately wanted to talk. Over 40 calls in a year. Hooker recorded everything. [142]

> *Oh my god, I cannot believe we did what we did. But we did. It's the lowest point in my career that I went along with that paper.*

---

[142] http://fearlessparent.org/why-is-thimerosal-still-in-vaccines-recording-1/

Thompson is stressed and wants to make amends, but he has to tread carefully. To begin with he confides in Hooker of a little known route through a backdoor CDC application process he can use to gain full access to all the data he wants, all the studies he wants, everything he needs to prove the extent of the fraud both men know surround the MMR vaccine. All within the rules. This is extraordinary access to the truth.

And like a wet dream for an untethered PhD who was hurting, like Hooker.

Thompson had secretly stashed a backup of over 10,000 documents and masses of computer files that the CDC conspirators had wanted destroyed. This is a treasure trove of information, like no other. True to his word soon as our whistleblower received Hookers data access applications at the CDC, he himself proceeded to filter this shattering story out to the world, keeping himself on the right side of the law. Whistleblowers take great risks and none more so than this.

This cache documents an unimaginable evil perpetrated on the human species. History, aka 'His story' will try to tell of Big Pharma's valiant efforts to save the lives of millions of tragic humans ravaged by disease, barely able to fend for themselves any longer, but it's all lies. Doctors destroy health at the behest of Big Pharma and Big Pharma is on the warpath.

The fraudulence CDC 'MMR is Safe' study had given the influential Institute of Medicine (IOM) the green light it needed to issue an inevitably fake report on the safety of MMR. Rumours away, the global media gobbled up the super science study findings like puppies in the yogurt tub and as a result the public were rallied into believing another conspiracy theory, each worshipper repeating the lie of the expert they heard speak before them. The prize for the pro-vax lobby at the end of this death game of Chinese whispers came in the form of the instant dismissal of 5,000 legal cases of vaccine damaged children, the victims and their families denied any crumbs of compensation for their injury, estimated to be £5 million each for lifelong care needs. A sickening obstruction of justice if ever there was one. Then, to complete the circle of deception the order came from the high priests to cut off any future funding looking into the dangers of the MMR vaccine.

With more science now settled, the ortho-docs settled on blaming genetics. Somehow this very dramatic elevation in brain damaged children is being passed not through the injecting of poisons into babies but down the generations in the damaged DNA of their parents. Faulty stock breeding in the last few years it would seem, since the 1980's when MMR was unleashed.

According to William Weil of the American Academy of Paediatricians in June 2000

> *The increased incidence of neurobehavioral problems in children in the past few decades is probably real... I work in the school system where my effort is entirely in special education and I have to say the number of kids getting help in special education is growing nationally and state by state at a rate we have not seen before so there is some kind of an increase. We can argue about*

what it is due to... the rise in the frequency of neurobehavioural disorders... is much too graphic. We don't see that kind of genetic change in 30 years. [143]

Bill Thompson languishes in no man's land; officially he has whistleblower status and a whistleblower lawyer. He should be subpoenaed to testify to these crimes but they don't want to do that. They can't sack him. He wanted to leave so they made it more attractive for him to stay with a pile of cash. So he still works for the CDC. He'll get due credit from the judge when the shit hits the fan but he has to live with what he did and so do a lot of other people. The mainstream media is silent on the biggest scoop since the last one they ignored. The MSM has been bought and paid for and is no longer relevant and should be treated with all due disregard. Journalists are duty bound to investigate the unexplained but prefer the role of explaining away what they haven't investigated.

This represents perhaps the most egregious fraud in medical history. Depending on how one views all the others we know about. And a cover up like no other. Well, lots of others! This is quackery on steroids. We get headlines about measles outbreaks here and there, and are taught to fear the next bogey virus as the talking heads and bleeding hearts blame the unvaccinated for outbreaks among **highly vaccinated** populations, without even blinking, while calling for more vaccines to keep us safe from the horrors of the past and others yet to be unleashed. And where is the truth?

If vaccines are so effective how do unvaccinated kids cause disease outbreaks among the vaccinated? What about those of us not boosted by needle, how come we aren't spreading measles, mumps and rubella?

You can watch the MMR story unravel in the film Vaxxed and I urge that. [144]

The Cochrane Library did some number crunching on all the MMR studies. We usually hear of this or that study proving this or that, well these guys add up all the relevant trials and present a more complete picture albeit based on discredited studies using laced placebos with selective end points and usually funded by industry. Nevertheless the findings speak for themselves.

We included five randomised controlled trials, one controlled clinical trial, 27 cohort studies, 17 case-control studies, five time-series trials, one case cross-over trial, two ecological studies, six self controlled case series studies involving in all about 14,700,000 children and assessing... safety of MMR vaccine.

And discovered that:

---

143 https://www.safeminds.org/wp-content/uploads/2013/04/Simpsonwood_Overview.pdf

144 http://vaxxedthemovie.com/
http://vaxxedthemovie.com/official-complaint-letter-to-the-CDC-10-14-2014.pdf

The design and reporting of safety outcomes in MMR vaccine studies, both pre-and post-marketing, are largely inadequate. The evidence of adverse events following immunisation with the MMR vaccine cannot be separated from its role in preventing the target diseases. [145]

The first MMR experiment on human children using the brand Trivirix caused so much meningitis in Canadian children in the late 1980's that it had to be withdrawn soon after launch. Regardless, rebranded as Pluserix, which according to the science of vaccines made it now safe, effective and necessary, the very same month it was pulled in Canada it was introduced into UK children. Of course in the real world over the next four years the outcome would be devastation as countless families had their children messed up. Pluserix was subsequently banned in the UK in late 1992 and those responsible were severely punished. Oh no, sorry, that was in one of my dreams, that never happens in the real world, here it is the parents who are blamed and many of them punished and the product moved on to bigger markets in developing countries with the help of UNICEF and others, where it remains, unleashing its inevitable anger and destroying lives. Because this is what they do for a living!

I think of Wakefield and a serious miscarriage of justice.

Which is not what this deluded science fiction vaccine fanatic and billionaire business magnate Bill Gates wants us to think, as captured by CNN in February 2011:

Dr Wakefield has been shown to use absolutely fraudulent data. He had a financial interest in some lawsuits. He created a fake paper. The journal allowed it to run.

All other studies were done showed no connection whatsoever again and again and again. And so, ***it's an absolute lie that has killed thousands of kids because the mothers who heard that lie, many of them didn't have their kids take either pertussis or measles vaccine and their children are dead today.*** *And so, you know,* ***the people who go and engage in those anti-vaccine efforts, you know, they killed children.*** *It's a very sad thing because these vaccines are important.* [146]

---

[145] http://cochranelibrary-wiley.com/doi/10.1002/14651858.CD004407.pub3/epdf/standard

[146] http://edition.cnn.com/2011/HEALTH/02/03/gupta.gates.vaccines.world.health/index.html

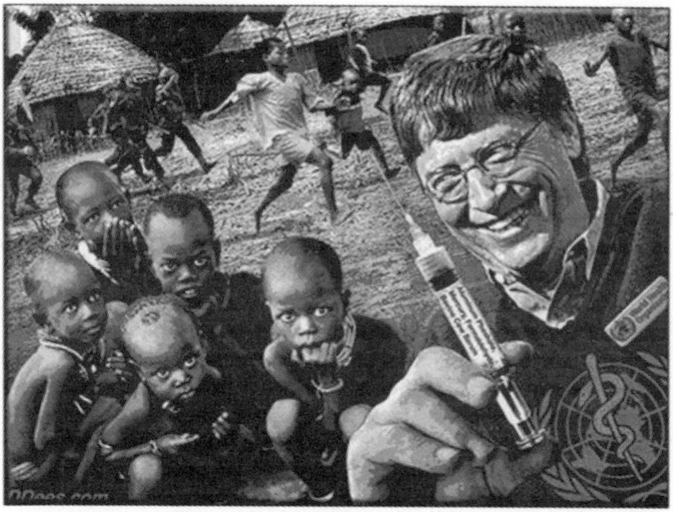

These vaccines are important so let's keep talking.
Image: D.Dees.com

A clear cut violation of the human rights of these girl children and adolescents. [147]

That's how a scathing Indian parliamentary committee describe the actions of The Gates Foundation funded HPV vaccine experiments on tens of thousands of tribal children in the country in 2009 using language such as *improper, unlawful, wrong doing, criminality, subterfuge and highly deplorable.* The Indian Supreme Courts are investigating after many of the children became violently ill following vaccination, and at least five died during these Big Pharma/philanthropist crimes against humanity. Undated consent forms reveal that illiterate parents were coerced into 'informed consent' with their thumbprints! Similar reports of medical fraud and mass casualties can be found wherever the vaccine gangs turn up to wipe out illness. Humans.

I apologise again for the price you paid for my dishonesty.
William Thompson in a text message to Andrew Wakefield

[147] http://164.100.47.5/newcommittee/reports/EnglishCommittees/Committee%20on%20Health%20and%20Family%20Welfare/72.pdf

Vaccines, Cancer, Contamination, Cover-up

Seeing, contrary to popular wisdom, is not believing. It's where belief stops because it isn't needed any more.
Terry Pratchet

Whatever billionaires want us to think these real life findings in real live people and animals are coming at us like a blizzard. And it's no small detail either that DNA damage is being done to the human being and our companion animals and experimental animals through imprinted foreign DNA which is passed down the line to offspring. We can see proof of this but we don't really know the half of it. We might want to reconsider our views on chiropractors and the Amish and other minorities of ridicule as one day humanity is probably going to need the pure unvaccinated gene pool of these people to rebuild what we are allowing those who we currently worship like gods to take from us. These communities don't see autism gone wild in their children and they have not gone extinct due to the terrifying multiple vaccine deficiency syndromes we are warned and warned and warned will wipe out humanity if we don't inject everyone urgently. [148]

This all started with the odd one and then 2 or 3 single shot vaccines. Given what we know about the polio vaccine this is troublesome enough. But today it's a full on assault as kids are bombarded unnaturally through their most fragile formative years, their immune systems forced to respond increasingly to multiple insults all at once. What are we to make of the super charged Special Brew of vaccines, the all new record-breaking 6-in-1 jab? Well why not; they got away with the cancer causing one-hit polio wonder jab and the 3-in-1 DTP and MMR vaccines turned out to be a really big hit! Would an even bigger needle hold more stuff? May as well cram as many in as possible! It's good for the science, where more is better, according to some scientists. The A380 of vaccines could be the *Super Vax-Max 10 in 1: An investment in your grandchildren's future.*

Check out this monster, brewed up in Vero monkey kidney cells with a bit of genetic engineering and poultry proteins to spice it up and not one but two kinds of nano particulate aluminium, a sprinkle of antibiotics, some yeast and a drop of formaldehyde. Shaken not stirred. Says it's for infants and toddlers to save them from diphtheria, tetanus, pertussis, hepatitis B, polio and disease caused by Haemophilus influenzae type b.

148 https://www.upi.com/Health_News/2005/12/07/The-Age-of-Autism-a-pretty-big-secret/UPI-68291133982531/

Diphtheria toxoid[1]	not less than 30 Interr
Tetanus toxoid[1]	not less than 40 Interr
Bordetella pertussis antigens	
Pertussis toxoid (PT)[1]	
Filamentous Haemagglutinin (FHA)[1]	
Pertactin (PRN)[1]	
Hepatitis B surface antigen (HBs)[2,3]	
Poliovirus (inactivated) (IPV)	
type 1 (Mahoney strain)[4]	
type 2 (MEF-1 strain)[4]	
type 3 (Saukett strain)[4]	
Haemophilus influenzae type b polysaccharide	
(polyribosylribitol phosphate, PRP)[3]	
conjugated to tetanus toxoid as carrier protein	approximate
[1]adsorbed on aluminium hydroxide, hydrated ($Al(OH)_3$)	(
[2]produced in yeast cells (*Saccharomyces cerevisiae*) by recombinant DNA technology	
[3]adsorbed on aluminium phosphate ($AlPO_4$)	0.
[4]propagated in VERO cells	

The vaccine may contain traces of formaldehyde, neomycin and polymyxin which are used during the manufacturing process (see section 4.3).

The electronic Medicines Compendium (eMC) [149]

I don't think that's a good idea.

They warm things up with what almost starts to sound cute, the 4-in-1 'pre-school booster' of diphtheria, tetanus, whooping cough and polio. It's not uncommon to get add-ons such as the trusty autistic MMR and whatever other shots they can make available during the doctor's appointment, or "health check", save you having to drag the kids back again. Often times and increasingly only hours or days after emerging from the safety of the womb (assuming mom hasn't been vaccinated during pregnancy that is, an increasing likelihood) and into the world of crazy, and way before the immune system is even ready for one dose, babies are being invaded intramuscularly by a vast army. Against what natural threats were these pseudoscientific plots formed? Such a coordinated multi-pronged viral attack would never happen in real life via the normal oral route let alone piercing the defence of the skin and must be viewed as either experimental, an investment in future markets or both. It is in our children and our animals where these things are being tested, and do you know what I think? I think they are working. To the crazies running the show this is a statistically significant aid to depopulation, dumbing down and full spectrum control.

That live vaccines cause the very diseases they are meant to prevent is written in the blueprint, which means diseases will never be eradicated only created! And they are churning them out!

---

149 http://www.medicines.org.uk/emc/medicine/33313

This Merck varicella chicken pox vaccine information insert warns recipients of the risk they pose by spreading the needle acquired virus onto others in the herd for weeks after vaccination.

> ***Vaccine recipients should attempt to avoid, to the extent possible, close association with high-risk individuals susceptible to varicella for up to 6 weeks following vaccination****. In circumstances where contact with high-risk individuals susceptible to varicella is unavoidable, the potential risk of transmission of the varicella vaccine virus should be weighed against the risk of acquiring and transmitting wild-type varicella virus.* ***Excretion of small amounts of the live, attenuated rubella virus from the nose or throat has occurred*** *in the majority of susceptible individuals* ***7 to 28 days after vaccination.*** *There is no confirmed evidence to indicate that such virus is transmitted to susceptible persons who are in contact with the vaccinated individuals. Consequently, transmission through close personal contact, while accepted as a theoretical possibility, is not regarded as a significant risk. However,* ***transmission of the rubella vaccine virus to infants via breast milk has been documented****.* [150]

So on top of all the other drawbacks, recipients of live virus vaccines become carriers of the disease. A fully 'compliant' child or domestic dog today can be given in excess of 70 vaccines for diseases they may never have come into contact with in their lifetime, or could instead in the event of infection be treated to aid recovery. So, rather than the unvaccinated being to blame for putting the vaccinated at risk, if that makes any sense, it is the virus-induced carriers who pose the greatest risk to others, particularly those who for medical reasons must not be exposed to vaccine-induced infection.

So much for the promise that vaccines would save us from disease!

Atypical measles (AMS) is a syndrome that may emerge following contact with the wild or live vaccine virus, and affects those who have been previously vaccinated with a killed measles virus, the immune system essentially misinformed by the dead invader. The physical presentation of vaccine-induced AMS is far more serious with a higher mortality rate and cases are being diagnosed many years after the original measles vaccine weakened the host. Measles-Induced Neuroautistic Encephalopathy is another creation of the vaxers and this has only been reported in children who have received MMR vaccines. [151]

With widespread administration of the measles vaccine, we expect that the incidence of modified measles will increase in the future. [152]

---

150 https://www.fda.gov/downloads/BiologicsBloodVaccines/Vaccines/ApprovedProducts/UCM123793.pdf

151 http://www.thelibertybeacon.com/measles-vaccines-part-i-ineffectiveness-of-vaccination-and-unintended-consequences-benefits-of-contracting-measles/

152 https://www.ncbi.nlm.nih.gov/pubmed/21228451

Herd Immunity
(Andrew Wakefield)

Herd Immunity is a term that is bandied around in defence of mass and mandatory vaccination. What is it and why is it important?

> *Let's set out a working definition of what Herd Immunity is at a functional level in the population: Herd Immunity is the presence of adequate immunity within a population against a specific infection that operates to protect those at high risk of serious infection and consequently, reduce morbidity and mortality from that infection.*
>
> *Now let's separate out Herd Immunity, comparing what it meant in the pre-vaccine era compared with what it means in the vaccine era, using specific infections as examples.*
>
> *Measles: Herd Immunity in the pre-vaccine era*

- *When measles first enters a population that has not been exposed to measles before, Herd Immunity is zero and there is, initially, a very high morbidity (illness) and mortality.*
- *This occurs in large part as a consequence of high dose exposure.*
- *High dose exposure occurs because, in the absence of viral immunity, viral replication is unimpeded in the multiple susceptible human reservoirs in which it thrives. High doses of measles virus are transmitted from one person to the next. Added to this, socioeconomic circumstances contribute to high dose exposure. This includes high population density (easy transmission) and poor antiviral defenses (e.g. low vitamins A, D, and C). An example is the ravage of measles in Confederate soldiers amassed in barracks and hospitals in the American Civil War.*
- *Over time, as measles becomes endemic (constantly circulating) in a population with typical 2-yearly epidemics, Herd Immunity increases rapidly. Natural exposure leads to long term immunity. Immunity limits viral transmission and opportunities for viral replication. Concomitantly, developed countries have experienced an improvement in nutritional status and consequently antiviral immunity. Dose of exposure falls and a dramatic reduction in morbidity and mortality is observed.*
- *As a consequence of natural Herd Immunity, in the developed world measles mortality had fallen by 99.6% before measles vaccines were introduced. A fall in morbidity will have paralleled the fall in mortality (mortality is the extreme of morbidity).* [153]

Another obstacle in the way of inducing herd immunity is list of exemptions for those of us with compromised immune systems, of who there are increasing numbers Practitioners injecting this MMRVaricella vaccine are warned to exclude anyone with:

---

153 http://vaxxedthemovie.com/notes-herd-immunity-andrew-wakefield/

> *A history of hypersensitivity to gelatin or any other component of the vaccine or following previous vaccination with blood dyscrasias, leukemia, lymphomas of any type, or other malignant neoplasms affecting the bone marrow or lymphatic system; or to individuals on immunosuppressive therapy (including high-dose systemic corticosteroids). Do not administer... to individuals with primary and acquired immunodeficiency states, including AIDS or other clinical manifestations of infection with human immunodeficiency viruses; cellular immune deficiencies; and hypogammaglobulinemic and dysgammaglobulinemic states.*
>
> *Measles inclusion body encephalitis, pneumonitis, and death as a direct consequence of disseminated measles vaccine virus infection have been reported in severely immunocompromised individuals inadvertently vaccinated with measles-containing vaccine. In addition, disseminated varicella vaccine virus infection has been reported in children with underlying immunodeficiency disorders who were inadvertently vaccinated with a varicella-containing vaccine, individuals with a family history of congenital or hereditary immunodeficiency, with active untreated tuberculosis or to individuals with an active febrile illness with fever, individuals who are pregnant because the effects of the vaccine on fetal development are unknown. If vaccination of postpubertal females is undertaken, pregnancy should be avoided for three months following administration.* [154]

Quite a list of potential exemptions outside of the growing resistance! And what of those individuals who don't yet know they are immune compromised? Cancer patients have cancer for years before diagnosis is confirmed, how many vaccines are safe for them? I say none but never mind at least the rest of the population is safe from viral infection thanks to the good old vaccine, right?

Vaccinations don't so much immunise against as sensitise to. Immune means immune as in exempt/resistant/protected from - not going to get - but that's not what we see. The CDC agrees that

> ***Transmission of measles can occur within a school population with a documented immunization level of 100%***. [155]

But even with that acknowledgement of vaccine failure they'll try and blame someone else...

> *Investigations of measles outbreaks among highly immunized populations have revealed risk factors such as improper storage or handling of vaccine, vaccine administered to children under 1 year of age, use of globulin with vaccine, and use of killed virus vaccine.* 152

Blame and fear.

---

154 httAps://www.fda.gov/downloads/BiologicsBloodVaccines/Vaccines/ApprovedProducts/UCM123793.pdf

155 https://www.cdc.gov/mmwr/preview/mmwrhtml/00000359.htm

> *If it turns out that vaccinated people lose their immunity as they get older, that could leave them vulnerable to measles outbreaks seeded by unvaccinated people - which are increasingly common in the United States and other developed countries.* ***Even a vaccine failure rate of 3% to 5% could devastate a high school with a few thousand students.*** [156]

This from fear mongering quack Robert Jacobson, director of clinical studies for the Mayo Clinic's Vaccine Research Group in Rochester, Minnesota. But he isn't referring to the well documented failure of the vaccines to protect recipients, and spread disease, and create disease, rather "the most important 'vaccine failure' with measles happens when people refuse the vaccine in the first place." [153]

If high school students have already lost their vaccine induced immunity and are at risk of devastation from measles, what is the point of the vaccines? Another hint at the malfunction of this process is the need to get a vaccine 'booster' next year, which suggests either the last one hasn't worked or we may have misunderstood how these jabs beat natural lifelong immunity! And consider, a boost to immunity can just as readily be obtained from contact with the wild virus or bacteria in the natural environment, as it can from the load of a needle. Yet we may be offered a dozen artificial boosters year after year and may even be invited to set up a direct debit or standing order for our loved one's annual toxin top ups. Vets are kind enough to offer this service to make it more convenient to treat Tiddles to his liquid cosh without really feeling the pinch yourself.

> *By signing up to our Pet Health Club you can make great savings on the annual costs of your pet's preventative health care. Additionally we will reward your loyalty with exclusive Pet Health Club discounts on food, microchipping and give you a free 6 month health check with the veterinary surgeon in between your annual vaccinations.*

The problem is that the UK has no transparent process for evaluating the effectiveness or cost effectiveness of vaccines. [157]

---

156 http://www.sciencemag.org/news/2014/04/measles-outbreak-traced-fully-vaccinated-patient-first-time

157 http://www.bmj.com/content/333/7574/0.7

And bad babies…

The government has never compensated, nor has it ever been ordered to compensate, any case based on a determination that autism was actually caused by vaccines. We have compensated cases in which children exhibited an encephalopathy, or general brain disease. Encephalopathy may be accompanied by a medical progression of an array of symptoms including autistic behavior, autism, or seizures. Some children who have been compensated for vaccine injuries may have shown signs of autism before the decision to compensate, or may ultimately end up with autism or autistic symptoms, but we do not track cases on this basis.

Tina Cheatham, US Health Resources and Services Administration, 2011 [158]

As reward for our general loyalty to the cause we are swamped with lies and deception. We've been guided to think that Shaken Baby Syndrome (SBS) is really more likely the fault of all those parents all over the world shaking their babies to a brain damaged death often, many parents say, soon after their baby was vaccinated. We are told by the name calling finger pointers that they shake their babies to keep them quiet. And as such our attention is guided away from the couldn't-care-less drug companies and their primitive concoctions, which they freely confess can cause vaccine-induced encephalitis and cot deaths and hundreds of other detrimental health effects. While they may be using less caustic terms as a way to describe the brain damaged children they are compensating, the vaccine courts have been quietly paying off autism cases for over a decade. Dr Viera Scheibner describes cot death as "a convenient waste basket in which to put vaccine damaged babies". [159]

With thousands of cases of SBS/Sudden Infant Death Syndrome (SIDS)/cot death or the upgraded and equally unscientific NAHI, Non-Accidental Head Injury cases recorded each year, through which typically the child has suffered encephalopathy/brain damage, which is a well documented and appalling effect of vaccines, one would hope that at least this cause might be considered and tested rather than ridiculed and rubbished. Is it credible science that leaves out some of the data? No, that's what science forbids but scientists are human and they love forbidden fruit. The establishment and its expert medical witnesses are infested with inflated egos and are at the end of the queue when it comes to humility, so naturally they point the finger at someone else.

Curiously this phenomenon of mums shaking their precious babies to the point of brain damage has gone international. That'll be the fault of the internet. Parents and the internet! I jest of course, the Joint Committee on Vaccination and Immunisation in the UK noted in 2001 with regard to the DTP/Hib vaccine that:

> *The overall pattern and type of suspected reactions in 2000 were similar to previous years, with the exception of an increase in the number of respiratory*

---

158 https://childhealthsafety.files.wordpress.com/2011/01/attkisson-cbs-hrsa-email-exchanges-autistic-conditions-vaccines.pdf

159 https://www.huffingtonpost.com/david-kirby/post2468343_b_2468343.html

reactions. Most of the increase appeared to be due to ***an increase in number of SIDS*** *and apnoea type reactions reported.* [160]

Does all this angry shaking cause respiratory reactions and sudden death? Unlikely piled on unlikely if you ask me. Nevertheless in the UK and US alone hundreds of parents and caregivers are now charged each year, with at least three on death row in the US. According to Deborah Tuerkheimer, author of 'Flawed Convictions: Shaken Baby Syndrome and the Inertia of Justice', there are 1,000 innocent Americans in prison for killing or disabling babies by vigorous, violent shaking. [161]

Incredibly the criteria for guilt in these trials rests upon the prosecutor proving a triad of physical effects: bleeding into the linings of the eyes; beneath the dural membrane; encephalopathy, which is damage to the brain affecting its function. And that's it! Deadly serious of course but certainly not proof of murders, which are essentially being diagnosed by doctors. But this is what's happening to keep hidden the vaccine effect. This is extreme internal brain disruption that doesn't involve a fractured or broken skull or trauma to the neck. It's a creepy thing to ponder but how do you do that with your hands in a fit of rage? And how do you validate such a hypothesis? Double blind placebo trial perhaps? It strikes me they have no choice but to stack up these ridiculous cover stories in order to keep the lie hidden. It's like a landfill of lies!

Dr Waney Squier is a world-renowned neuropathologist, at John Radcliffe Hospital in Oxford, just about. For years she gave expert witness in prosecution of the accused baby shakers, but upon recognising the folly in the quack-pot theory she switched sides. Her credentials are impeccable.

Once I came here I specialised in baby brains. I have looked at thousands and written more than 100 medical papers on normal brain development and what happens when things go wrong both in pregnancy and after birth. In the past 15 years, I have investigated many unexpected deaths.

She is no longer sharing her expertise and simply speaking her truth; in doing so she has blown the whistle and has become an enemy of the state. As such she is also an enemy of the state of mind of others and an honorary conspiracy theorist. She had argued in over 200 legal cases in the UK and the US, occasionally, in a "manner in which" the General Medical Council disciplinary panel deemed unacceptable, to suggest that the triad of symptoms taken as a sign of child abuse may have other causes. D'y think? I think shaking is the least likely but it is the most talked about, while vaccines are the most likely and the least talked about. This is more science fiction than fact, making this just another unproven unlikely medical theory with as many critics as implications.

Waney Squier's radicalisation in honour of the truth led to her being struck off the medical register in March 2017 by these high priests of drug medicine. A High Court

160 http://parentsandcarersagainstinjustice.weebly.com/uploads/2/5/2/8/25284293/04_jcvi_meeting_04th_may_2001.pdf

161 http://www.medilljusticeproject.org/2013/12/10/hot-spots/

judge ordered her reinstatement six months later citing "serious irregularity" in the GMC case, but she was nevertheless banned from appearing as expert witness in brain damaged baby cases for three years. Silenced in court! This of course does the opposite of protect the public since it was the public she was assisting against the state machine and its evil mechanisms. But it isn't about protecting the public is it, or that would be the outcome.

The GMC medical panel chairman was a retired RAF wing commander. The panel further comprised of a retired geriatric psychiatrist and a retired senior policeman. Like that rock band: the Status Quo!

And to maintain the status quo top spot: a cover up. "I still feel that it's not safe to give an opinion, so I can't risk my job by giving evidence in court", says Irene Scheimberg, one of the few experts in this field in the UK who had dared to speak in defence of the accused, but seeing the way others are treated no longer feels it's safe to do so.[162] It's 2017 and we are living a lie.

Dr Squier is appealing but whatever the outcome we can see how the chilling effect will continue playing its part. And more and more innocent parents and carers and nanny's will be left prey to a criminal injustice system that has eliminated the opposition, leaving them with no one to speak in their defence.

The vaccine schedule is protected for now but its days are numbered.

In 2009 Judy Mikovits, PhD in microbiology and biochemistry, announced to the scientific community her groundbreaking discovery that a significant number of patients suffering with Chronic Fatigue Syndrome, M.E., autism, Parkinson's and cancers, were also harbouring a group of xenotropic murine-related viruses, known as XMRVs', which had at some point somehow transferred from their natural reservoir – mice - into humans, and may be suggestive of a disease link. This revelation, as a potential link to a cause and effect and a cure, could and should have been announced to the world as a significant medical breakthrough potentially affecting hundreds of millions of people. And this could have restored some credibility to the shattered reputation of the medical profession for whom most diseases and cures are a mystery. But this was all spoiled the minute Mikovits uttered that one fateful word central to her findings.

Vaccines.

And with that all hell broke loose on the brave Dr Mikovits and another illustrious career was forced head first down the toilet.

> *When they destroyed all of our work, and discredited everything I or Frank Ruscetti had ever published, and arranged for the publication of my mug shot in Science, the NIH [National Institute of Health] very deliberately sent the*

162 https://www.newscientist.com/article/mg23230994-100-evidence-of-shaken-baby-questioned-by-controversial-study/#bx309941B1

message to researchers everywhere about what would happen to any honest scientist who dared ask those important questions. [163]

The ortho-docs and their well oiled machine had gathered around Mikovits like a gang of football hooligans. She was threatened and ordered to destroy her data. Indignant, she refused to bury the truth and was then arrested for supposedly stealing data from her workplace, fired, charged and imprisoned. While she was out of the way her data really was then stolen and has been hidden from the world ever since, to protect us from uncomfortable truths. Freed but accused she was gagged by order of the court for the next four years until the charges were dropped and the gag order lifted. But by then she's a quack, the vaccines are safer than ever because another quack has been routed from the holy order, and I'm a fairy. In reality the cat is out of the bag and everyone knows that the viruses are swarming out of the vaccines.

- ***The xenotropic murine leukemia virus-related virus (XMRV) is undoubtedly the most controversial human virus since its first detection in human samples in 2006.*** *The combined results suggest (1) that XMRV was recently transmitted from mice to humans, either from a single source, or at least from a single (sub) species of mice, and (2) that all XMRV-positive individuals known today were infected with this newly emerged virus only recently, as a very high sequence identity is normally only seen after a direct retrovirus transmission.*

  Among the biological products, ***vaccines that were produced in mice or mouse cells are possible candidates that warrant further inspection.***

  Whatever the mechanism of XMRV cross-species transmission from mouse in humans, the possible spread from human to human forms a major health threat. [164]

- *The most likely mode of XMRV transmission points to mouse-derived biological products.* [164]

- *There is potential biohazard risk from this virus for humans. Moreover, the fact that productively infected cells... have spread infection to other cell lines, raises the possibility that laboratory workers could have been unknowingly exposed to the virus... the possibility of infection by XMRV (or other xenotropic MLVs) in humans (particularly in the laboratory setting) should be considered. At a minimum, standard biosafety precautions for handling xenotropic viruses as well as screening of laboratory cell lines for infection with xenotropic MLVs is important.* [165]

---

[163] https://vimeo.com/146831570

[164] https://www.ncbi.nlm.nih.gov/pmc/articles/PMC3109487/

[165] https://www.nature.com/articles/emi201425

- *Virus-based vaccines are made in living cells (cell substrates). Some manufacturers are investigating the use of new cell lines to make vaccines. The continual growth of cell lines ensures that there is a consistent supply of the same cells that can yield high quantities of the vaccine.*

  In some cases ***the cell lines that are used might be tumorigenic****, that is, they form tumors when injected into rodents.* ***Some of these tumor-forming cell lines may contain cancer-causing viruses*** *that are not actively reproducing.* ***Such viruses are hard to detect*** *using standard methods. These* ***latent, or "quiet," viruses pose a potential threat, since they might become active under vaccine manufacturing conditions****. Therefore, to ensure the safety of vaccines, our laboratory is* ***investigating ways*** *to activate latent viruses in cell lines and* ***to detect the activated viruses****, as well as other unknown viruses, using new technologies. We will then adapt our findings to detect viruses in the same types of cell substrates that are used to produce vaccines.* ***We are also trying*** *to identify specific biological processes that reflect virus activity.* [166]

I blame the mice. And their parents.

Whatever, this is what we get back from allowing age old theories to dominate long past sell-by-date and to direct our health goals. But the good news is we have reinforced that life saving lesson: **all the vaccines are contaminated**. Go science!

Mikovits and her small research team found that at least 30% of the vaccines are contaminated with these mouse viruses which are appearing in a very high percentage of people with certain, modern diseases. Dr Mikovits asks, "How many new retroviruses have we created through all the mouse research, the vaccine research, gene therapy research? More importantly, how many new diseases have we created?" [167]

Always good to ask but I think we have a pretty good instinct that it's way too many.

When you look around now you see cot (vaccine) deaths, SIDS, schizophrenia, skin allergies, food allergies, dyslexia, stuttering, [168] tics [169] & tourettes, **A**utism**SD**, 'special needs', epilepsy, handicap, ADD/ADHD (Attention Deficit Hyperactivity Disorder - whatever that might be - it's a most confused category in which they dump the super sharp kids who are bored to distraction with mainstream teaching alongside those they vaccine damage) and the less overt learning difficulties and behavioral abnormalities and neurodevelopmental disorders, to low grade or full blown encephalitis, M.E., cancer and others yet uncategorised. They'll insist they

---

166 https://www.fda.gov/biologicsbloodvaccines/scienceresearch/biologicsresearchareas/ucm127327.htm

167 https://www.organiclifestylemagazine.com/vaccines-retroviruses-dna-and-the-discovery-that-destroyed-judy-mikovits-career

168 https://iaomt.org/TestFoundation/pdffiles/vaccinesafety.pdf

169 http://fearlessparent.org/wp-content/uploads/2016/04/Thompson-transcript-recording_04_Fearless-Parent.pdf

don't know where all this stuff came from while insisting the vaccines are keeping us safe!

Where else did this explosion in brain damage and immune suppressed illnesses, allergies and multitude syndromes arrive from in recent years? Corresponding needles of unsafe, untested, unproven neurotoxins and heavy metals or just one of those things? Is it really worth the risk or better to chance a natural immune boost of Mother Nature's pure infections and lifelong protection that you can safely then pass down to your children? The older generation is of course being struck down with Alzheimer's, Parkinson's and dementia which are often linked with suspect vaccine ingredients. Of course there are other sources. We're in the age of aluminium after all with an insidious drip-feed from cook wear, baby food, food wrapping and underarm deodorants. Armpits loaded with aluminium nanoparticles are like one of those events waiting to happen! Then there's the incessant geoengineering of the skies, more commonly known as chemtrails, which contain aluminium. [170]

Chris Exley is a professor in bioinorganic chemistry based at Keele University, he reached some quite radical conclusions. I say quite because he had to tone it down and leave something out. See if you can spot what:

> *Environmental or occupational exposure to aluminium results in higher levels of aluminium in human brain tissue and an early onset form of sporadic Alzheimer's disease.*
>
> *The genetic predispositions which are used to define familial or early-onset Alzheimer's disease also predispose individuals to higher levels of brain aluminium at a much younger age.*
>
> ***Aluminium is accepted as a known neurotoxin, for example being the cause of dialysis encephalopathy, and its accumulation in human brain tissue at any age can only contribute to any ongoing disease state or toxicity.***
>
> *There has been a strong link between human exposure to aluminium and the incidence of Alzheimer's disease for half a century or more. However, without definite proof, there is still no consensus in the scientific community about the role of this known neurotoxin in this devastating brain disease.*
>
> *The latest research from my group, published in the Journal of Trace Elements in Medicine and Biology, makes this link even more compelling. In my view, the findings are unequivocal in their confirmation of a role for aluminium in some if not all Alzheimer's disease.*

---

170 http://www.geoengineeringwatch.org/lab-tests-2/

> *This new research may suggest that these genetic predispositions to early onset Alzheimer's disease are linked in some way to the accumulation of aluminium (**through 'normal' everyday human exposure**) in brain tissue.*
>
> *We should take all possible precautions to reduce the accumulation of aluminium in our brain tissue through our everyday activities and we should start to do this as early in our lives as possible.* [171]

A profound perhaps logical conclusion. We should be aware of all potential sources but we're sticking with the aluminium in vaccines partly because wherever you look it's like everyone is afraid they'll be struck down if they speak ill of the vaccine. Vaccines are a common denominator young and old, but shuuush! Blame the baby, blame the budgie but don't mention vaccines. The very principle of inoculating someone with an artificial boost should be debated openly and honestly but we are so far from that place. We are no longer dealing with the principle of immunisation; we are dealing with big business in the hands of extremists and with corruption and negligence on an unprecedented scale. Of course they don't want to talk about it!

Vaccines have become one of those taboo subjects around which there is simply nothing more to know. The experts and the repeaters know it all yet are desperate to stifle the inquiry of others, while protecting a ruthless band of thugs working tirelessly to steal our natural individual immunity and sell it back to us crude and inferior and mass produced.

Our ancestors weren't just experts at making spear heads, jewellery, clay pots and pyramids they were experts at surviving viruses too using all the wonders of the natural world. For millions of years the human child has beaten all comers naturally using an ancient biologically programmed immune system. Only in recent years have we been persuaded to stop believing in ourselves and programmed to believe we now need Big Daddy's boosters to help keep us going. It makes no sense and what of our future if we carry on believing that longevity is another needle away? How many needles can one infant take? Think about that or they will keep them coming.

In the UK even before Wakefield sounded the alarm decent non-medical citizens were also raising concerns regarding the safety of vaccines in the exploding 1980's schedule. We are now going to see for ourselves how these very real concerns for the safety of children were received and addressed by the top medical experts at the heart of the vast vaccine programme. We've touched on some shocking details already and this is more of the same. Deep and dark at the highest level. At the end of the day it is the medical people at the CDC and the Joint Committee on Vaccination and Immunisation etc that clear the way for all the vaccines and the cancer drugs. Here the buck stops.

When I tell regular people that these top medical professionals are the real terrorists they look at me with concern. For me, mostly, with not a thought for the

---

[171] https://www.hippocraticpost.com/mental-health/strong-evidence-linking-aluminium-alzheimers/

ramifications of such a reality, which it seems most people *know* is simply not true. Doctors save lives so it must be a conspiracy theory. That's the programming. In the next couple of chapters I will give you a feel for how we come up with such theories. It actually takes a lot more courage to deny the truth of what's going on here.

This first exchange regarding the pertussis/whooping cough vaccine took place at a meeting of the JCVI. Don't get bogged down with all the high titles. Where a bunch of Dr's, Mr's and PhD's meet regularly in private to pave the way for more of the same there is no brilliance and no genuine oversight, this is classic status quo disguised under acronyms.

> *If the public was given a risk ratio - any ratio – they would still see it as a scientifically proven risk. It was therefore preferable not to use insecure figures if possible but to stress the benefits from vaccination.* [172]

During the 1980's the JCVI and the National Childhood Encephalopathy Study (NCES) were juggling well over a thousand vaccine related legal claims and they were desperate for someone else to blame. Dozens of these, "vaccine-associated cases" of brain damaged children who had been hit with the triple vaccine in the week prior to the onset of their neurological illness were children who, our experts claimed, had a "history of neurological events before immunisation **which indicated possible prior abnormality."** So it's not really the vaccine's fault. [173]

Bad babies.

Science is good in the right hands but this is not good. What is it they say about informed consent? And it's not just the one bad apple it's the top layer of the cart and the rot is dribbling on the rest.

This inflated meeting of medical minds in 1987 between the Committee on Safety of Medicines (CSM), the JCVI and the Joint Sub-Committee on Adverse Reactions to Vaccines and Immunisation gives us a flavour for the real intent. Headed with the warning 'COMMERCIAL IN CONFIDENCE. NOT FOR PUBLICATION', we learn

> *The CSM had called for ARVI's advice about updating the statement made in the 1981 report on Whooping Cough (HMSO)* ***about a possible link between DTP immunisation and serious neurological illness, it had been hoped that by this means of 'discovery' of all the relevant JCVI, CSM and ARVI documentation on whooping cough vaccine could be avoided.*** *However… it was already clear that nothing could be done to avoid discovery.* [174]

---

[172] JCVI Meeting 3 November 1989: http://webarchive.nationalarchives.gov.uk/20130123173003/http://www.dh.gov.uk/ab/DH_095169

[173] https://parentsandcarersagainstinjustice.weebly.com/uploads/2/5/2/8/25284293/17_csm_jcvi_arvi_3rd_oct_1986.pdf

[174] (4. item 5.1 Whooping cough disease, vaccination, vaccine damage.)
http://parentsandcarersagainstinjustice.weebly.com/uploads/2/5/2/8/25284293/22_csm_jcvi_arvi_6th_july_1987.pdf

Not so much concern there about blood leaking from baby brains more about the truth leaking and spoiling the illusion. Still not a conspiracy?

A year prior, they discussed in another private meeting how they disapproved of

> *… the use of the term 'brain damage' in reference with the whooping cough vaccine which the public might consider as a permanent entity, the public may also not understand the significance of febrile convulsions.* [175]

Brain damage is another of those terms that I think speaks for itself, but in this field of compartmentalised medicine everything is made more confusing. In the mid 1980's with the new wave of children whose brains had been damaged by doctors, partly out of desperation but equally from that difference of opinions that makes us all unique, a whole library of phrases, reasons, excuses and even a scattering of science emerged to mask the reality of what was going on. In 1985 the Japanese Journal of Medical Science and Biology published a startling and sickening early warning:

> *Administration of* ***the pertussis vaccine causes a variety of untoward reactions in children****. The most distressing reactions are* ***encephalopathy*** *and* ***neurological disturbances*** *which have occasionally been observed and in rare cases produced* ***severe brain damage*** *and* ***even death****.*
>
> *Although there have been numerous reports on the biological activities and toxic substances of B pertussis cultures and of pertussis vaccine, there is little information concerning the possible factor(s) responsible for* ***postvaccination encephalopathy*** *or neurological disturbances.*

Fcuk! Now what? Pull the vaccine? Nah!

> ***A major reason why such an unfavorable situation has lasted for a long time may be the total lack of an experimental model for studying the postvaccination neurological complications****.*

So they decide instead to continue the search for that special laboratory animal to replicate the vaccine damage they have caused in children and take it from there. This is where science really comes into its own, by finding answers to the hard questions and making stuff safe that shouldn't even be on the market in the first place if it isn't!

Here's what the geniuses came up with:

Suckling mice, fresh into the world of the warped, were injected "intercerebally" (into their baby brains) with a dribble of the whooping cough vaccine and soon after they were killed, thus: "Exanguinating from both the carotid and jugular cut with a pair of scissors." Seriously, obliviously to their drift from humanity, using a pair of

---

[175] https://parentsandcarersagainstinjustice.weebly.com/uploads/2/5/2/8/25284293/12_csm_jcvi_arvi_7th_feb_1986.pdf

scissors the life-saving vivisecting scientists took off the heads of our fellow earthlings "harvested" the brains tested them against the saline control mice and discovered a pattern of brain damage, not dissimilar to that caused in the children.

> ***A significant increase in the mean brain weight of the mice inoculated with the vaccine****… the brain swelling reached the maximum on day 1 and persisted for at least 5 days. A 6 to 12% increase in the mean brain weight was induced by injection of the vaccine.*

Bingo! Let the well crafted science speak!

Now we pull the vaccine, right? Wrong! Wake up! Only in the world of crazy could such a conclusion as this be reached: they ignored the results. Having got their scientist approved confirmation of a brain damaging vaccine they decide instead to stick and search some more, concluding in a kind of scientist plea to fellow researchers everywhere:

> *It is important to develop a useful animal model for evaluating neurological complications following vaccination with pertussis vaccine.* [176]

Status quo still top of the charts! That was 30 years ago and the search continues for that special little magic mouse to save us from all ills.

The CSM itself is on record accepting that a "prima facie case" may exist between the DTP vaccine and "serious neurological illness" and admit that "the vaccines could cause **complex febrile convulsions**", which "**could result in permanent handicap**" yet they roll out the vaccine regardless. [177] We are meant to be confused by this medical research process of course and anyone who says any of this makes sense is a fool.

The cover up queen at the CDC Julie Gerberding tried not to admit in a CNN interview in 2008 what she knows as well as anyone about vaccines causing autism in healthy babies, while confessing that "complications from the vaccine… can certainly set off some **damage**" in children with an underlying mitochondrial disorder and that "some of the symptoms can be symptoms that have characteristics of autism". The "characteristics" of disease become the disease when? After legal proceedings are over or when the parents are too exhausted to fight any longer? Mothers have been reporting these characteristic signs of damaged children for decades and there we have it: a criminal confession!

Noteworthy in that stunning public announcement is her acknowledgement that if a child when attending for vaccination "has **what we think is a rare** mitochondrial disorder… anything that stresses them creates a situation where their cells can't

---

176 https://www.jstage.jst.go.jp/article/yoken1952/38/2/38_2_53/_pdf

177 (7.1 Whooping Cough Vaccine) https://parentsandcarersagainstinjustice.weebly.com/uploads/2/5/2/8/25284293/19_csm_jcvi_arvi_6th_feb_1987.pdf

make enough energy to keep their brains functioning normally..." [178] And the vaccine sets off that bomb.

In this interview I hear that brain damage/autism is caused by vaccines and I calculate from this that children with undiagnosed mitochondrial disorders/dysfunction need to be exempt the injections and urgently. Like duh! But how?

Based on what I have studied I think the mitochondrial disorder is likely caused by the vaccines and gets worse in some kids the more vaccinations they have, and since they haven't done any studies to prove otherwise I'm sticking. The ortho-docs will continue to twirl around in the middle of the circle with their eyes wide shut like kids in the playground, pointing the finger of blame at genetics, parents and the fatally flawed children they've damaged. And eventually they'll be found to be correct if we allow this to continue another generation - it will be all our fault and our genes will be screwed.

After several years of Alice being poked at hopelessly by ortho-docs, we left them to poke at other people and went to see a doctor of functional medicine who carried out an organic acid test and found this mitochondrial dysfunction. Since the mitochondria generate energy for every cell in the body and are malfunctioning, increasing the demand, as the ortho-docs suggest with their graded exercise ideas, can be so devastating for M.E. (Myalgic Encephalomyelitis) patients. Lucky she had no more vaccines in the meantime eh, as some of these doctors suggested she must, to "protect" her from the flu and shingles! Really lucky. We suspect the last vaccine they hit her with as a teenager, for meningitis, is what tipped her over. Soon after this she deteriorated, her nose started to bleed regularly, she began suffering with abdominal issues and then steadily all else fell apart. She later landed an M.E. diagnosis, kids less developed cop for 'autism' but it's the same type of disrupted methylation cycle and reduced glutathione levels causing oxidative stress and often caused by the same antagonists causing similar damage and requiring the same kind of treatment protocol. The meningitis campaign was launched in the UK in 1999.

> *The majority of the safety experience with Meningitec comes from a **single study** conducted in the United States... in which Meningitec was compared with [**another vaccine**]. Infants in this study received Meningitec or [other vaccine] on a 2, 4, 6 month schedule, **along with routine immunisation** with either DTP/Hib... or DTPa... The infants **may also have received other routine childhood vaccines**.* [179]

What a mess. This widely used vaccine was later withdrawn in the UK and the vaccine schedule changed. They planted their bombs and ran away to hide!

But here's the kicker. According to some, mitochondrial disorder affects around 1 in 4000 and is described officially as rare, others, based on more recent information

---

178 http://adventuresinautism.blogspot.co.uk/2008/03/julie-gerberding-admits-on-cnn-that.html

179 http://experimentalvaccines.org/wp-content/uploads/2014/12/Meningitec.pdf

think it's more like 1 in 50, but these are still estimates. Mitochondrial disorder is like autism and M.E/CFS etc and become labelled as such because we all respond in our own way to infection, toxicity and deficiency. Some may remain subclinical and undetected for decades; others suffer their pains daily while tormented by the wounded egos of a broken medical profession at war with these victims of their incompetence. [180]

We discovered in our journey that there is no reliable or approved means of diagnosis for human mitochondrial disorder using the lab animal technology that helped get us into this global health crisis. Mitochondrial disorder is another of the many unknowns that characterise orthodox medicine, but that doesn't matter because what we are told by them now is that anyone with a dysfunction in the mitochondria is at risk of vaccine-induced brain damage. These high risk categories are stacking up like doctor-induced diseases.

This on the face of it deflects attention from the perpetrators, but until they can actually diagnose mitochondrial disorders and then rule them out, then this danger is another unknown and they need to inform everyone they hope to inject that everyone is at risk of brain damage and that 'rare' can quickly become common and that none of this is based on science but theory.

However this brain damage is dressed up by the conspirators and whatever it is blamed upon, it often follows vaccination and it stunts the growth of whole families and causes suffering we cannot comprehend. A prima facie case is usually what kick starts a criminal prosecution, as those accused of shaking their babies to a state characterised by damaged brains can testify in droves.

For many years the fake health guardians at the JCVI have been working to a goal of more vaccines and less information. In 2001 with the world focussing its attention on that conspiracy theory about a James Bond super villain hiding in a mountain lair in a land far, far away controlling a war of terror on his laptop, the medicine men over here were promoting 3-in-1 vaccines as superior science. In fact the science was non-existent, they were merely restricting parental choice in order to increase sales because "It was felt that, should single vaccines be introduced, parents would inevitably pick and choose. This would result in reduced update of full required course..." [181]

By 2010 with the patent on Osama Bin Bogeyman expired, the easily led had their attention turned to quack bashing instead. While they were throwing rotten eggs and insults at Andy Wakefield, (who was at that time actually suggesting concerned parents use the single measles vaccine as an alternative for their babies until the MMR questions were resolved, which they never were) the JCVI baby killing conspirators were outlining their enthusiasm to boost vaccine uptake further by

---

180 https://www.huffingtonpost.com/david-kirby/the-next-big-autism-bomb-_b_93627.html

181 (7.2.4). http://parentsandcarersagainstinjustice.weebly.com/uploads/2/5/2/8/25284293/04_jcvi_meeting_04th_may_2001.pdf

quietly introducing the 6-in-1 special into the kid's schedule. This was guided by a Department of Health Market Research study. Given the passage of time and the weight of evidence Wakefield has evolved his thinking on all the vaccines and now thinks even one is too many.

A single dose vaccine would be a reasonable compromise you might think, but none of this is reasonable. Instead of allowing parents this choice, the UK government guided by the experts running the JCVI (who work together with vaccine makers) quickly pulled the single measles vaccine from the market forcing concerned parents to either overdose or face accusations of neglecting their children.

The Market Research study report, which wasn't meant to be shown to us plebs either, was headed 'Market Research 2010 Childhood Immunisation Programme: Attitudinal Research into Combining 12 and 13 Month Immunisations'. This incredible insight into the inner workings of the medical establishment was only released to researcher and author Christina England under via the Freedom of Information Act (FOIA) and would otherwise have remained hidden from the public. This also helps us paint our picture on informed consent.

> *It is also clear that* ***offering parents detailed information,*** *and flagging up changes, can generate anxiety where it is not warranted. In light of this, it seems sensible to introduce the combined schedule as far as possible* ***without announcing it explicitly as a change.*** (Conclusions and Recommendations: 6)

To secretly give the children lethal poisons!

> ***Offering parents a choice between the two schedules could generate more questions than answers, and seems unwise. It might also risk compromising current understandings of the vaccination schedule as 'just what happens', and reframing it as optional, which could negatively affect vaccine uptake.*** (Conclusions and Recommendations: 5)

See their priorities? Regarding the tear-off sheet on side effects:

> *There are diverging views on when the sheet should be given to parents; on balance it seems wise to hand it out immediately before vaccination, so that parents* ***feel they have been given advance warning, but do not dwell on the content to the extent that they begin to worry.***
>
> *Finally, it is important that the information given by health professionals is* ***pitched at the right level****. Clearly, the JCVI information prompted questions among many respondents, but was useful for reassuring some, particularly those with a more pragmatic view of immunisation. Information at this level needs to be* ***carefully tailored*** *by health professionals according to*

> *the* ***attitudes*** *of individual parents. If in doubt,* ***we would suggest keeping it simple****, as outlined above.* [182]

The truth is the truth. If it isn't the truth it's a lie.

There are thousands of associated studies and in-house exchanges that expose these people and the products they peddle for what they are and we have some juicy stuff to come plotting the full extent of the cover up and the deception and leaving no room for silly coincidence theories. The conspiracy is proven. I've experienced first-hand what it takes to be charged with a conspiracy and this would be a prosecutor's party. And when taken as a whole there is no hope of revealing a picture of safety, efficacy or necessity in the middle of the scheming, but either one of these essential elements improperly established and the science is out of the window. Necessity takes us to the heart of the problem. A picture paints a thousand words, right? Let's take look at necessity.

In assessing the rise and fall of any communicable disease, it is essential to examine its background of secular and cyclical trends. Historically, the dominant and obvious fact is that most, if not all, major communicable diseases of childhood have become less serious in all developed countries for 50 years or more. Whooping cough is no exception. It has behaved in this respect exactly like measles and similarly to scarlet fever and diphtheria, in each of which at least 80% of the total decline in mortality, since records began to be kept in the United Kingdom in 1860, occurred before any vaccines or antimicrobial drugs were available and 90% or more before there was any national vaccine programme. [183]

Gordon T. Stewart Department of Community Medicine, University of Glasgow. 1981.

---

[182] https://parentsandcarersagainstinjustice.weebly.com/uploads/2/5/2/8/25284293/13_mar_res_childhood_immun_prog_attitudinal_research_combining_12_and_13_month_immunisations_june_2010.pdf

[183] http://jech.bmj.com/content/jech/35/2/139.full.pdf

Unnecessary Evil

There has been a steady decline in infectious diseases in most developing countries regardless of the percentage of immunisation administered in those countries.
WHO, World Health Statistics Annual, 1973-76, Vol.2

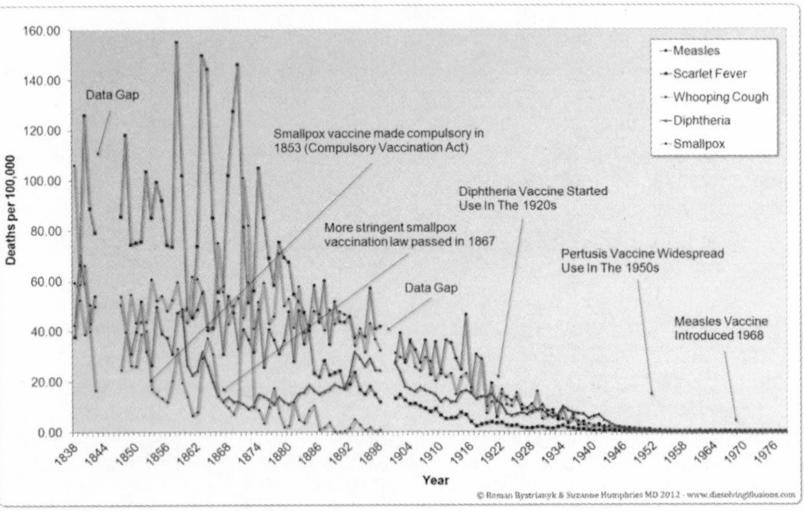

184

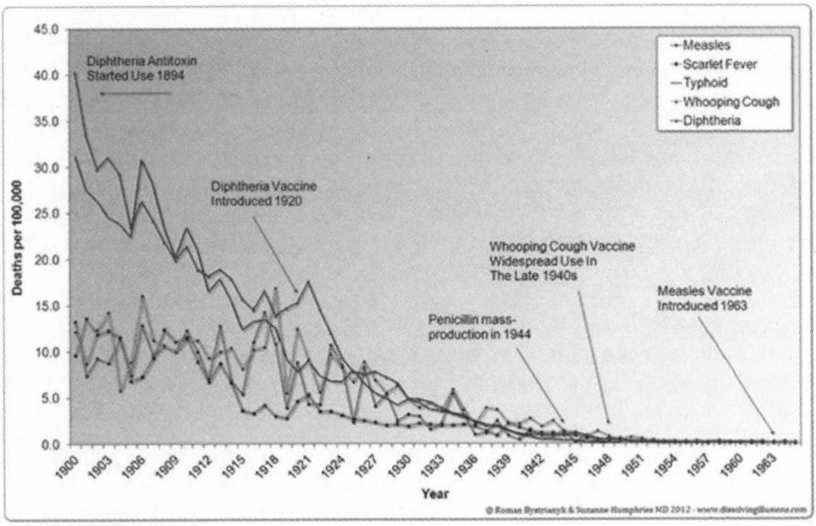

185

---

184 England & Wales Mortality Rates. http//vaxinfostarthere.com/did-vaccines-save-us/

185 US Mortality Rates. https://childhealthsafety.wordpress.com/graphs/#MortUK_USA_Aus

Makes you wonder, huh? Covering up the open sewers and separating the water supply and the industrial human masses from toxic filth from the late 1800's onwards did this, alongside natural building herd immunity, and not the addition of injectable toxins. All the official data from this time in our recent history and the witnesses clearly paint this picture. The way we lived and died in the very recent past paints not such a pretty picture, but seeing so graphically how we revolutionised social living, sanitation and disease control, well that does.

So, if vaccines aren't necessary then safety and efficacy are surplus to requirements and that's quite apt given what we are learning about safety and efficacy.

When you properly investigate vaccines, from the half told story of Jenner's cow pox claims to the clamour for anti allergy vaccines, you can't ignore the intriguing 'Leicester Method'. When we look at this story we realise that vaccines have been an issue for what seems an inordinate length of time, but it's much more than that. This proves there is another way.

From the heart of the public resistance in the English east midland town of Leicester at the end of the 1800's the people were elevating the vaccine issue beyond anything witnessed before or since. The poor working people had been bearing the brunt of the vax fanatics and they were rebelling over the loss of freedoms and at the harm the compulsory injections were doing in their communities. We are again at that point in the cycle. The turning point.

At the pinnacle of this social revolt in 1885 an estimated 80,000 - 100,000 protestors from anti-vaccine leagues across the country gathered in Leicester to protest what they had experienced for nearly 100 years - the increasing aggressive vaccine programmes that saw thousands arrested and many voluntarily imprisoned for resisting and refusing to submit their infants to the vaxers. This international uprising was built in no small part by the Leicester Anti Vaccination League formed in 1869 and according to one record of this rebellion; it "came to have an influence out of all proportion to its size". I can't do justice here but for a statistically significant self regulated social experiment Leicester stands head and shoulders above the rest and is irreplaceable evidence that we can do better than vaccines, when we choose.

The Leicester Method was simple and beautiful. It relied on the cooperation of everyone working in the interest of each other and the vaxers told where to shove their lethal potions. With the vaxers warning of epidemics for everyone, in Leicester by 1887 the vaccination coverage rates had plummeted to 10% yet the death rate from infection was zero.

A sign of the times

Enforcing the Vaccination Laws.

Photo of an abortive Sale at East Croydon, May 3rd, 1907.

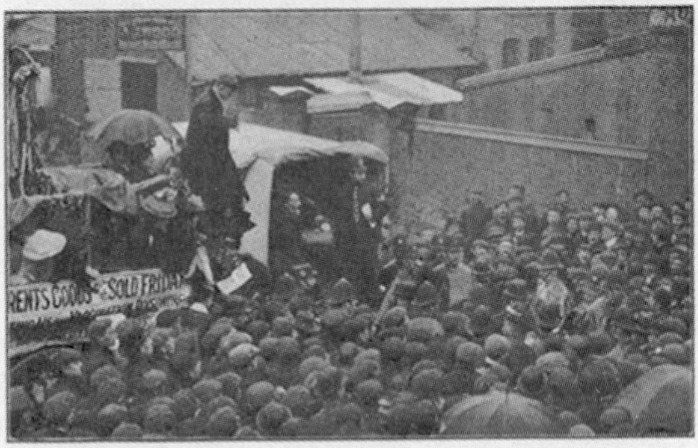

The Clerk to the Croydon Magistrates stated that over two thousand Vaccination Summonses had been applied for in Croydon. During recent years, six distress sales and attempted sales have been held, involving hundreds of cases of Fines and Costs. About fifty Croydon fathers have gone to prison rather than have their children vaccinated, or pay monetary penalties imposed.

The last decade has witnessed an extraordinary decrease in vaccination, but nevertheless, the town has enjoyed an almost entire immunity from small-pox, there never having been more than two or three cases in the town at any one time. A new method for which great practical utility is claimed has been enforced by the sanitary committee of the Corporation for the stamping out of small-pox is one of the least troublesome diseases we have to deal with. The method of treatment, in a word, is this:- as soon as small-pox breaks out, the medical man and a householder are compelled under penalty to at once report the outbreak to the Corporation. The small-pox van is at once ordered by telephone to make all the arrangements, and thus, within a few hours, the sufferer is safely in the hospital. The family and inmates of the house are placed in quarantine in comfortable quarters, and the house thoroughly disinfected. The result is that in every instance the disease has been promptly and completely stamped out at a paltry expense. Under such a system the Corporation have expressed their opinion that vaccination is unnecessary, as they claim to deal with the disease in a more direct and a much more efficacious manner. This and the widespread belief that death and disease have resulted from the operation of vaccination, may be said to be the foundation upon which the existing opposition to the Acts rests.

"Anti-Vaccination Demonstration at Leicester", The Times 24, 1885.

The role of the scientists and assorted experts is to replicate. Go on then! The survival of Leicester's brave citizens continued to surpass all expectations from there on and the dire medical predictions of the worst epidemic ever just around the corner for those who rejected diseased injections never came to pass. Elsewhere the vaccinated suffered significantly elevated death rates.

> *Leicester had less than one-third of the cases of small-pox and less than one-fourth the deaths in proportion to the well - vaccinated Birmingham; so that both the alleged protection from attacks of the disease and the mitigation of its severity when it does attack, are shown not only to be absolutely untrue, in this case, to the absence of vaccination.* **J.W. Hodge MD describing the 1891 – 1894 smallpox outbreak in the Vaccination Superstition 1902.**

> *Not only may well-vaccinated towns be affected with small-pox, but the most thorough vaccination of a population that is possible to imagine may be followed by an extensive outbreak of the disease. This happened in... Mold, in Flintshire... [in 1893] Leicester with a population under ten years practically unvaccinated, had a small-pox death-rate of 144 per million; whereas Mold, with all the births vaccinated for eighteen years previous to the epidemic, had one of 3,614 per million.* **William Scott Tebb, MD, A Century of Vaccination and What It Teaches, 1898.**

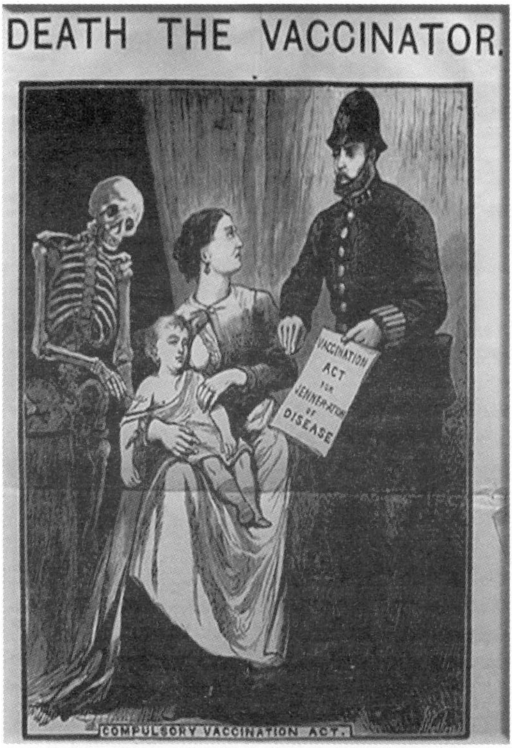

We can tell ourselves and each other that they wouldn't do harm to our children but that doesn't change the fact that a great deal of harm is being done to our children, and why? When a baby gets infected naturally with a communicable disease, his immune system responds through a sophisticated chain of reactions that generates a permanent key to that disease DNA. This is a lesson in life and as old as the beast and as efficient as life itself. I think it's always best to do it as nature intended and to do it with the very best of intention.

Vaccines intercept this natural process and add that toxic mix of live or killed viruses, matured in animal and human body parts, mixed with proteins from other species, killed bacteria, genetically engineered DNA and RNA fragments and chemical preservatives, injected into the muscles, the blood, the brain and the baby. This entire process is abnormal: square peg, round hole. The use of a needle bypasses natural immune defences, which in turn disables the necessary immune response through which these intricate systems learn to communicate and construct DNA access codes, mount a defence and strengthen. The crude tinkering of the quacks sends everything out of sync and deprives the body of its survival driven instinct to naturally imprint life-long immunity in all its unimaginable complexity.

Mass vaccination is a man made attempt to play god and get us to pay them for their service. We hear the rhetoric and rely on wishful thinking. They are seeking to conquer the human being and to replace our innate infection response with a seemingly endless bombardment of artificially imposed genetically modified viruses and a hopeful immune reaction determined by aggressive drug company vaccination schedules.

Who invited these people anyway? I don't remember all these diseases or any others wiping out my classmates in the 70's and 80's when this insane clamour to invest heavily to save every child from every ill gripped the controllers of orthodox medicine. What I do clearly remember was scheming to drag a dose out long enough to get me into a second week off school instead of the 3 or 4 days I needed to recover from the measles, chicken pox or tonsillitis. The need to prevent every ill is subjective, the desire is financial and it's based upon made up science.

Through the fog of two world wars and a heap of hype the vaxers had regained control of the agenda and Leicester had succumbed. It's 2001 at the Joint Committee on Vaccination and Immunisation and it's the same old story.

> *A large outbreak of tuberculosis had occurred in a Leicester secondary school.* ***Most of the affected... had been previously immunised with BCG.*** *There therefore appeared to be a high risk rate despite the use of vaccine. It was noted that despite the incomplete, and variable, efficacy of BCG vaccine in trials across the world, no new candidate vaccines appeared better than the existing BCG in animal models.* ***JCVI was content to await further evidence.*** [185]

What that says is the bargain basement technology did ok in some iffy animal tests and kinda passed the loaded clever sounding over-costed double-blind clinic trial process, so it makes no difference it doesn't work in children in the real world 'cos science is science and science keeps things nice and orderly.

Currently, the United States has the safest, most effective vaccine supply in its history.
CDC 2011

185 (10.2) http://parentsandcarersagainstinjustice.weebly.com/uploads/2/5/2/8/25284293/04_jcvi_meeting_04th_may_2001.pdf

Licence to Kill

Key elements of the immunization schedule – for example the number frequency timing age at the time of the administration of vaccines have not been systematically examined in research studies. Few studies have comprehensively assessed the association between the entire immunization schedule [of 69 doses up to 18 years of age in the US] or variations in the overall schedule and categories of health outcomes, and no study has directly examined health outcomes... No studies have compared the differences in health outcomes... between entirely unimmunized populations of children and fully immunized children. Experts who addressed the committee pointed not to a body of evidence that had been overlooked but rather to the fact that existing research has not been designed to test the entire immunization schedule.

Committee on the Assessment of Studies of Health Outcomes Related to the Recommended Childhood Immunization Schedule; Board on Population Health and Public Health Practice; Institute of Medicine. 2013

With all this vaccine damage you'd think the vaxers would be under some kind of pressure from litigants and lawyers and sure enough they were. But of course they had a different sort of solution to the problem in mind to what we might hope.

In the US drug companies had manipulated themselves liability protection under the National Childhood Vaccination Act 1986. The Vaccine Damage Payment Scheme (VDPS) is a provision of the welfare system in the United Kingdom and mirrors this rather attractive good business model which is predictably being rolled out globally. What this does is ensure that the ever escalating bill for vaccine damage is essentially sent to the parents of the vaccine damaged children and taken from the poor people's pot. The drug companies found themselves so bogged down by victims of the vaccines prosecuting for compensation that they bullied the US Congress to change the law to let them off the hook so they could concentrate on making money and not worry about legal disclosure and spending the wealth on hopelessly defending the dodgy science in endless court cases. And we can clearly see how they've loaded up the vaccine catalogue since the cost and the strain of quality control was lifted from their shoulders and the whining victims told where to go with their crackpot conspiracy theories.

During 1986 the JCVI were on hand for any troubles their friends in vaccine production might be having.

> *22 million doses of DTP were manufactured annually in the United States prior to difficulties concerning whooping cough vaccine and litigation. Since 1985, the price of vaccine has risen from 40 cents per dose to $ [unreadable] in 1986 and is expected to rise to $11 per dose. Litigation claims per year have risen from virtually nil in 1978/79 to over 219 in 1985, claiming [unreadable] billion dollars, and litigation suits follow a similar pattern. The total amount claimed has likewise greatly increased.*
>
> *... out of court settlements had not been included in these figures.* ***It was difficult to protect manufacturers against such heavy compensation***

claims. The situation has been aggravated by an organisation called 'Dissatisfied Parents Together'. (6.2)

The Hawkins Congressional Commission suggested that ***claimants might go into a system with a panel and if accepted*** *would be given an award of $1 million or alternatively accept court settlement. There was also a Bill before the American Government which suggested that punitive damages be done away with and that damages for pain and suffering only be awarded.* [186]

You can see when someone's actions are from the heart and maybe even recognise a necessary in an evil, but this is all about screwing kids and serving self. It was difficult enough already to prove vaccine injury when the defendants have failed to do any scientific studies on the long-term effects of their vaccines. The victim stories are therefore easily dismissed as anecdotal or incidental because there are no scientific trials to back them up or to compare to. And who will stand up to defend the poor victims placing their career on the line, facing demonisation, death threats and death?

This vaccine feeding frenzy fully took off in the few years after the licence to kill was in place. It was clearly planned. Hundreds of new vaccines are now being unleashed upon humanity, including HIV, DNA viruses, equine encephalitis virus and other encephalitis causing viruses, new influenza vaccines, respiratory viruses, vaccines for emerging diseases and agents of bioterrorism, human papilloma virus, herpes simplex, cytomegalovirus, new smallpox vaccines, childhood viruses, new rotavirus vaccines and chimeras using spliced genes, genetic modification and body parts and fragments you didn't even know existed. You know that money talks when it can buy exemption from justice for taking the health and destroying the future of young children and their families. You also now have absolute confirmation that there is no science to defend.

Vaccines are the final frontier in resource exploitation. A wide scale human mining operation of our own creation and maintenance. The numbers tell anyone who is paying attention that this is finite and they are going to extremes to exploit it to the max before it just like everything else exploited for money becomes so sick and depleted it is no longer viable. And why not! We seem to like them, there are no advertising costs, no marketing costs and no liability and by cramming multiple vaccines into each shot the overheads have come right down too. They use the principle of science to launch their product and science fiction to defend it; they use governments to sell their product through acts of terror paid for by the public which are promoted vigorously by the discredited mainstream media and self-service cancer charities.

Checkmate. This is a good business to be in.

---

[186] (6.1, 6.2) June 1986 http://webarchive.nationalarchives.gov.uk/20120503091024/http://www.dh.gov.uk/en/FreedomOfInformation/Freedomofinformationpublicationschemefeedback/FOIreleases/DH_4135306

Minutes of the JCVI meeting of May 5 1995 record the modus operandi brought to light by What Doctors Don't Tell You in complaints to the Advertising Standards Authority.

> *HEA MEASLES/RUBELLA CAMPAIGN REPORT: The HEA [Health Education Authority] did acknowledge the view that* ***the TV advertising had been a little frightening, and also that not enough information on the possible side-effects of the vaccine had been provided for some people.*** [187]

We can see how injecting babies with poison to make money based on lies could fit into the category of an evil crime. I tell you now you stand up in the dock and admit to the judge and jury that propaganda you have been spreading among vulnerable people instilling fear in order to manipulate them into handing over their babies, you're going down for a long stretch, sucker.

With no liability for killing people and making people sick (which is good for future business and so cutting more corners is a must) and capacity to cram even more vaccines into each needle, this thing is only going to go in one direction until we say no more. Then we can do great things with science and nutrition and repair some damage.

With the Dr's, Mr's and PhD's fronting this grotesque scam at the JCVI playing dare with the devil, we haven't a hope in hell if we play along. I hope they enjoy it there.

> 1990. ***The Chairman said that Departmental officials had recently met vaccine manufacturers who were keen to be informed, in confidence, of the outcome of JCVI discussions which might affect their own plans. Agreement was sought from the committee on the appropriateness of a summary of such discussions, cleared by the Chairman, being provided to manufacturers. The Committee agreed to this.*** [188]

Groups of people representing a criminal drug syndicate in secret negotiations with government officials and health professionals regarding a dangerous, covert medical agenda, each party in cahoots with mainstream media agents-of-deception using terror tactics against vulnerable citizens, each with a clear understanding of how much damage the vaccines are doing (ignorance being no defence anyway) and in full knowledge of how despicable they are. If this isn't a criminal conspiracy what is it?

Seriously, when we talk about conspiracies it's this kind of thing we mean. There are plenty of them but does it get more evil? To continue dismissing what these people

---

[187] (6.5) May 1995. http://webarchive.nationalarchives.gov.uk/20120907200905/http://www.dh.gov.uk/prod_consum_dh/groups/dh_digitalassets/@dh/@ab/documents/digitalasset/dh_117393.pdf

[188] May 1990. https://parentsandcarersagainstinjustice.weebly.com/uploads/2/5/2/8/25284293/02_jcvi_meetings_4_may_1990.pdf

are doing as some kind of fantasy is a personal choice. I think it's good to know what's being done to us and to our animals in our name and at our expense so we are certain of the facts before we choose to be part of it or not.

This cache of official documents have been mostly removed from government websites but are stored for all to see here. I look forward to a jury seeing them.

www.iamkeithmann.com

http://parentsandcarersagainstinjustice.weebly.com/uk-government-removed-documents.html

http://webarchive.nationalarchives.gov.uk/20120503091024/http://www.dh.gov.uk/en/FreedomOfInformation/Freedomofinformationpublicationschemefeedback/FOIreleases/DH_4135306

Quack: an ignorant, misinformed, or dishonest practitioner of medicine

In 2011 the US Supreme Court ruled that vaccines were "unavoidably unsafe" and reaffirmed the earlier legal exemption for vaccine makers stating that there should be no more litigation. In people speak 'unsafe' means dangerous; high risk; life threatening. Where vaccine profits are concerned it's a free for all, but this is all you need to know for that not to matter. All the responsibility falls on you and again it's not me saying that it's them, so you need to get this right. And you need to tell everyone you know because most people are still unaware that the definitive legal advice on vaccines is the same as for tobacco, radioactive waste, second-hand syringes, rusty razor blades and predatory paedophiles. Keep well away from young children.

Of that unwanted list, curiously it is the vaccines that cause the greatest number of child victims and the one we willingly induce. In some places of course vaccines are mandated and they would like to force them upon us all from cradle to early grave. We need to wake up and shake up and fast.

The globalists are circling the human wagons and picking off one group at a time with their quack jabs. They have killed over 40,000 military personnel in recent years with the anthrax vaccine alone and forced hundreds of thousands of others into vaccine-induced syndromes, such as that they call Gulf War Syndrome, "to protect them from chemical weapons". It's a given that soldiers sign their lives away to corporate agendas, but any mass vaccine experiments with trusting human beings is sickening. Kids are being rounded up at birth particularly in the land of the free, which is the globalist model for the world, where they can be denied a state education and medical care if they refuse to be injected with every disease and poison combo on the pharma schedule, to *protect* them. They are trapping health care workers who in exchange for keeping their jobs have to agree to be injected with last years flu and a whole mess more which will make them flu carriers and may destroy their health, to *protect* patients.

It's the taxpayer who is now responsible for compensating the victims of vaccines, which are not even tested to the same dangerous, shoddy standards of the pharmaceuticals, and that's not so reassuring when we look at the damage they do! They get to dodge complying with these self-serving regulations by classifying this stuff in syringes as biologics. New name, new rules. Well, no rules really. No placebo trials needed to measure toxicity or effectiveness of this stuff cos vaccines are just a good idea, always have been always will be. And anyway they've been passed through lab loads of mice and monkeys so hey, whiz it up them kids.

Some vaccines appear worse than others and demonstrably affect more recipients in the short to midterm but who can quantify the long-term impact of those appearing more benign in the here and now? Certainly not the drug companies, they have washed their hands of all responsibility thank you very much. *You deal with it, it's yours, you consented.* Any practitioner could easily find what I can find but they get paid to write prescriptions and make referrals to colleagues and to sell products not to do research. And where are they going to find the time to do that and why would they bother and what are they going to do with all this information if they do the research? A Wakefield? Not on your Nelly! They'd end up in the do-do and just now business has friends in high places and business is booming.

It is incredible but should by now come as little surprise to hear that the kings of the castle at the Centres for Disease Control in the US actually hold patents for more than 50 vaccines and associated products and services. And the CDC itself buys billions of dollars worth of vaccines from the makers and sells them to the public health service. Conflicts of interest all over the place! So the CDC benefits and the public pay the price. The CDC is responsible for vaccine safety oversight, which they failed at, while benefiting to the tune of nearly $5billion annually from the sale of its vaccines. This was always going to turn out messy.

To get a flavour for some of their investment portfolio we can find CDC patents for vaccines for flu, rotavirus, hepatitis A, HIV, anthrax, rabies, dengue fever, West Nile virus, group A strep, pneumococcal disease, meningococcal disease, RSV, gastroenteritis, Japanese encephalitis, SARS, Rift Valley fever, and chlamydophila pneumoniae, nucleic acid vaccines for prevention of flavivirus infection, Zika, tick-borne encephalitis virus, yellow fever, Palm Creek virus, and Parramatta River virus, and more. The full list of the CDC products can be found here: [189] [190]

The CDC also has several patents for administering vaccines via aerosol delivery systems. This is a valuable step forward, potentially cutting the cost of all those needles and even less scary for the kids. Yeah! Maybe they'll mix it with the chemtrails and deliver it from the sky!

---

[189] https://www.google.co.uk/search?tbo=p&tbm=pts&hl=en&q=vaccine+inassignee:centers+inassignee:for+inassignee:disease+inassignee:control&tbs=,ptss:g&num=100&gws_rd=cr&ei=I6DiWMnTGeuWgAb0kaXADQ

[190] http://www.greenmedinfo.com/blog/examining-rfk-jrs-claim-cdc-owns-over-20-vaccine-patents

Before we move on try this for curious. Take the word vaccination and a calculator and appoint the number 6 to the letter A and work through the alphabet adding an additional 6 to each letter as you go. B =12, C =18 and so on. I = 54, N = 84, O = 90, T = 120, V = 132. Add up the numbers in the word VACCINATION. See if you see what I see. If you are keeping up with the story so far you probably have an idea what it will add up to. The answer is on page 412.

It has been demonstrated that inflammation may contribute to epileptogenesis and cause neuronal injury in epilepsy. In this study, the prevalence of antibodies to simian virus 40... a kidney and neurotropic polyomavirus, was investigated in serum samples from 88 epileptic children/adolescents/young adults.

A significantly higher prevalence of antibodies against SV40 was detected in sera from epileptic patients compared to controls. *Specifically, the highest significant difference was revealed in the cohort of patients from 1.1 to 10 years old with a peak in the sub-cohort of 3.1-6 years old.*

Our immunological data suggest a strong association between epilepsy and the SV40 infection. [191]

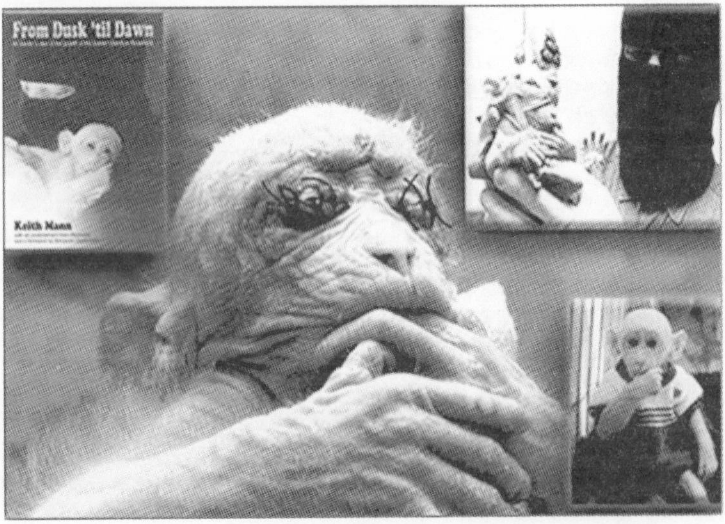

This is Britches, the Animal Liberation Front poster boy from the cover of my first book. He was a stump-tailed macaque used in some freaky experiment in the 1980's similar to the polio experiments of 30 years earlier. Today they are using the very same animals in the very same way to the very same end. Our acceptance of this defines not intellect but insanity.

---

[191] https://www.ncbi.nlm.nih.gov/pubmed/25598431

Setting the Stage

Because clinical trials are conducted under widely varying conditions, adverse reaction rates observed in the clinical trials of a vaccine cannot be directly compared to rates in the clinical trials of another vaccine and may not reflect the rates observed in practice. **FDA.gov**

My medical records arrived a few weeks after asking, but not a word about vaccines. Funny that. They will cling onto my criminal record way past my death but I was never officially vaccinated! Polio happened before I was age 2 but only notes from age 2 were included in my little bundle of photocopies at 50p per page. I wasn't surprised material was missing, more so that I got anything at all. I know better by now which is why I promptly set about my own vax inquiry, but I still felt let down. It's as if all the talking ends once the vaccines have been delivered. So, those bright sparks who put the SV40 cancer causing virus into me soon after my birth in 1966 have no way of monitoring any long-term effects. Such as cancer. I went to the GP surgery to ask of the absent notes and all I got from the receptionist were shrugged shoulders and informed that records aren't usually kept that long if at all because they aren't necessary because vaccines are safe. Words to that effect. It takes a hopeless leap of faith to reach such a conclusion and there is no point in any further discussion so I returned to my desk.

What did stand out in notes between doctors from 1969 through to 1973 were the constant references to enlarged lymph nodes and tonsils.

June 24 1969. Aged 3. Dr Murthy notes:

> *He looked well but had a cough... He had a few palpable glands in the neck.*

March 9 1972. Aged 5. Dr Buston:

> *On examination he looked well. He looked rather thin but his weight at 44lbs. was within the normal range for his age. A few small lymph nodes were palpable in his neck and his tonsils were moderately enlarged but no other abnormal signs were found.*

October 24 1973. Aged 7. Dr Chowdhury:

> *He has recently broken his right clavicle and is now receiving treatment. He has been seen by Mr Burns, who thought he was quite normal and so has been discharged from the Psychology Department. On examination he looked alright. No apparent abnormality could be detected in any system apart from a few enlarged lymph nodes.*

My mum recalls this lymph node thing being an issue for many years. She also recalls quite clearly the immediate effect the polio vaccine had on me and relayed to me often over the years how worried she was for me at the time. Seems to have had quite a lasting effect! She is 88 now and proud to see what I have turned these conspiring events into. She feels some guilt for the vaccine knowing what she now knows but it ain't her fault. It wasn't easy to know what was going on back then and we had less reason to mistrust the medicine men, but that trust has been abused.

While I am here, another albeit unrelated event of this period is recorded for posterity within my early medical records. Mum remembers clear as day the early morning of Xmas day 1972 when my brother and I got up very early to try and ambush Santa only to find we'd missed him. He had been though, and he'd left us a pile of wrapped up stuff, so we set about Xmas early before the parents woke. What happened next I don't quite believe to this day but, because it was 2am and we were cold, we decided to set fire to the Xmas wrapping paper heaped in a pile in the middle of the living room floor, to warm up! Don't try this at home.

Doesn't it burn!

In no time the carpet, sofa and living room were well alight as we tried hopelessly to pour first cups and then pans of water on the rapidly growing flames. But the water wasn't coming out of the taps quick enough and we failed terribly and that was pretty much the end of our Xmas. It was good while it lasted, which was about half an hour. But we did get to meet some firemen. I recall being carried on my dad's shoulders early Christmas morning back through the sodden, thoroughly gutted living room and kitchen. Financially we never really recovered from that and all I had to show for it was burnt Ted, my teddy bear who survived the blaze, and who I'm pretty sure the police took in a raid, some years later, on some place I used to live over some arson attack they blamed me for. Not sure quite what role they suspected Ted played but his ear was fire damaged and they had precious little else to go on so I can kinda see the point of holding him in the hope he might be evidence, but what gets me is he was never returned. They kidnapped my teddy bear!

Maybe when they let those guys out of Guantanamo Terror Ted will show up.

Dr Rowlands 1973:

> *I am pleased to say that Keith's chest is very much better after he has been on continuous Penbritin. The only problem now appears to be pyromania. I gather their house was burned down some time ago and there have been a few fires in the flats where they live and Keith may well have something to do with it. His mother says he had not been seen again by Mr Burns.*

I admit I was a busy child. Mr Burns was a psychologist I was sent to over some issue I had with my dad, or rather he had with me. He concluded from my assessment that I was "quite normal." Funny that, as I'm now seen by some as a bit deranged. My Dad would not allow them into his head.

I was also something of an escape artist from very early on and would often be found out of my cot. Once, at just 6 months, I got out of the house and halfway down the street before I was captured and returned home by a neighbour.

Arson, escape, enlarged lymph nodes and vaccines all returned in later life!

Gifts one and all. I have a happy recall.

Anyway, I digress but this should get us back on track. I've talked a lot about the dark side and it's time to look at how we can turn what we have learnt to our advantage and recover this situation. Not quite done with vaccines so don't get too comfortable!

By the middle of 2016 Alice and I had reached a significant and considered conclusion. We, and just about everyone everywhere treating cancer has got it wrong. The essence, as viewed by many of those working with the natural world to heal the host, of deterioration caused by deficiency and toxicity, remains as an impenetrable fact. But the cancer, which we were about to very successfully and very rapidly eradicate, is something else. This was a very significant observation, and pivotal in my recovery from cancer.

The individual is handicapped by coming face to face with a conspiracy so monstrous he cannot believe it exists.
Edgar J Hoover (1895 – 1972)

The Shape Shifting Microbe

- Progenitor primordiales -

(roughly translated: a biological ancestor from our earliest stage of development)

All of the old menaces like typhoid, smallpox, measles, scarlet fever, whooping cough and diphtheria have become minor causes of death. The chance is very remote that any of them will ever again assume sufficient importance in the mortality tables seriously to affect the general death rate.

Dr Louis Dublin, 'Better Economic Conditions Felt in Fewer Deaths', Berkley Daily Gazette December 27, 1935.

I love solving a mystery and a bit irony, and there have been an awful lot of powerful moments in this journey that have stopped me in my tracks and sent a chill down my spine and later made me laugh like a fool, and this has it all. When it first dawned on me that what we had uncovered in our search for cancer's Holy Grail involved a similar impossible shape shifting principle that makes debunkers throw tantrums at David Icke, I nearly choked.

I've followed Icke's work for some years and have witnessed the strangest reactions when sharing the findings of a man so mild. People can be fun! I understand where he's coming from. I like his thinking as he thinks for himself and is brave enough to speak his truth. That truth causes irrational behaviour. I think he makes perfect sense and he thinks it makes sense to follow the evidence of inquiry to wherever it may lead, instead of this thing we like to do where we go so far and then park up some place in our comfort zone with the information that provides us most comfort.

So for anyone who doesn't know of David Icke it is necessary for me to say a few words of introduction so we are on the same page. My page.

In the early 1990's David Icke was going through his awakening and trying to bring to light another way of looking at the world. A former professional footballer and well-known public figure Icke had a media platform through which he was able to express his vision of the world.

I discovered from the work of Icke and Nassim Haramein [192] and others that we are living through a long predicted process of accelerated conscious evolutionary development on the planet. We don't think about it and barely know it but we are spiritually awakening at an unstoppable speed. We are evolving into higher energy, new dimensions where the old ways struggle to ground themselves, where we can begin to see through the fog, where the lies become transparent as the veil lifts. You can see all around this process in action as the more evolved among us begin to shine and glow, love and grow. And those who can't let go of the old ways cannot hide their struggle to hoard more money and more stuff, to control and deceive. Others less clingy appear to be able to see more of the spirit world and more UFO's and crop formations, but we don't have to, it can still be a whole pile of hoaxes, to fool us all to think about things, if we prefer.

---

192 https://resonance.is/

David Icke is a researcher and a political commentator. What he'd discovered and was trying to share with the rest of us did not represent what most of us thought the world looked like and what he had to say did not go down especially well. We collectively, in the UK at least, did what most modern humans do when confronted with new ideas: we reverted back to the playground and lost ourselves in a name calling frenzy. Even his children at school were targets for roaming bands of bigots who seek to limit the topic of conversation. I didn't know what David Icke was talking about then and was so wrapped up in my own world that I never made the time to listen, but bullying makes me uncomfortable and this thing about assassinating the character of someone to drown out their message doesn't sit well with me either. I was keen as mustard many years later when downtime was forced upon me and I began by digesting David Icke's book 'The Biggest Secret' which really focuses the attention.

The Icke bashing is ongoing in spite of the wealth of evidence that already proves much of what he says to be the correct, such as the fact we are controlled by an evil intent with an obsession for everything including our hearts, minds, souls and children, one that will stop at nothing to get its way. These people we can see for ourselves are at war with humanity and the animal kingdom and do despicable things to serve their ends and for the most part the collective turns a blind eye to the worst excesses of our leaders, with the less evolved among us using their example as a kind of guide. That is until someone like David Icke draws our attention to it and then the collective without taking a moment to consider or do any research loses the plot with him! It was David Icke who warned over a decade ago that they would next seek a war with China and Russia as they wound down in the Middle East. Nut job.

The one area of David Icke's research that really messes with the collective ego is the idea that non-human intelligence plays a role in organising human affairs and keeps us in conflict and struggle. We like to think we are the top of the food chain but we are the main course! There are good and bad aliens involved in our evolution, recorded in a story long told by human civilisations much more in tune with the reality of the natural and supernatural worlds than the one we have created that tunes into reality TV. We see politicians on our TV screen but hidden from view there are many layers of influence with persuasive financial clout who pull their strings and make them dance. This must be obvious by now? For those who are able to see past the Prime Minister to the possibility of a hidden hand it is here we usually rest our inquiry, at 'capitalism' or the Tories. Yet according to Icke, who didn't park up, at the top of this pyramid of control of the big money and the big people is an off planet, or non-human entity with designs on Planet Earth and a depopulation agenda. These persons of dubious heritage want it all and operate through those major consumer powerhouses of food, drugs and petrochemicals and politics as they seek to consolidate global control into a one world government. Seems clear to me that's what's forming! Certainly the way human affairs are managed is anything but humane and I reckon 'human' is too much a part of humane to be so irresponsible.

The Reptilians Icke made popular are the Annunaki of the Sumerian library. They are described as another dimensional entity with some control over events in this 3D world, particularly through politics. It is said this race of beings are absent the genes of empathy, which may explain the extreme cruelty we see, the lack of resolution and no remorse. Modern religious texts refer to the Devil or the Jinn misguiding humanity. The older native traditions describe the god creator as the gods (they) who arrived on the Earth around 200,000 years ago and genetically upgraded the pre-human to be me and thee. Three million years of ape - then boom - the moon, in the blink of an eye. Science has even begun to catch up, discovering that indeed something did happen with our DNA around this time to transform - not evolve - it from that of our primate brothers. We can always find answers when we look beyond what we are told to look at and if we look for the ever elusive missing link in our evolution beyond the walls of our imprisoned mind we can find that connection from whence we came. We don't have to accept it, we can continue the search. We do like a good search!

These are spectacularly consistent witness descriptions of the history of humanity told by ancient cultures scattered across continents. Few scientists would dare even postulate the deliberate nature of this gene splicing event that left us with two fewer chromosomes than our supposed closest ancestors. The monkey's have 48, we have 46! Happy to maintain a belief that one day science will find the missing link it thinks exists in a hole somewhere, but how does the scientist theory of evolution account for all that disappearing DNA? [193]

We do not now have to believe either in God or evolution as dictated by those who guide our beliefs. Same applies in cancer treatment and in the principle of immunisation – there are other ways to think. The third way I prefer for the stack of evidence that points at it. I got irritated waiting for the elusive missing (bit of bone) link, which was my preference through my formative years as opposed to the Bible story which always confused me. But no one mentioned that by necessity there needs to be not just one (bit of bone) but so many cousins of this missing link to fill the gap in the monkey-moon story we could be searching forever. Which is how they want it!

What Icke is sharing is a story complied from modern human history as told by well informed human civilisations smart enough to figure how to make this information available for us to decipher when we are ready, so we might grow. Well we are ready and when we look we will see that something incredible is happening and we have a more important role to play than simply denying everything and poking fun.

We could find, if we look at all this with an open mind, that all we have left of the story we have been told of simple beings coming down from the trees and building spaceships, or made in the hand of God five thousand years ago, are beliefs. We like to glory in our ability to reason but we could sometimes do a bit better.

On the surface we may see humanity being dragged into a living hell and that appears to be the plan. But in fact we are taking ourselves there, and no matter who

[193] http://www.pnas.org/content/88/20/9051.full.pdf

is pulling the strings, it's for us to fix. Ordo Ab Chao they call it. Order out of Chaos. Look around! Chaos is a picture painted for us in the daily news but these are the dying throws of this monster and it is we who will bring order from the chaos. Away from the news a beautiful world is forming like a seed sprouting through the earth, the seed of which will be a grand old oak, as we begin to awaken in greater numbers when we've suffered enough, just as Ickey has been saying we would when everyone was laughing at him just 25 years ago. Stood his ground, told his truth and who's laughing now?

I am.

Because this is funny.

Serious as cancer but still funny.

And it's about shape shifting cancer causing microbes.

Bear with me. I appreciate this will all be a bit far out there for the uninitiated but what David Icke refers to is merely an energetic 'shift' of shape, and when you weigh all this up his explanation of hidden influential entities may be less far out than mine! He talks a lot about how everything is simply a form of energy, with forms vibrating to their own resonance, the slower denser forms we can see, and the lighter beings we can't. We rock and mock like something demented when we hear about power trippy reptilians morphing from ET into human form, but what we are not hearing is how this is a vibratory transition and may be only temporary 'witnessed' and not physically felt. This change of appearance or switching between channels or dimensions takes a lot of energy, apparently. But what would I know?

Well we did some research and our findings served me very well as we got some pretty useful insight on some real shape shifting. Before attempting to address the spread of my cancer we had come to realise that cancer is caused or better said spread by a resourceful germ more technically referred to as a pleo or polymorphic microbe known as *Progenitor primordiales* as described by Royal Rife in the 1920's. They are also known as *Progenitor cryptocides*, microsomes, chromatin granules, little bodies, scintillating corpsules, mycrozymas, bion, endobionts, somatid, and so on. We're sticking with microbes but that's not what's most important. What matters most is that we pay attention to them and their role in the spread of cancer.

The human body is said to be 90% microbes and 10% human cells and microbes are the best hope this earth has when it comes to cleaning up the mess of oil spills and nuclear waste and keeping our biological innards clean, so we have reason to make note to consider these chaps and their role in our world. Some microbes feed off the waste of other microbes and on down the food chain and they all live happily ever after when the neighbourhood is orderly, but where there is disorder there is disease. The disruptive microbes (the cancer microbes for example) become dominant and spread cancer.

Pleomorphic and polymorphic mean to change shape. Shift. From one form to another. Significantly our cancer bug grows through cycles of change in form **into bacteria or virus or fungus and** back again dependent upon his environment. We can see this happen thanks to the work of independent research scientists such as Gaston Naessens and Raymond Rife, who I'll come back to, and Elmer Nemes. These men developed microscopes so rare in this field there have only ever been a handful.

These instruments are the work of genius and brought into view for the first time life at that miniature level, as we can see from these extraordinary images captured by Dr Elmer Nemes in the 1950's. The story of Nemes follows the pattern of innovators in this field but his story is even less easy to track. What we can record is that he developed the Nemescope which was able to magnify **live** specimens in excess of 3,500,000x. Today's standard optical microscopes operate below 2,500x while electron microscopes can see dead material at magnifications around 160,000x. This Nemus device was by far the most powerful ever invented, it was stolen in 1960's and Nemus was later killed, but by pure fluke these images are from a set of around 50 that represent all that survived and it doesn't take a trained eye to see the potential in thinking beyond the limits of the settled sciences. [194]

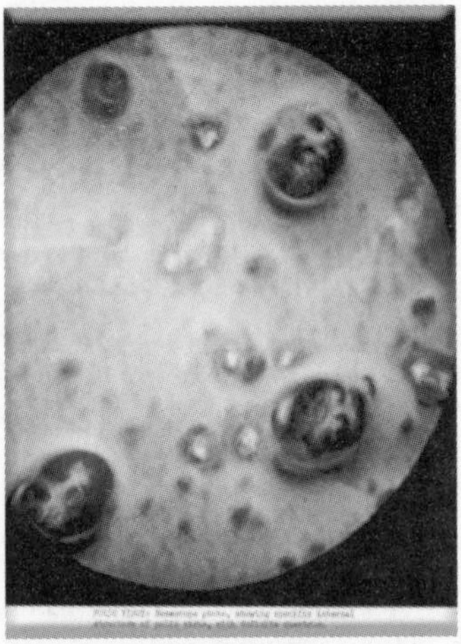

The polio virus

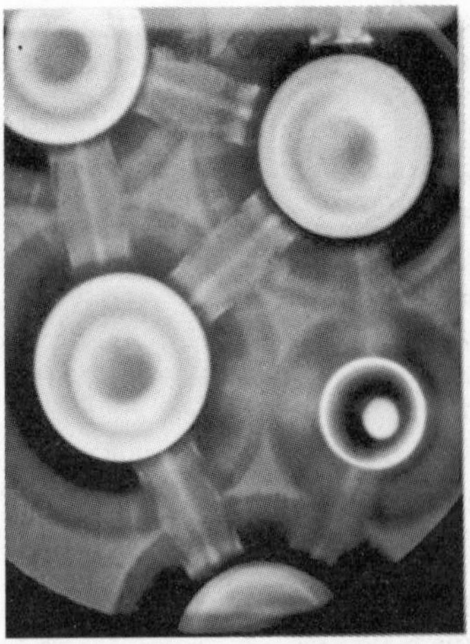

Taken in the 1950's at 3,500,000x magnification. Described as the lines of force between atoms

[194] https://www.lesscomplicated.net/philosophy/category/nemescope

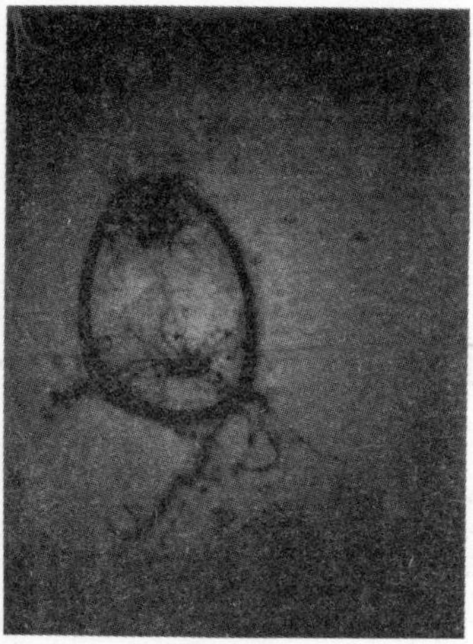

Cancer virus

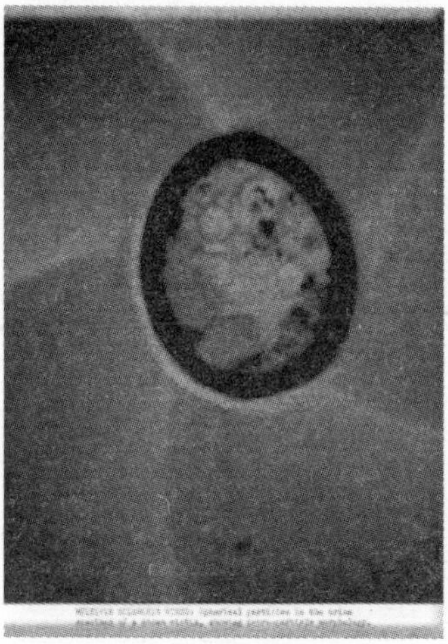

Multiple Sclerosis virus

Life down there in the micro-universe involves real life shape shifting perhaps better described as the accelerated evolution of germs.

Our French genius, Gaston Naessens, a former haematologist now in his 90's who knew there was more in the unseen, went his own way and designed his vision to record the 16 phase life cycle of this once hidden microbial killer he named the somatid. The first three stages of this growth cycle he describes as in unison with the host cell (living happily ever after). Once the burden of disease or deficiency weakens the immune barrier and the conditions deviate from the lessons learnt from evolution, a growth opportunity opens up for our lowly microbe. If nothing changes in the way we live to change this process, he settles into the new more toxic environment OK, he will adapt and soon figure how to incorporate himself into the DNA code of the weakened cell, replicate the damage and proliferate. With continued deterioration in the real world of our innards this guy is heading for the big time.

Tumours.

Acidity is a critical factor in this process. As the internal pH steadily acidifies the microbes do this shape shifting thing to adapt. Evolving to exploit the newly formed uninhabited territory they thrive and spread out of control and soon become a pest. When alkalinity is restored the microbes retreat and cannot re-establish occupation unless conditions revert.

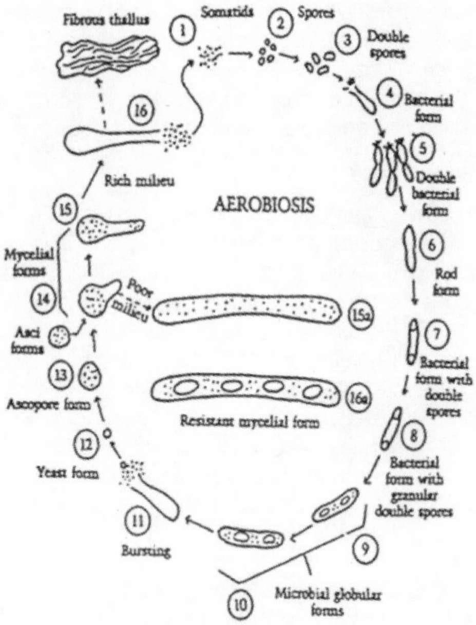

Gaston Naessens Somatid Cycle

Naessens and other leaders in this new science may not all meet on the fine details but all agree with the old ways of healing where reversing the disease environment facilitates the reversal of the disease process. It should be noted that the status quo sides with monomorphism, which is no shape shifting. Nothing changes, everything stays the same. A virus is a virus. A fungus is a fungus. And a mind made up is a mind made up.

But this isn't about them any longer, we've moved on.

This is about Keith Mann and the Shape Shifters.

Ohh, there's a band in there somewhere, set to knock the status quo off the top spot?

The role of these microbes are not so much a mystery to the orthodox, but like most significant mould-busting discoveries it was put to one side in deference to more commercially-viable theories about tumours, animal research and patentable poisons. And the success of that is clear for all to see, even if the microbe isn't! It doesn't really matter to us that we can't see the cause of our disease as readily as we can see the symptoms when they show up, because what we are able to prove is that by adjusting our internal environment we can genuinely affect those symptoms and force the microbe into retreat. Let's call him Marvin for the sake of our story. Marvin the shape shifting microbe.

Are we having fun or what? This is how science should be taught!

Reading all about Marvin really struck a chord and completed the circle of our understanding of what cancer is and how it spreads. I could never quite wrap my mind around the notion of size when I hear of microbes and atoms, viruses and microns. I can't for the life of me bring into view the size of the universe or trillions and trillions of anything but I am sure of one thing, and that's this teeny little fella is a very big deal.

The research of Dr Royal Raymond Rife in the 1920's, through who the cancer microbe has come to be associated, was followed by Dr Virginia Livingston-Wheeler and her team and reflected earlier pioneers in the field such as Antoine Bechamp, MD (1816-1908), Claude Bernard (1813-1878), Robert Koch in the 1800's, Professor Günther Enderlein and Dr Peyton Rous and Dr Alan Cantwell and Gaston Naessens more recently who are still holding the fort with many others in between. In 1890 Scottish pathologist William Russell described them as the "cancer parasites". In this disparate community there is a clear consensus on the role of the microbe. The earlier research established a microbe as a cause of TB and later a cause of cancer. Crucial to our understanding is that they typically originate and establish within the host (or in more recent times may be injected by doctors and nurses) but they will only thrive when conditions suit.

Louis Pasteur was a fierce rival of Pierre Antoine Bechamp and is well known for his plagiarism of the work of others, but it was Pasteur and his germ theory that won the day and as a consequence the science of healing lost out to targeted drugs and a scourge of 'incurable' diseases. Pasteur got the accolades for claiming that disease came from out there, from unknown germs moving in. Someone else to blame is always good. We like that and it sat with the times, as human society gathered from the wilds and became more condensed in shitty cities festering germ conditions, the germs found a home. Pasteur thought we could kill all the germs and live happily ever after, but Pasteur was barking up the wrong tree and so it remains as we follow the leader to poison the invader with the products of death and merrily deride all notion of healing the host. It is easier to pop that pill on the face of it, in the short-term at least. There's less to worry about, no need to figure out bothersome and unnecessary chores like changing our lifestyle and giving up those things we have long enjoyed, the things we were enjoying when our immune defences broke down, when we created a niche for and 'got' cancer.

Funny, we are programmed from pre-school to pension to work hard study hard and train hard in order to achieve greatness. And the harder we work study and train the more we achieve. We hear how it will surely come to pass that the lazy among us and those who don't contribute as they are expected to will fail and even bring down the rest of us! Yet when it comes to the most important duty of them all, that is to protect, nurture and nourish the very temple in which our eternal being is able to experience this life at all, the very same experts take over our responsibilities and insist that the least we do the better!

The view of these microbe researchers is that the textbook programming of what is and what isn't possible prevents establishment microbiologists and bacteriologists and all the other boxed off specialists from seeing something they haven't been trained to see or to even look for (not that the equipment is up to it). This sounds unlikely but this is perfectly normal as we are as easy to program, train and control as the dog and just as easy to misguide. And even when something like the truth is discovered, as happened here, such as a shape shifting cancer causing microbe, there are few brave enough to face to the ridicule, isolation and career stunting manoeuvres that follow, so they tip toe quietly along the party line, pay the mortgage and brush aside the most important discovery since DNA as 'debris' or artefacts or something that just happens to be there. Another coincidence theory! Nothing to talk about.

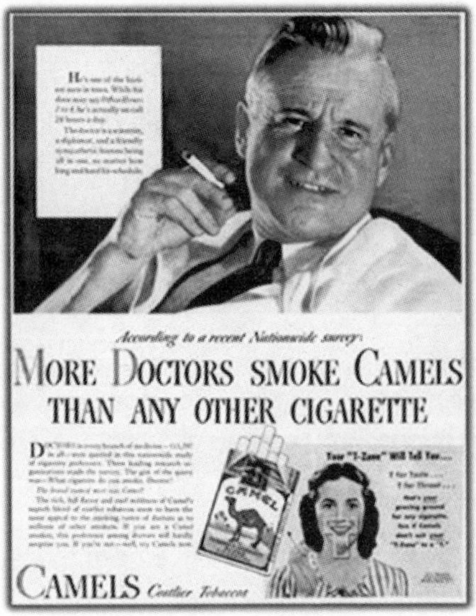

There are no exceptions to this rule I can find in any of the great discoveries of our time or any time. We would do well to remember the not so long ago when experts denied manned flight was possible, when medical experts insisted that breaking the 4 minute mile would kill anyone who tried, when doctors promoted cigarettes and politicians warned us of dire consequences if they didn't go to war to get rid of those dastardly weapons of mass destruction that the intelligence experts knew all about in Iraq.

Will they ever apologise for getting it so terribly wrong so often?

More well-paid experts decided there was no risk, based on their idea of sound scientific research, of feeding herbivores to each other. Soon after we got Bovine Spongiform Encephalopathy or rather cows did, mad cow disease they called it, more like mad scientist disease if you ask me, and that led to the human variant Creutzfeldt-Jakob disease (vCJD), something else targeting human development. Our brains do seem to be a focus of our science experts! And it was experts who assured us that statins and Vioxx, lead paint, DDT, asbestos, mercury, and a host of other toxic gack now proven lethal were safe. Isn't it curious how illness and death follow these health experts around like a dark shadow, the very people who get paid to keep us healthy!

In the 1800's Hungarian born Ignas Semmelweis was a pioneering physician who met the wrath of fellow doctors and surgeons for inviting them to consider washing their hands in the time between fishing around inside their patients, as a way to prevent them spreading disease. Smart, you might think, and indeed Semmelweis had proven this simple solution to the spiralling mortality rate in hospitals where patients were begging to be cared for by this gentleman. But the self-styled experts can be very blinkered and as history records many patients lost their lives at the hands of the quacks of the day who thought they knew better. And in order to prove their superior knowledge they turned on Semmelweis and battled like soldiers to keep that hive mind locked. The good doctor eventually suffered a breakdown following years of bullying by the medical experts around him.

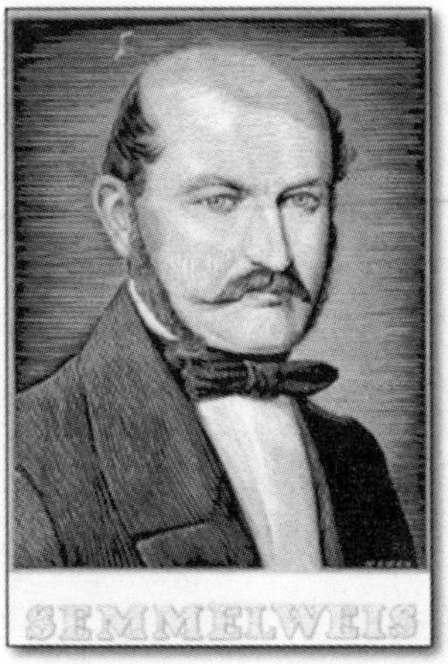

Tragically, Semmelweis died under suspicious circumstances an object of scorn in a mental institution. He could be considered a conspiracy theorist of his time, believing that others were conspiring to keep the truth from coming out. As if! It was many years after his death before the weight of evidence had submerged them and the medical marvels were forced to stop spreading disease with the blood on their hands. They continue to kill more people than any other profession, mind you, but now they wear gloves. Is that medical progress or what criminals do?

The 'Semmelweis effect' is a metaphor for the knee jerk reaction many of us exhibit when offered new ideas or even direct in yer face irrefutable evidence, if it contradicts entrenched beliefs or old rules. We only have to look at how whistleblowers are treated to see how the truth is received. It is never with open arms, more often with clenched fists and gritted teeth, threats and retribution.

Penicillin sat on my shelf for 12 years while I was called a quack. I can only think of the thousands who died needlessly because my peers would not use my discovery.
Dr Alexander Fleming (1881 -1955)

Dr Virginia Livingston, like most, was into her animal experiments and as we can see they do the opposite of deliver good health. Penicillin actually kills guinea pigs. Get that! Somehow we have allowed this primitive practice to persist into the age of microbe biosciences, quantum physics and the microchip. In fact it is expected of the greatest thinkers, and unless your new idea or product has been forced through a lab full of animals first the scientific community will not even look at you. But even when it has been so "thoroughly tested", if the results challenge conventional wisdom or the requirements of those funding the trial they will simply be ignored or discarded irrelevant. We can compare to insurance cover where the policy provider will often find a way to invalidate your loyalty.

Nevertheless, from such, Livingston made some quite revealing observations.

> *After years of research, I consider the potential for cancer in chickens to be almost one hundred per cent. That is, most of the chickens on the dining tables and barbecue grills of America today have the pathogenic form of the PC microbe, which I contend is transmissible to human beings. This is not to be confused with the dormant form of the PC in the healthy, high-immunity human being; the PC viral forms in chickens are already pathogenic, generating malignant cells and already forming tumors. Not only that, but*

many of the chickens processed for human consumption have already displayed tumours both visible and invisible to the naked eye.
Dr Virginia Livingston-Wheeler - The Conquest of Cancer

Dr Virginia, as she was known to her colleagues, was central to a network of like-minded researchers, mostly women. She was an advocate of cancer vaccination coupled with a nutritional foundation and she employed such a protocol on her patients. She was also pretty scathing of conventional treatments and soon slipped from favour.

A major discovery I made in 1974 has a great bearing on our treatment program and has already influenced cancer research throughout the world. This discovery was that the microbe P. Cryptocides secretes a mammalian hormone called choriogonadotropin (CG). This is important because CG is a hormone necessary for life itself to begin. It has been shown by Hernan Acevedo, Ph.D., that all cancer cells contain CG regardless of whether they are animal or human. The CG in the cancer cell is located in the nuclear membrane, the cytoplasm, and the cell membrane. It is postulated that the P. Cryptocides may have hybridized with the mammalian nucleus and imparted to the latter the ability to produce CG. In other words the DNA of the P. Cryptocides may act as a kind of fertilization of the human or animal cell to initiate an abnormal cell replication known as cancer.

There are four sources of CG in the human being: the sperm, the trophoblast, the bone marrow, and the cancer cell (via the P. Cryptocides microbe). Unless CG is controlled by antibodies, white cells, and dietary factors, it can continue to reproduce activity indefinitely in an uncontrolled way. The reparative cell is also controlled by CG. All productive life, whether of the fetus in utero or of the cancer cell is controlled by CG. It is therefore, the hormone of life and the hormone of death.

That is when the sperm enters the ovum, the secretion of the CG by the P. Cryptocides microbe envelops the new life cell (zygote) so that the mother's immune system does not reject the fetus. The placenta is coated with CG, protecting the fetus from the mother's immune system and the mother from invasion by the fetal cells. Therefore when one considers that the P. Cryptocides microbe is carried by human sperm and is required for every new life to evolve and survive (because it is the source of the CG), it is not difficult to understand how this potentially killing but also reparative microbe exists in all human cells. However the microbe remains dormant until our immune system becomes so weak as to let it gain a foothold at which time its secretion of CG allows a tumor to grow. [195]

Livingston seemed to have got her lead from Rife, as most have, and she was able to isolate and replicate. She found that our cancer microbe can be good or bad dependant on the food he has to eat and this is a recurring theme with the researchers in this field and there is no escaping this reality. This sounds like

[195] Dr Virginia Livingston-Wheeler - The Conquest of Cancer

something we might see for ourselves in our kids. And she is clear that while the removal of the tumour may slow the disease, it is not enough.

> *Immunity is the answer. If the patient's immune system is not at maximum strength, the smallest tumour completely removed will not prevent other tumours arising in other parts of the body. [P. Cryptocides are] an essential but dormant part of all cells, only activated to repair cell damage. After the repair it returns to a resting state in a healthy cell, where it remains dormant again. A strong immune system controls this process. However when immunity is suppressed or weakened, it proliferates and allows cancer to gain a foothold.* 195

Dr Alan Cantwell details in 'The Cancer Microbe' something interesting he found in the cells of autopsied medical victims who had been treated conventionally

> *[some]... with massive doses of antibiotics for weeks before death: the antibiotics failed to kill the cancer microbes. I saw the microbes in tissue that had been burned with massive doses of radiation therapy.* ***I saw the microbe thriving in cancerous tissue that had been blitzed with chemotherapy; the cancer cells were destroyed but the cancer microbe remained. Nothing fazed the cancer microbe: not surgery, not radiation, not antibiotics, not chemotherapy. The cancer microbe was indestructible!***

There are differing views on whether the cancer microbe evolves in the weakened cell or moves into it once it becomes weak but either way our role is to make it inhospitable again and repair the cell. Indestructible microbes are another recurring theme that come up in this early research but remember this only relates to orthodox treatments targeting cells and tumours.

If we follow the principle and process of evolution we see single cells shifting shape into all the forms we see in the world. The cancer tumour begins its life as a micro-organism, mostly invisible, its evolution to the point of cancer diagnosis is said to take 10 – 15 years and more depending on many variables. Mine took nearly 5 decades from the first cancer causing attack. This is a simple evolutionary process that can be sped up and slowed down in the lab and in the real world.

I read it over and over. In the lab they make cancer and make it grow quicker, and slower. They make cancer, we make it stop!

There was something of a competition building through this experience of my protocol design, a kind of mounting of momentum with so many crucial elements adding overall value beyond their individual worth. As we were approaching this cancer thing from all angles and had these microbes in mind we found this next element by no coincidence. I do agree there are occasional coincidences but I don't think this was one of them leading as it would to a very important tool for my kit.

In view of the minimal impact of cytotoxic chemotherapy on 5-year survival, and the lack of any major progress over the last 20 years, it follows that the major role of cytotoxic chemotherapy is in palliation. Although for many malignancies, symptom control may occur with cytotoxic chemotherapy, this is rarely reported and, for most patients, the survival in those who obtain a response is rarely beyond 12 months.

The Contribution of Cytotoxic Chemotherapy to 5-year Survival in Adult Malignancies
The Journal of Clinical Oncology, 2004

A Cure for AIDS

There are no specific diseases, only specific disease conditions.
Florence Nightingale (1820 -1910)

There are some bold claims made within these pages and why not? It's my party! What if I was to tell you not only have I healed myself of cancer but we could do it with AIDS too? We haven't tried but why not, because the doctor says it's not possible?

According to this recent US Patent, No 5,139,684:

> *It is now well known in the medical profession and the general public that blood collected in a blood bank from a large number of donors may be contaminated by contaminants such as bacteria, virus, parasites or fungus obtained from even a single donor. While screening of donors has done much to alleviate this problem, the screening of donors can and does miss occasional donors whose blood is unfit for use. When this occurs and the unfit blood is mixed with otherwise usable blood, the entire batch must be discarded for transfusion purposes. Because of this problem,* ***the present invention has been devised to attenuate any bacteria, virus (including the AIDS HIV virus), parasites and/or fungus contained in blood*** *contributed by a donor* ***to the point that any such contaminant is rendered ineffective for infecting a normally healthy human cell, but does not make the blood biologically unfit for use in humans.*** *Similar problems exist with respect to the treatment of other body fluids, such as amniotic fluids. The treatment method and system is also applicable to mammals other than humans.* [196]

There is a lot of really useful information in that paragraph.

This patent was issued on August 18 1992 two years after the invention was (re)discovered in a laboratory. Proof of concept is essential in acquiring a patent and for something as significant as this blood cleaning device and the bold claims made, one would expect that proof of concept was clearly provided. It is and it is crystal clear. A device with the potential to cleanse the life blood of the body would be beneficial to anyone, but to someone in a diseased state whose blood and organs are sick this could be a life-saver. I had a blood/lymphatic cancer but all cancers need a blood supply to feed from. Dirty blood. SV40 is a virus that corrupts DNA and causes cancer. Dirty vaccine! So let's get one of these and clean my blood, see how the cancer likes that!

Never before a fan but I'm getting into patents.

---

196 http://patft.uspto.gov/netacgi/nph-Parser?Sect1=PTO1&Sect2=HITOFF&d=PALL&p=1&u=%2Fnetahtml%2FPTO%2Fsrchnum.htm&r=1&f=G&l=50&s1=5139684.PN.&OS=PN/5139684&RS=PN/5139684

It was a simple test tube experiment with HIV-1 virus infected blood that led two researchers at the Albert Einstein College of Medicine in New York City in the spring of 1990 to observe the death of the virus, by running a very low voltage electrical current (50-100 microamperes) through blood. What this shift of energy does, it appears, is disrupt the protective protein coating of the virus, destroying it. This discovery could be as significant as anything we might care to mention. Sliced bread? I don't think so. I choose electricity.

Blood letting stems back to ancient Greece and continued through medieval Europe, the intention being to balance the bodily *humors*. In this practice blood would be drained from a diseased patient in order to rid toxins and hopefully restore health. The principle persists and the practice is now much more user friendly, thankfully. No blood coming out of anywhere! Not with our model of health anyway, the orthodox will today place a patient whose kidney's no longer serve their purpose onto dialysis so the blood can be cleaned through a sort of laundry:

> *You need dialysis if your kidneys no longer remove enough wastes and fluid from your blood to keep you healthy. This usually happens when you have only 10 to 15 percent of your kidney function left. You may have symptoms such as nausea, vomiting, swelling and fatigue. However, even if you don't have these symptoms yet, you can still have a high level of wastes in your blood that may be toxic to your body.*
>
> *In hemodialysis, a dialysis machine and a special filter called an artificial kidney, or a dialyzer, are used to clean your blood. To get your blood into the dialyzer, the doctor needs to make an access, or entrance, into your blood vessels. This is done with minor surgery, usually to your arm. The dialyzer, or filter, has two parts, one for your blood and one for a washing fluid called dialysate. A thin membrane separates these two parts. Blood cells, protein and other important things remain in your blood because they are too big to pass through the membrane. Smaller waste products in the blood, such as urea, creatinine, potassium and extra fluid pass through the membrane and are washed away.* [197]

This is daily. Forever! A cure is not the goal of this intervention, only maintenance of the status quo.

The microcurrent of this invention does not affect the natural biology of the blood only the germs that don't belong and it is thought it can kill cancer cells that are within the blood. I was irreversibly curious when I read all this and set myself up for all or nothing. And well, just, wow!

This early patent I quoted was for a device that would clean the blood outside the body or require an implant. Neither was a draw, they were costly and invasive. A step forward nevertheless, but the next leap in the evolution of this technology came quickly as a bright spark by the name of Bob Beck D.Sc. got wind of this miracle in

[197] https://www.kidney.org/atoz/content/hemodialysis

the making and set about designing a DIY upgrade. We now have a neat little device that can be worn on the arm and provide the same unparalleled deep cleansing service. [198]

I have two.

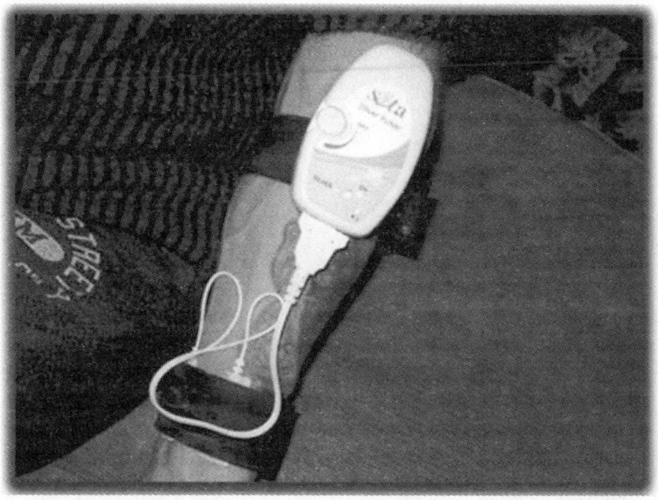

I hope you are paying attention because it's with these little ideas that big things can happen.

Clean the blood by deactivating the pathogens and the immune system has a chance. Work with the immune system and the odds go through the roof. This serves to strengthen those cancer defences that have been weakened by generations of insult. Imagine in cancer a struggling immune system isolating the debris from dirty blood into one place, forming a mass or tumour. We can dissolve that tumour back into the blood with radiation and chemo in the faint hope the problem has gone away, or we can clean the blood to help stop the formation of tumours in the first place.

All the free thinkers and researchers in this awakening are singing from the same song sheet about frequency, vibration and energy. Tesla, Rife, Michael Tellinger, [199] Georges Lakhovsky,[200] Icke, John Hutchinson.[201] Always the in thing! Unwinding the Bible creation story we can see reference to this precious knowledge at the moment 'God **said**, "Let there be light"'. If we read between the lines in the encoded biblical story of the spoken word we can see that sound frequency came first! It is the

198 http://www.bobbeck.com

199 http://michaeltellinger.com

200 https://educate-yourself.org/be/lakhovskyindex.shtml

201 http://www.hutchisoneffect.com/Research/pdf/TheHutchisonFile.pdf

foundation of everything. Everything is made up of atoms. Electrons of energy rotate around the nucleus of atoms at particular energy or frequency levels and the dance of the atoms creates frequency. Disrupting that song and dance with an incompatible frequency field or instrument and everything from 500,000 tonne skyscrapers to wine glasses to microscopic no weight microbes can be molecularly disrupted. Nothing is immune to the right frequency, right?

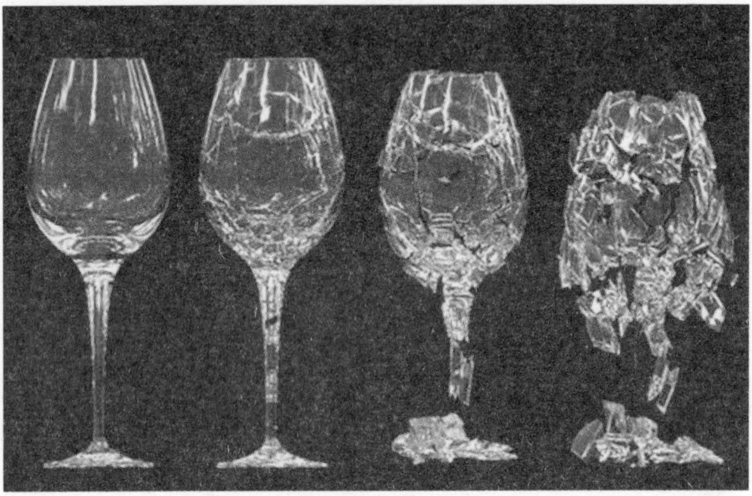

Use energy wisely and we can do magic!

So, under the surface of the skin the blood flows through arteries and veins and it is said every minute all the blood has circulated around our body. With two electrodes strapped over the ulnar and radial arteries closest to the surface of the under side of the wrist and running a microcurrent on a 9v battery, anything passing by that doesn't belong can't physically tolerate the microcurrent/3.92HZ energy signal it generates and is eliminated. It's quite logical and observable.

The micro-pulsing blood cleaner/Sota Silver Pulser is the size of a small mobile phone with a couple of wires and electrodes to slot under a wrist strap. I wear it under my sleeve like a fat watch. Anyway, don't get too excited if you think this is the magic bullet that saves you the trouble of repairing the mess your innards are in and giving up the addictions, it ain't. The immune system needs to be restored in treating cancer successfully and I found this to be a unique aid in that regard, but it isn't the answer to cancer alone or even all the viruses, in our experience.

The current is palpable to the wearer and has the effect of making your fingers vibrate. This can be adjusted to lessen the pulse but it needs to be felt. It can get intense with a new or recharged battery or freshly salted water-dampened electrode 'socks', to encourage conductivity, and makes typing and cooking impossible, but it's safe. Unless you try to type or cook.

Views differ among researchers as to the exact mechanism of this destructive process but we believe it is the microcurrents that do the damage and the 3.92HZ (½ of the Earth Schumann frequency of 7.83 Hz alternating electric current in which the cycle of polarity change happens 3.92 times a second) is a carrier wave for those microcurrents. I understand enough to know it makes sense to me.

The remedy in my opinion, is not to kill the microbes but to reinforce the oscillations of the cell... the main thing is to produce the greatest number of harmonics possible.

Georges Lakhovsky (1869-1942)

Switching it on. Switching it off

The organism has remained an unclassified mystery due in part to its remarkable pleomorphism and its stimulation of other micro-organisms. Its various phases may resemble viruses, micrococci, diptheroids, bacilli, and fungi.
Dr Virginia Livingston, Dr Eleanor Alexander-Jackson 1969

That August, of 2016, I added a homeopathic antidote to begin correcting the vaccine damage affecting my lymphatic system. However unconventional and unlikely that sounds to a trained mind, mine was the choice of an open mind. My nosode was formulated with the help of VEGA/EAV, and a qualified homeopath. We paw over how easily we could have missed this link to the legacy of the cancer causing polio vaccine.

By the beginning of October I was starting to feel quite ill again with nausea made worse with the slightest exertion and I was angry and irritable as hell. I have experienced disappointment, upset, elation and shock in my life but I don't really do anger yet this was off the scale! But this was what I'd been waiting for all these years. These were novel symptoms for me and they came and went at my command. And we knew in this moment that we'd cracked it. For two months we had been building the protocol by introducing a mosaic of elements to correct the imbalance in me and push back cancer with NK cell support, various nutritional supplements and other immune support, saunas, magnesium/bicarb baths, Trojan horse shots and not least this £300 Sota-crafted device [202] and their £300 Magnetic Pulser. Soon enough all hell let loose on my cancer and healing accelerated to the point where due diligence to the speed of this microbe devolutionary process became all that mattered. The question itself had evolved from if I can cure cancer, to how quickly do I want to do it! There is nothing in the world to compare with this feeling. We had stopped cancer from growing, the night sweats gradually stopped and we would soon see the tumours actually reverse en masse. The process is inevitably slow for impatient humans, particularly with an indolent, slow growing cancer but the speed of demise in this moment in time is of little consequence. There are few words to describe the feeling of discovering and managing a cure for a disease you have been assured will kill you. Awesome, elated, alive and love are some that come to mind.

Intense lower abdominal cramps can be a sign of toxic elimination and were the first physical sign for me. As my detox peaked I could barely walk due to the tension and could be found curled up on the sofa groaning and laughing like a fool at my achievements. I felt sick on and off and exhausted. And edgy and ravenous. I shifted between dreadful and thrilled. Had we achieved a miracle or made things worse? The battle with the mind was in full swing. And then returned night sweats that the regular doctors automatically assume are disease progression. The night sweats weren't the drenchers I had experienced with disease progression in 2012/13 and following the failure of chemo in early 2016 but nevertheless I needed to wash the bed sheets daily. At my next two hospital appointments I'd get that all-knowing

---

[202] http://www.cytodoc.co.uk/Sota

expert look that says 'poor, poor deluded you' when I told them my sweaty nights were merely a sign I was in a healing reaction. They had never heard of such a thing and were of course having none of it and I didn't expect them to, but the proof is in the pudding and we have free will to take it or leave it. I know what I'd do if I got cancer. The sweating soon stopped as did other novel detox symptoms.

In the first few days I could only manage an hour of this blood cleaning before I had to switch the thing off and then gradually I'd feel a little better. It was against all the odds but so perfectly tuned is this protocol that at the flick of a switch I was suddenly in complete control of disease die off and of my recovery! Pulling back on any elements would of course have the same effect, some sooner than others, but why would you? No broke no fix. I was managing a truly awesome reconstruction project. This is not for the faint-hearted, the professional non-believers and the fanatical sceptics; this is the real deal and comes highly recommended.

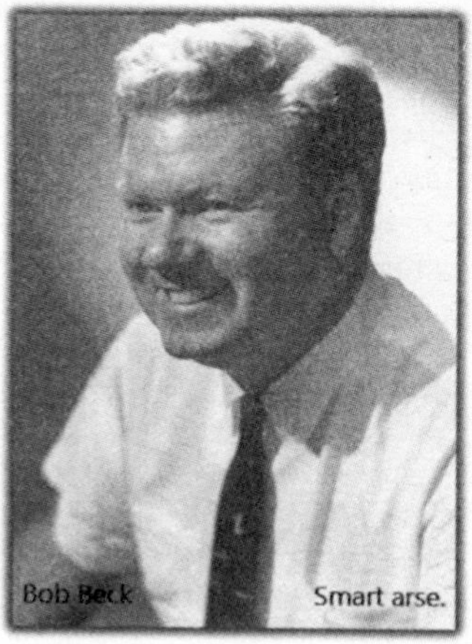

The Magnetic Pulser works in synergy and is the next essential in our box of tricks. Bob Beck found that the microbes hide in the organs and specifically the lymphatic system which can become sluggish so the Magnetic Pulser works on them while we work on the rest of the clean up. Sota teach us that "The Magnetic Pulser generates a pulsed electro-magnetic field that helps to balance the body's natural electricity."

It sounds simple but the best ideas usually are. This equipment is simply brilliant. Let them deny. Tease it out of them! They have all their chemo, radiation and bone marrow to transplant so why do they care? You go do, this is our organic chemo! Our package carries elements that do more than just shrink the lumps, nor do they kill any healthy cells! We hold the magnet paddle over anywhere on the body we wish to re-energise, shall we say, such as the liver, to allow our orchestra to drown out the bad guys hidden deep within and help to recover diseased tissue by raising the voltage of the cells. We might refer to these as our orchestral manoeuvres in the dark! I pulse during enemas. Lie on my side with the paddle positioned at my target organ and chill out for 15 minutes with coffee sloshing. I was actually listening to OMD at the time it dawned on me that was what was playing out in my innards!

We followed the sheer logic of this technology, concluding this fit perfectly with our understanding of what cancer is and how to tackle it. With the host (I'm your host) in a positive or proactive state of immune restoration and detoxification, the disease cycle is broken and the microbes stop producing. Supported, cells can repair and revert to normal. In an oxygenated state the cancer microbes revert or die. I like the way that works, it makes sense. This is my kind of evidence based medicine and I am hooked.

In the mix is a third Sota device for making ozone water as a further aid to detoxification. And when the blood device is not deployed cleaning blood it can be adapted to make colloidal silver, a natural antibiotic that we are using in our Trojan horse to kill microbes! No joke. Sota is single minded in this package design. The equipment is simply designed and practical with a great deal more potential than another 50 year cancer war. And no dreadful side effects.

Managing a self-inflicted detox is another necessity for surviving cancer. It's a given that the diseased body has to be replaced with a healthy body and there is much more to a diseased body than you might imagine, revealing some creative elimination techniques, such as rage. This can be uncomfortable and unpleasant but healing reactions come in short bursts and soon pass. The young Max Gerson lost patients to the overload of poisons leaving the body once he kick started their immune defences, unravelling disease and breaking down the tumours, until he deployed enemas to help the liver flush it all out in a regular orderly fashion. We have no concerns in this regard now because we have learnt from the work of others but tumour lysis can sabotage the best cancer treatments without the best detox. This most commonly occurs following the nuclear impact of chemotherapy and mostly affects patients with high-grade non-Hodgkin and Burkitt's lymphomas, acute leukaemia's and other bulky or rapidly growing, treatment-responsive solid tumours. The orthodox will hook you up with their dialysis in the event your chemo treatment finishes off your kidneys.

The logic of a bulky quick dying cancer burden causing an overload I get, but it's baffling to me how so much toxic waste can be stored or where exactly it is in cells or how it fits in among the piles of other stuff crammed in there yet its heavy presence is undeniable. What I can see clearly now is how I built this load up daily over many years and how I eliminated them daily and I am absolutely certain we need to carefully consider both these mechanisms. Then the storage bit will be resolved, naturally.

Over the days and weeks and months of regimented supplements and enemas, pulsing and juicing, bathing, saunas and rebounding, my lymph nodes all began to slightly shift shape. Some of these tumours begun to narrow, some softened or would feel tender to touch, some flattened then narrowed, others seemed to separate into smaller parts as they proceeded to dissolve. There was no consistency in this process and it was tricky to judge. I was sure until the next day when my mind would say *"nah, it's the same, you are imagining it"*. It does that. But after a week and then a month and more toxic dumping and undeniable shifting of tumour shape and size it was game over for the mind. It doesn't feel right calling it a miracle but it was miraculous.

I had been assured by orthodox cancer experts and a million hangers-on to their word that this was simply not possible, that my health would never return and that there was no natural way of removing cancer tumours. Not now, not never. When it does happen it will be a pharma invention that does it. I think that view is pretty much a given for most of us, right? If chemo can't do it then you need to get your affairs in order because there is nothing else in the specialist's bag of toxic treatments. And of course there can be nothing else or the medical school debts, the long work hours and sleep deprivation, the state of the nation's health service and its health – it's all for nothing. Especially when the solution is so simple and cannot be owned!

My once bulging lymph nodes used to meld into one another like a range of hills or mountains with no sign of gaps. But we had made them shrink and fall apart and they would eventually feel like they'd come loose of the chain. This process begun within days of initiation and accelerated as time went by. At the 2 - 3 month mark there was a general and widespread cancer kill evident with the 'stubborn' tumours in decline along side those that begun to regress early in the process. We believe the NK Cell Activator and the mushroom were key to this but all elements are essential in the rebuilding process.

To welcome in 2017 I amused myself by chasing tumours around under the skin like tadpoles with no tail trying to count what was left. This had been near impossible with so many and feeling them grow had caused some level of anxiety but we had changed all that. I once counted over 70 externally forming the hills but as time and disease passed away and as some tumours dissolved completely I'd find others underneath the surface layer, also now themselves wriggling about and struggling to survive. It took a few weeks of steadily increasing the time I wore the blood unit to the point where I could spend all day with it on and pulse all I wanted. I would alternate with a sauna one day and bathing the next. As the tumours dissolved away, the toxic dumping became a much less intense experience. I must stress the need for the maintaining the working protocol long past no sign of disease. We are layered with toxins and this material becomes unravelled bit by bit, with breaks, seemingly random periods of time when nothing happens. You may wonder if you are fully healed. You most likely aren't but continue doing what you are doing and eventually those layers can be cleared. This can be expected to take two years or more after we see no evidence of disease. The body when given what it needs will do just what Max Gerson found it will that is clear out a layer allow you to recover and go again every few weeks. We sped up this process with the MannIcure, stopping cancer growth in days and forcing healing every few days there after. I would get maybe two day of recovery and then another round of toxic dumping, mostly beginning later in the day and on into the night followed by obvious tumour shrinkage a few days later. Some nights I had no choice if I wanted to sleep but to do an enema at 2am and almost instantly the irritation or shaking which was keeping me awake would ease.

The angry rage lasted for weeks and was by a distance the most intimidating aspect of the detox, eased greatly by increasing enemas to one every 4 hours when things got really intense with some back to back if the first didn't really help. Curious, but two like this can have a significant effect. The detoxification process turned me into one of those people you don't make eye contact with. I don't suffer fools for long and may consider a second chance, but I'm not a fool. Still, it takes an awful lot to press my button and make me an angry person but not so much during my healing where this button of mine was pressing itself. I couldn't drop a spoon without snarling and was snapping at Alice and the dog for no reason. And as for those irritating low paid telephone stalkers who were unfortunate enough to have called during my time of rage trying to sell me stuff, well - don't call me! Ever. Gerson warns of the healing rage but no one can prepare you, or your family, for what those words on paper translate to in real time. I can't adequately describe this feeling except to say the less anyone says to you while you are going through this the better!

The left brain points a finger at the placebo effect when confronted with anything like this, or wishful thinking. Instantly into a box shut the lid, no discussion, no debate - untested by a left brain test so it must be a trick of the mind, the placebo effect. I believed for all I'm worth that Gerson would heal my body of cancer and that chemo would remove all visible signs, for a while, but neither came to pass. I was naturally cautious and wasn't sure of our MannIcure, but that worked like a dream. Don't most of us go into chemo believing it is going to work? That's an awful lot of energy believing in the process yet what do we see when the process ends? And what do they know about placebo anyway – they killed it!

I may have been lightening tempered with Alice but this was a two Mann dream and knowing what it meant she was glorying in the state I was in too and had no choice but to take it. Careful what you wish for eh! I'm not sure what the dog was thinking about all this but this is where he comes in and his story is important so we're going on another apparent diversion, although it isn't. None of my diversions from cancer to cure are missing the point and if you think they are then you may be missing the point.

Ten outbreaks of poliomyelitis caused by pathogenic circulating vaccine-derived polioviruses (cVDPVs) have recently been reported in different regions of the world.

Most cVDPVs were recombinants of mutated poliovaccine strains and other unidentified enteroviruses. The goal of this study was to investigate whether these... can act as recombination partners of poliovirus... The co-circulation in children and genetic recombination of viruses... can lead to the generation of pathogenic recombinants, thus constituting an interesting model of viral evolution and emergence. [203]

---

203 Published 2009. http://journals.plos.org/plospathogens/article?id=10.1371/journal.ppat.1000412

The Dog
(our little helper)

Darkness cannot drive out darkness; only light can do that. Hate cannot drive out hate; only love can do that.
Martin Luther King Jr. (1929 – 1968)

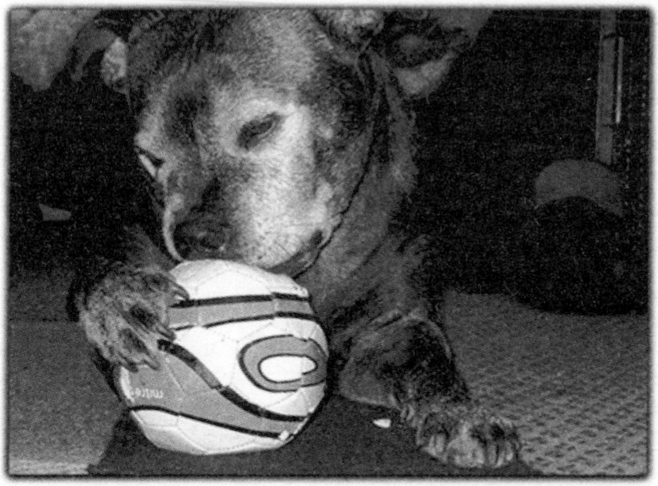

As I gradually found space in my new life to think beyond being ravaged by cancer I began mapping my journey into something for everyone. The story began as a simple 'carrot juice cure' and rapidly became something so awesome to surpass even that. As if discovering cancer in vaccines, a clear conspiracy to cover it up, microbes in cancer cells, hopeless cancer treatments and a cancer cure wasn't enough to be processing, I found myself being jostled by the dog to hold on a minute.

With words pouring out of me as readily as dead cancer, our beautiful 12 year old boy Taz was struck down with an aggressive cancer of his own. Wasn't so much our dog as we were his people. When we moved into our flat seven years earlier he was a neighbour's dog who loved a fuss when we met in the hall. Nothing compares to a dog that likes a fuss! Soon we would find him sitting outside our door wanting more of the Manns. Once he'd been invited in and found his way onto our sofa he quickly adopted us and essentially moved himself in permanently, nipping home to eat and on time for his regular early morning walks and returning when he was ready. This dog was loved everywhere he went, he now had two homes and three times the love. He loved our sofa and had never been allowed in bed with his peeps before! The first time he was invited to get on the bed he wee'd himself a dribble in excitement as he ran around the bedroom unsure how to cope! He was an almost human, highly sociable and loved up mutt who would actually purr if you only looked at him adoringly and he was living the dream. Taz liked to be cosy and comfortable and we were indoors a lot just now and we're the kind of people who think every home should have dogs on the sofa. We were his dream come true and he ours. A timeshare dog oozing love! He's also a big tough Staffie and he knew it and he had a lot of attitude towards other dogs and cats and foxes and this created something of an issue when walking him.

His dad was an early riser and would come and get Taz from our flat and take him out before light and avoid meeting other dogs. This was deliberate; the dog was unhinged in the wilderness. Foxes couldn't be avoided and cats creeping home after a night on the kill took their life in their hands as our little helper patrolled his streets. By default this left me with the later walk when of course I'd bump into people, with dogs. Me and psycho-on-a-lead would be found walking around the perimeter of the park with all the fun happening in the middle where all the normal dogs play together in the big puppy playschool. I told him when he's gone I'd get a dog who was less angry than him so we could hang out with the others. He was one of them that knew what you were saying and could decode spellings but warning him he was to be replaced with Fun Bobby never changed a thing. A personality transplant at the doorstep turned him from a teddy bear indoors to a thug outdoors. His dad was happy for Taz to chase the foxes and cats early in the morning and it was, I admit, funny to watch this mass of muscle take off like his arse was on fire when he had something to chase. He was the opposite of a whippet but he'd put his heart and soul into this hopeless pursuit, and being drawn to the underdog I could feel in me a longing that one day he might just succeed. But alas it wasn't to be as I am in control of my primitive aggression and I don't like hunting, so with me on a walk if he even looked sideways at a fox he would be scolded. Poor thing was ever so confused! Or pretended to be.

Anyway seven years on our Taz got cancer and did he! Grade 4, mast cell cancer, which is very aggressive. Spring 2016 a tumour in his chest quickly reached the size of a golf ball but then disappeared. A few months later it came back only this time there was no stopping it. This type of cancer is erratic so this was normal.

This lump got so ridiculous so fast and Taz was physically struggling and couldn't lay on his chest. We got him to the vets, primarily for an X ray to see if there was any point in putting him through surgery. The vet rang while he was under anaesthetic and said the tumour was literally erupting and it was surgery or sleep. They needed to know now! We said go ahead and do him. Don't do him in! Do him.

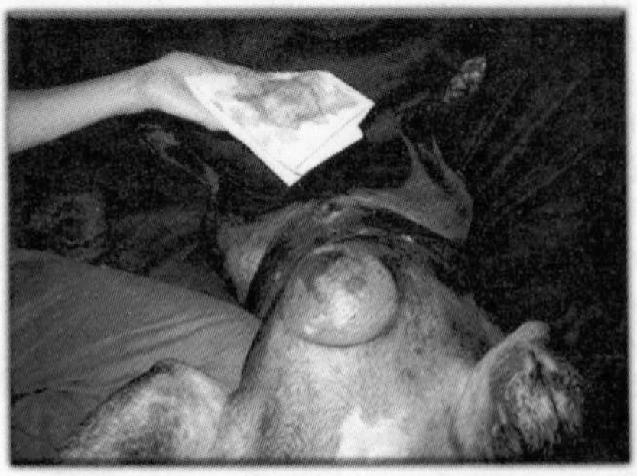

We then waited anxiously as they spent over 4 hours inside the chest cavity of our boy removing this tumour and ideally a clear margin around it. Somehow he was back home that night very sorry for himself exhausted, sore, stitched up and stapled. It *looked like* a very professional job.

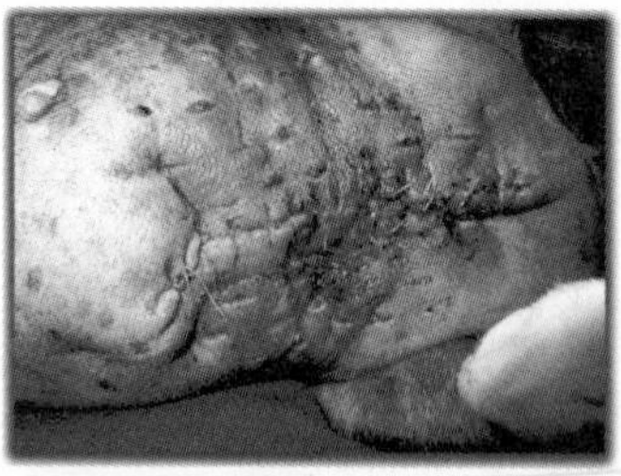

Successful surgery, tumour gone.

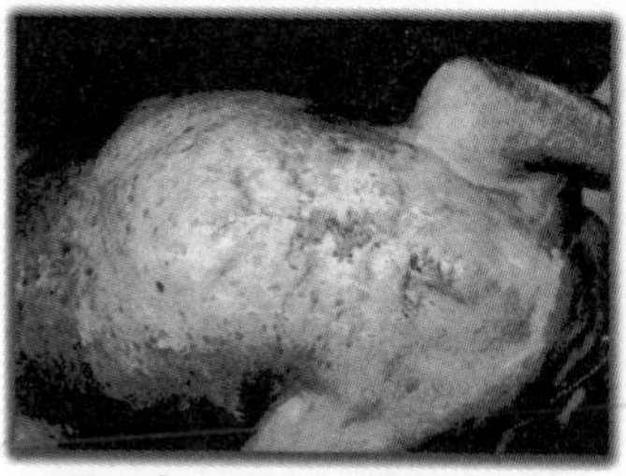

But the patient still has cancer.

We now had this added challenge of keeping the stitches in place for the next few weeks until the hole sealed, but we did. We also now assumed full custody since he barely left anyway and couldn't really get upstairs and needed intensive care. We added supplements, quercetin to control the mast cells, probiotics, colloidal silver and Barley Power. He continued to enjoy a carrot juice and his apples and he healed well but his prognosis was awful and a few months was all he had if we didn't magic up a solution. For an elderly dog of this size he was lucky to be here at all apparently. I don't buy that; I think we have become accustomed to them not living long because that's the world we have been creating.

Taz also had a small tumour on his paw which had apparently irritated him since he was aged three. It drove him nuts at times and for as long as we knew him he nibbled at it. It would come and go but stayed for the past two years. Such was the location it couldn't be surgically removed. We would later find this was a cancerous tumour. We cleaned up his diet, cut out the crappy tinned dog food and grains that are increasingly problematic in animals causing allergic reactions and histamine release. This type of cancer can be influenced equally by grains, pesticides and by artificial food-like products, such as those affecting human health. He went raw and organic.

We knew we had another big challenge in this unchartered territory. For our part we had as much experience with 2nd time cancer in a dog as in a Mann but nothing to lose or gain except time with our friend. And cancer is cancer right and restoring balance is what we do to resolve cancer, right? Truth is Taz was an experiment for his whole life and for our part in this we would be too late to save him, but for as long as we could see some hope we would do what we could. He and I were now entangled in a cancer experiment together and we both discovered information you may find helpful.

Left to heal from surgery in his basket, which was now in our living room, he bounced back very quickly and started to sing and purr like he used to. Nursing him as he physically and spiritually climbed out of his post-op stupor and back to being a full size, full on puppy was another magical experience. We knew we weren't out of the woods due to the initial Grade 4 diagnosis and terrible prognosis, and we still had this irritating little tumour on his right front paw, which was inoperable, right? Well that depends who you ask. We asked the vet to remove that while he was under. No can do said the expert. Have to take the leg off. So he kept the irritating little tumour on his paw.

I get it, it was in the shin of the paw so surgery was out of the question, but that doesn't mean we stop asking questions. In this case the cancer in the dog was not going to be cured but the tumour in the paw, small as it might be, has a lesson to teach us.

I was going through my peak of high strangeness at the end of 2016 with sweaty nights and all manner of unusual, smelly, angry things going on and I wasn't sleeping. In fact I hadn't really slept for months but I didn't seem to need it and I didn't really care because I knew what it all represented and I had energy and a new life opening up for me. Ideas were coming out of me like explosions! One of them, at all hours of the morning, was to leave the flat to go scrumping which is apple harvesting to the uninitiated. We had over time used a lot of sour green apples in my juices as they are a necessary ingredient of Gerson's therapy. An apple a day keeps the doctor away! In the juices they aid the enzyme release of the other ingredients.

Anyway we had to cut back to fund our big project which on balance meant fewer apples. Except I knew where the good apple trees were. And it was Autumn. Who doesn't! Can't miss 'em. Not strictly organic by the rule book as they don't have costly official certification but they aren't sprayed and I'm not sleeping and these are free apples. We are being charged for the word organic while the poisons come free! It might sound silly but I'm a crackpot and that's what we do best, so I harvested hundreds of apples during the wee small hours of October, November and December 2016 clambering through fields and hedges with a bursting rucksack and I feasted on my hoard like I never grew up. Apple sauce with everything because I could.

Just a few weeks earlier I was pondering dying for the first time in my life. Now, 5am on those dark, crisp and quiet winter mornings so few of us really experience and I was climbing trees and chuckling quietly to myself! I laugh to myself more than I know. I've always climbed trees, as a kid for bird's eggs, then later in life to set up nesting boxes to help the birds. Now I had the tingle of life about me like never before. It was never quite dawn as I crept about but it was dawning on me just what we'd done. Every time I allow myself the space to think about it I get a tingle of life, like a rush of gratitude. My store of energy was coming back in leaps and bounds and I noticed I had my walk, my purposeful spring in my step. I am alive and my brain is ahead of my body. That's why I get up early, fit it all in! In truth I still had to focus on healing and on Alice and our boy and all the rest of it before I was going up any mountains.

If you want to find the secrets of the universe, think in terms of energy, frequency and vibration.

Nikola Tesla (1856 -1943)

Black Salve for Cancer Tumour Removal (in our dog) (from herbs) [204]

During the surgical procedure, natural barriers that contain the tumor to a region of the body are breached, enabling cancer cells to escape their original confinement and spread to other parts of the body. Surgery also induces immune suppression while initiating an inflammatory cascade that provides the cancer cells with biological fuel to propagate. Surgery inflicts a wound on the body that requires healing. The body secretes growth factors to facilitate healing. Unfortunately these same growth factors also stimulate tumor cell growth. Unless proper steps are taken before surgery, cancer cells can spill into the bloodstream from the surgical margins and establish colonies in other parts of the body.

Bill Falloon of the Life Extension Foundation in Knockout by Suzanne Somers

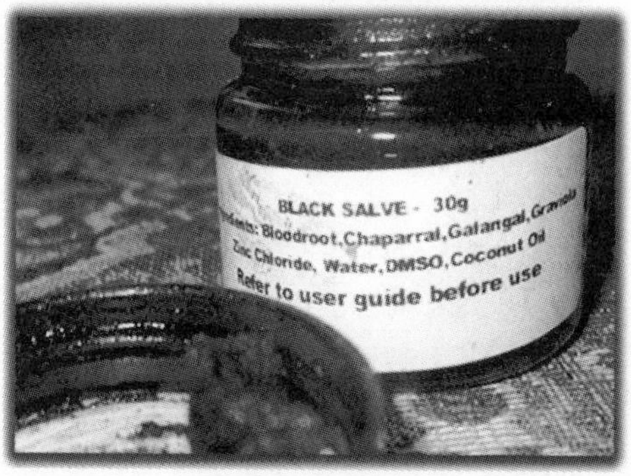

Ok it's November 22nd, two days after I begun applying black salve on this cancerous tumour on the dog's paw. **Black salve** (means *to save)* and is otherwise known as escharotics or botanical surgery. Take note, this herbal paste **will safely extract any surface-based malignant tumour complete with roots all within hours or days, from any host. The same applies to tumours under the skin surface.** If it ain't cancer there will be no reaction. I know because I did it. Anyone who says it doesn't work either didn't do it, is attached to a belief, or has a vested interest in maintaining the status quo.

Our dog's paw was wrapped in a bandage at night and removed the next day. I did this for two nights in a row. That 2nd morning I got up at silly o'clock and was fumbling through the dark for my sofa space to set up a much needed enema before I went raiding the apple trees. Next to me is Taz wrapped up in his bandage all bullied and bruised and probably in need of an enema himself but, well not so sure how to manage that without a garden and all manner of chaos so we didn't go there. Anyway, when I finally switch the light on I see a very, very sorry-for-himself looking dog tangled in bits of bandage and acting like he did something wrong. The tumour in its entirety was gone! That included the roots. There was something of a nice looking deep bloodless hole in his shin where the tumour once was, but the salve had pulled it all out and the dog ate the tumour.

Even he liked to recycle. Cat poo, too, occasionally.

---

[204] We get our black salve from: https://lozzswellnessstore.co.uk/

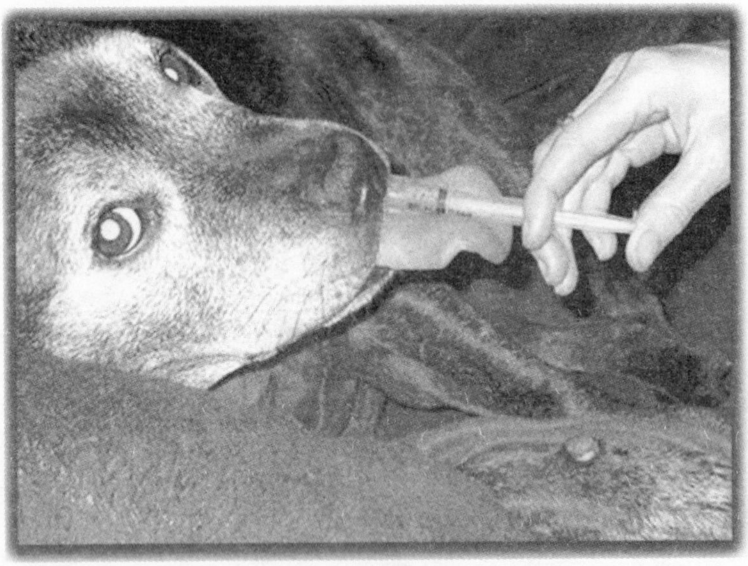

Taz recovering from surgery in October 2016 with carrot juice via syringe, save him getting up! The medical experts said the raw looking tumour you can see on his right paw was impossible to remove. But look at this.

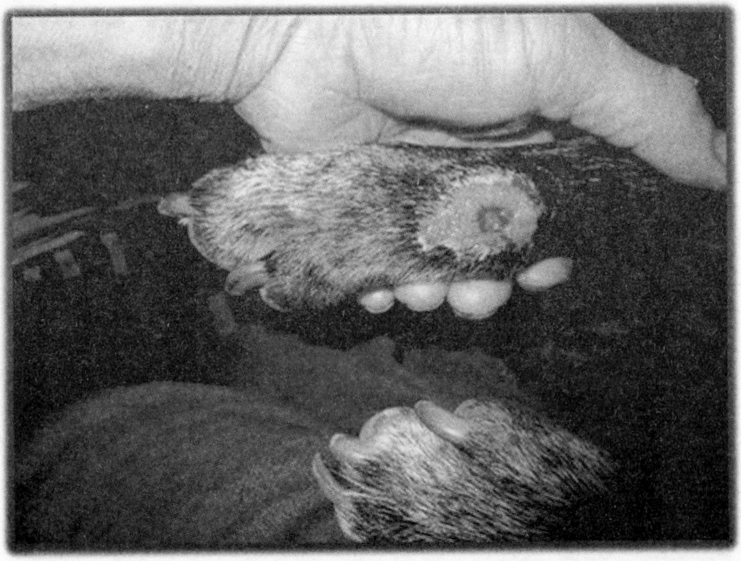

No tumour. Roots and all neatly removed with two applications of black salve.

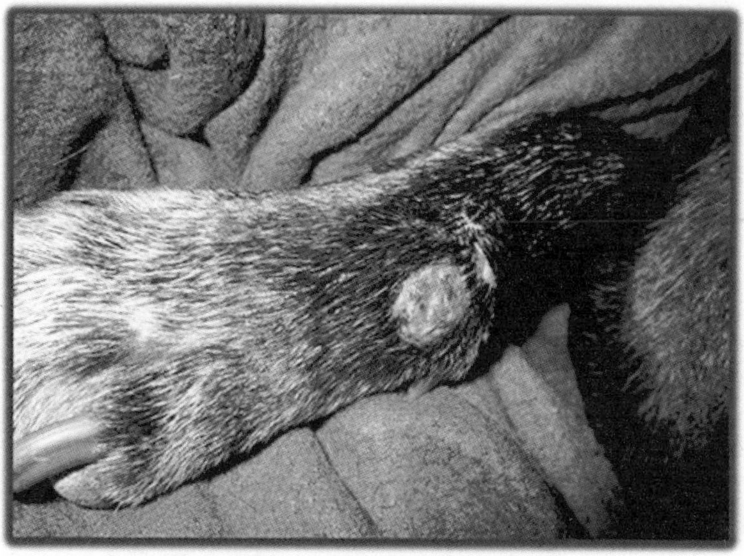

Two weeks later the wound is healing well.

This Native American treatment is simple and ingenious and has stood the test of time. They've made cancer today so complicated and unnecessary. Let's be clear this is not a cure in itself, but salves were being used to remove surface tumours long before the drug companies crushed the competition. Remember we always need to clean up our internal environment to bring full-body healing, but it is entirely possible to debulk cancer mass by removing the accessible tumours such as this with no need for surgery. This herbal paste reacts with cancer cells and only cancer cells. It sticks to them down to the roots, forms a crust at the surface and appears to suffocate the tumour which the body forces out until it completely emerges and detaches itself and can be painlessly removed.

Be warned this simple action may lead to a deeply empowering experience. I approached it with full consideration to infection control and pain management.

Once I'd helped heal this small wound I tried the salve on other little lumps he had. There were fatty lumps and another bulge at the site of the microchip but neither of these had that cancer feel about them and sure enough there was no reaction. Later we found other small tumours developing on his chest which were cancerous but were under the surface of the skin. Salve isn't designed for this but three of these responded excellently and again came away complete, **from under the skin**.

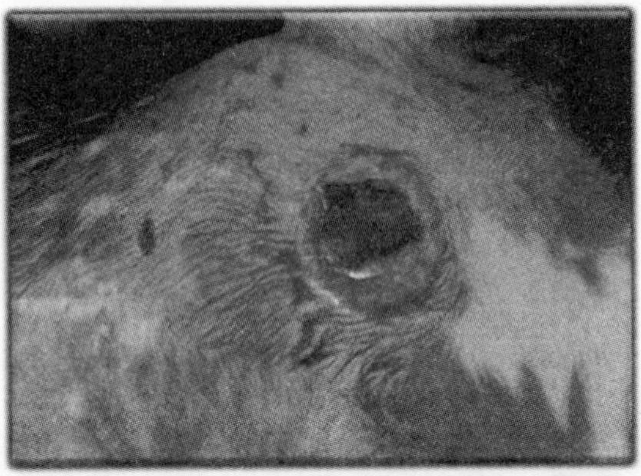

Salve crust attached to sub-surface tumour it is 'working out'.

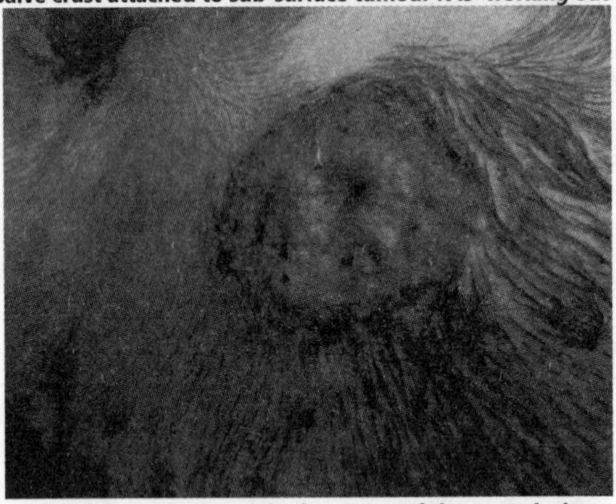

Hole left by tumour root in the centre of the wound where I was able to 'suck' out the growth attached to the salve.

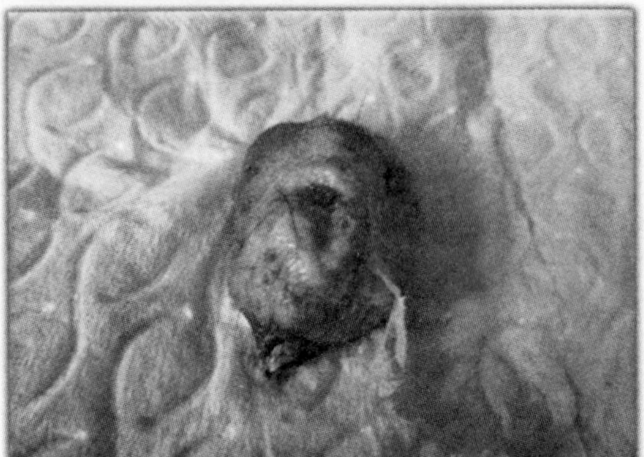

Excised tumour face up stuck to salve with V shaped root.

Clearly there should be some pain or burning during this tumour removal process, especially where the skin is breached, but none of this fazed our boy. Taz had a high pain tolerance and hurt more when a voice was raised than when crashing through brambles and into barbed wire fences.

Over the coming months we spent every available minute focussed on that dog as we knew his time was limited. Thing is, he did sleep a lot. The puppy we met a few years before was now ever grey day by day and was steadily slowing down, with increasingly decreasing walks, but he was the same intensely loved up mutt and a delight to be around. Watching him launch himself from his back feet in the air one minute to snoring on the sofa, to dancing in front of the fruit bowl drooling when invited for an apple was a treat to behold! Not so much a launch in later years more like a walrus trying to right itself.

We syringe fed him carrot juice, nursed him like a baby and fed him his supplements with a view to boosting his immunity, but the cancer just kept coming. How do you detox a dog with recurrent cancer and a massive tumour burden? We didn't have the time to figure this out. We were chasing the devil and the devil was running around in circles and as fast as we could extract one tumour and heal the wound, another would show up. The wounds healed flawlessly with daily sprays of 3% food grade hydrogen peroxide which again he didn't even notice, even on open wounds.[205] His paw never bothered him again after the hole healed and the large surgical scar across his chest healed perfectly too.

All credit to the veterinary team for the job they did with that operation but his records later confirmed what we weren't told at the time that they couldn't get a clear margin of tumour because of its depth, so there was always this stuff sloshing around in our dog and this thing on his right shoulder in the photo below was it already showing through. We pulsed this for 2 or 3 hours a day and within a week it had dropped and hung like a bag of fat but it was too big to get on top of with our limited tools and time. Smaller tumours or more resources: different matter.

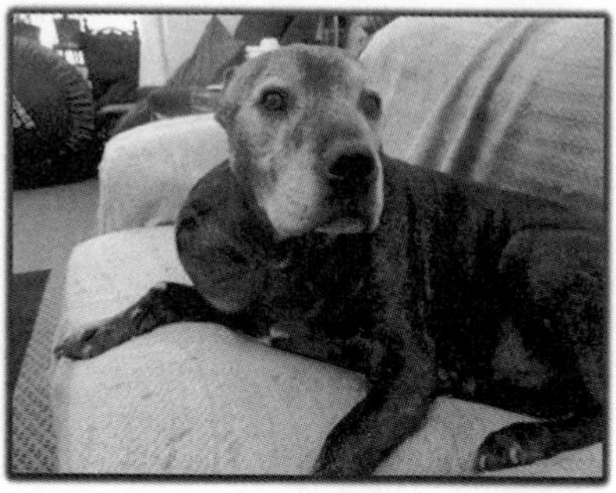

Taz with his post surgery tumour mass

Acute trauma recovery is where orthodox medicine excels but aside from that we are on our own. Three months after they cut out one huge lump the second big one mushroomed on his neck and we were in a worse place. All the supplementary support in the world wasn't going to save this dog if we didn't get rid of that. They may have recovered him briefly but more surgery was not an option and cancer would ultimately kill him.

205 http://www.bobbyshealthyshop.co.uk/Hydrogen-Peroxide.php

So we loved him and did all we could. We couldn't save him but we have witnessed others achieve great success with their animals following similar protocols.

Taz died at home quite peacefully in July 2017 age 12. He was a healing dog who snook into our lives and was always a couple of days ahead, at least.

It never occurred to me at the time but with hindsight I am left wondering how he filled up with so much cancer as all mine was leaving.

It's the kind of thing they would do if they could.

It hurt terribly losing this bundle of love but it was an honour to meet him.

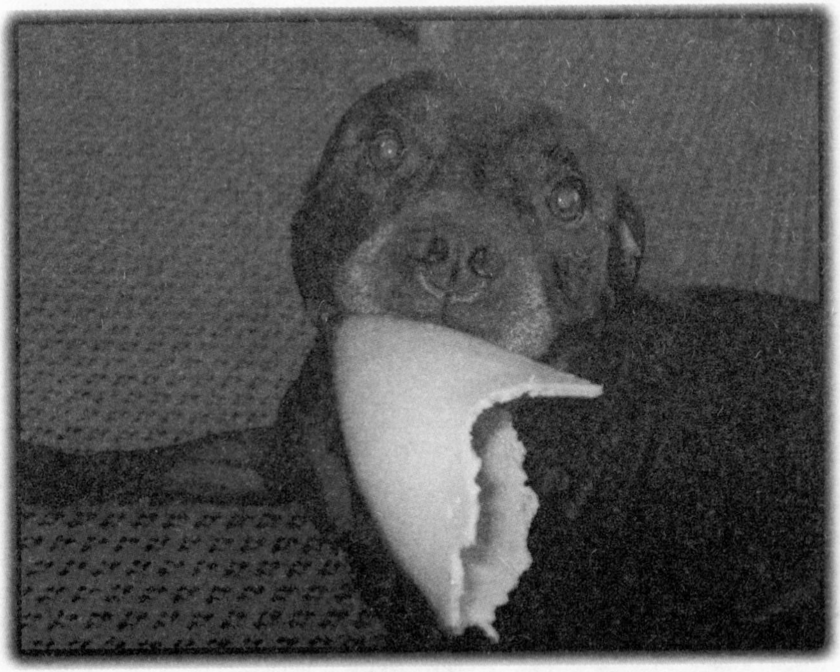

What football?

Vaccines, Vivisection & Vets
(from Taz with love)

This idea that escharotics can "draw out" cancers from underneath the skin is preposterous.
Stephen Barrett MD, Quackwatch

It always bothered me that our boy not only had cancer but had cancer from age 3. A week after he'd gone and we'd buried him and when the crying became more manageable I got an urgency about my day to apply for his records from the vet. Which I did. We liked the vet, she liked the dog, she quickly replied and readily complied, "please accept my deepest condolences for your loss of Taz. You must devastated. He was such a great dog".

We are and he was. In my hindsight moment I've realised that this whole thing was a set up. The dog was in on this from the very start, he and I were going to go through this cancer thing together and he was guiding me through his experience to weave in the vaccine experience of our animals and the power of the herbs. Sounds silly? I'm full of it. Taz came into our lives with purpose and a medical history; it records that vaccines don't discriminate and his story is your story.

We have a tendency to blame breeders for the state of dog's health and I think it's a given that by narrowing the gene pool by design we allow dysfunction to manifest in designer breeds. And while I'm not a fan of breeding dogs with so many dogs homeless, that's a separate issue. Selective breeding cannot explain the general breakdown of the health of our companion animals and the huge rise in allergies they face and I think we should be looking closer to home for answers. Like at the 'jabs' we load them up with.

The following is Taz's veterinary record. This typifies a normalised pattern of behaviour and what many view as a classic case of cause and effect. This vet responded to my request with all due courtesy but she was oblivious to the grave harm her jabs are doing and was equally ignorant of necessity, which must be established first and foremost.

The early months of his life are missing as he was with another vet, so his capture is first recorded 17th August 2005 age 4 months. This day he is injected with Merck's Nobivac 4in1 DHPPi + L2. This represents **D**istemper, **H**epatitis and **P**arvo viruses and includes among other things thiomersal/mercury @ 0.1 mg and gelatin, sorbitol, pancreatic digest of casein, disodium phosphate dihydrate, potassium dihydrogen phosphate. These core vaccines are recommended by the makers to be repeated **every three years**. The **Pi** element is Para-influenza vaccine which they say may, **"reduce clinical signs** of canine para-influenza infection and... **reduce** viral shedding. Duration of immunity has not been demonstrated". The **L** is **2** types of the leptospirosis bacteria (of which there are 250+) – "a single **annual booster dose is recommended"**. He was also given frontline, a chemical spot on pesticide flea killer and his 'health check' described him as "all well".

31st January 2005 he gets Nobivac DHPPiL2 again and another hit of mercury. Next visit in Feb 2007 he is injected with Nobivac DHPPiL2 again including mercury and described again as "all well". Two months later they record what they describe as a "compliance" issue following a missed appointment for another vaccination. August 2007 his dad complies and he gets a Nobivac rabies shot with aluminium phosphate Al3+di-Sodium hydrogen phosphate, and another dose of mercury. In November they note he is "all well" but now he has become "timid". A week on they again bemoan "compliance" over another missed vaccine appointment. I think the time has come they start complying with us. Next visit in March 2008 age 3 he is for the final time in his life assessed as "all well", albeit with some "intermittent lameness" in his hind leg. Another Nobivac PPiL2 vaccination is given including the mercury.

Next visit in July 2008 he gets a passport to travel to Spain with his dad and another Nobivac aluminium/thiomersal vaccination for rabies. April 2009 is the next visit and guess what? Yep, Nobivac DHPPiL2 combo with mercury, and some pesticides. They now record "slight amount of hair loss on dorsum and ventrum" (back and belly). Seven months later they find "patchy low grade bilat [eral] symm [etrical] alopecia occurred last year also? Possible hypothyroidism" has also now set in and they note that "taz seeks warmth" which he did.

Next visit is April 2010 when he is treated to more pesticides and Nobivac L2 with mercury. May 2011 he is injected with vaccination boosters Nobivac PPiL2 with mercury. Seven months later they note he has now developed a "mass on right point of shoulder with mid dorsal cyst present for many years. mass has appeared recently solitary SQ fatty feeling 2cm dia".

At his next visit in June 2012 they record he is "very scared in here". And he had every right to be! He is again injected with Nobivac PPiL2 + mercury, and more Advocate/pesticide now to be applied to his skin monthly. Do the way these injections make him feel instil that fear? We have moved in next door by now and have thoroughly informed his dad on the other side of the vaccine industry and he has stopped injecting his dog. Most people react like this once fully informed. His next visit is July 2013 when he is given more anti-insect pesticides (he had no more after this date) and they note: "taz has been scratching and this has become progressively worse. evidence of previous chewing of feet but no current open sores. however thickened erythematous area on ventral thorax, with evidence of excoriation of nipples, thickened erythematous, alopecic elbows."

Far from protecting this dog from disease this dog was falling apart. This was an increasingly unhealthy animal and he should not according to the vaccine makers have been vaccinated at all for that very reason, yet this was what I would describe as a caring veterinary practice where we were comfortable that they knew how to treat an animal.

I see estimates that vets generate around 40-50% of their income from vaccine sales, but this example with one dog suggests it may be more than that. Especially taking into account the money they make from vaccine damaged animals needing to return within days, for a drip maybe, or antibiotics, with kidney failure, with allergic reactions or to be put to sleep. On which there is a growing market. And it may not be within days, as there appears to be no cut off point after which vaccines have not done damage. I take into account the next time our boy attended the vet. This was three years later with a mass of cancer and now needing surgery costing £2,700 + three lesser bills. Did the vaccines cause or contribute to his cancer? Pretty much all Taz got from the vets for the first 7 years of his life was a bombardment of no less than 40 vaccinations including at the very least 11 hits of mercury some supercharged with aluminium, a pile of pesticides and deteriorating health checks. This only stopped because we forced the issue and it would have continued until our dog died.

The vets are happy, the customer did right by their little piggy, and piggy is in the middle. But the customer was duped and piggy is at risk. Would anyone in their right mind and in full disclosure give their consent to be injected through the skin with this amount of mercury? I don't think so.

But it isn't just that, is it? Most of these vaccines are the multi-dose, meaning for each 6 in 1 insult 6 viruses or bacteria have been nourished into life on the rich nutritious living innards of six different animal species. So in one needle we may find a bewildering assortment of ingredients such as formaldehyde, genetically modified wotnots, hydrolised gelatine, polysorbate 80, MSG, the heavy metals, and crucially we get the inseparable DNA of cat and mouse brains, rabbit nerves, dog and monkey kidneys and so on.

If you think about it, as we now must, this sesame street soup of DNA stealth viruses and who knows what else living in the microscopic world, forms the element of the vaccines we *want* for our companion animals. I say we. The implanted viral antigen (such as parvovirus) being grown in this soup, is the active ingredient that is supposed to generate the appropriate antibody response and from that comes protection from the wild disease. Aside whether that theory is even valid, this one vaccine ingredient alone is of course a DNA time bomb.

During this series of experiments on our dog he developed skin and food allergies, his thyroid flagged up, he lost hair, he grew multiple lumps, he became timid and he limped. And he got cancer. Of course it wasn't anything **at all** to do with **any** of the vaccines because vets sell vaccines and vets love animals and according to the manufacturer's data and vaccine inserts there are no such side effects to look out for so they simply cannot be there. See the plain and simple logic? And if there are any changes seen in the victim in the time after vaccine, there are always coincidences to explain them away. Once upon a time that worked, but we're waking.

In WDJ's [Whole Dog Journal] opinion (and that of the experts we consult), annual vaccination for most canine diseases is unnecessary and potentially harmful. Dog owners should avoid employing those old-fashioned veterinarians who recommend annual vaccines. [206]

---

[206] https://www.whole-dog-journal.com/issues/13_8/features/Over-Vaccinating-Your-Dog_20036-1.html

Pesticides, in pets?

We have a multi-billion dollar industry that is killing people, right and left, just for financial gain. Their idea of research is to see whether two doses of this poison is better than three doses of that poison.
Glen Warner, M.D. oncologist.

We *may* come into contact with any mercury our animals are fortunate to excrete after vaccination but we would be *unlikely* to avoid the pesticides. These chemical spot-on products are well known for the damage they do, as is their purpose after all. As example the Canadian Pest Management Regulatory Agency recorded 4,726 incidents for cats and dogs related to topical flea treatments between 2009 and 2013 including 1,188 dead cats and 872 dogs.

Earlier the Environmental Protection Agency (EPA) compiled a damning report after investigating over 44,000 adverse reactions to pesticides in pets during 2008 alone including 600 deaths. The system for reporting and recording adverse events to pesticides and vaccines and drugs is not like wearing seat belts, these are voluntary schemes and it's our responsibility to report them and these statistics always represent only a tiny fraction of the true impact.

Not only are the numbers unacceptable and apparently an unknown so too is the damage they do.

> ***... the data we now require to determine the safety of these products for pets do not accurately predict the toxicity seen in the incidents that took place.*** [207]

This suggests the modern science of toxicity and safety testing is unable or unwilling to predict that poisons are poisonous when it really matters.

They highlight yet another problem, this time with what are described as the inert or filler ingredients in these products.

> *Formulant ingredients, commonly known as "inerts", provide a solvent for the insecticidal active ingredient and aid in dispersal of the product. These ingredients were discussed during the review process and it was felt that they* ***contribute to toxicity*** *reported in some incidents. Because these ingredients are considered* ***confidential business information****, they are not reported here but* ***should undergo continued evaluations****.* [207]

What's that say? Secret and dangerous, need to keep doing studies. It's the MO of the status quo.

---

[207] https://www.regulations.gov/document?D=EPA-HQ-OPP-2010-0229-0023

We are all exposed to this stuff once it's squirted onto the skin of our animals but especially while attempting to heal yourself naturally using the MannIcure or any like protocol extreme caution is called for in respect of these poisons.

I see an incredulous Charlotte Gerson at the idea of putting anything onto our skin we would not eat.

The EPA goes further by bringing to light the very real concern of cross contamination of these **neurotoxic** pesticide sprays. Yes they get into the blood of the parasites we want to get rid of, but they also get elsewhere. These adverse events include reports of the canine range of flea products leading to cats suffering "more deaths and major incidents than dogs".

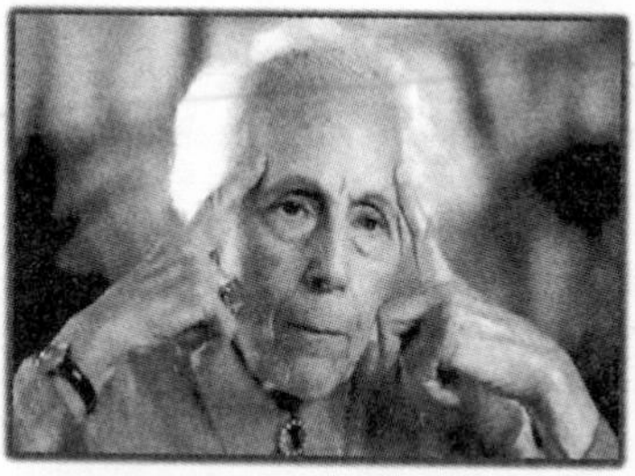

Incredulous Charlotte Gerson

If you think that represents stupid science then what about this:

> *The companion animal safety studies rely upon Beagle dogs, but* ***Beagles were not a sensitive breed for predicting adverse incidents in dogs*** *as shown in the incident analysis.* [208]

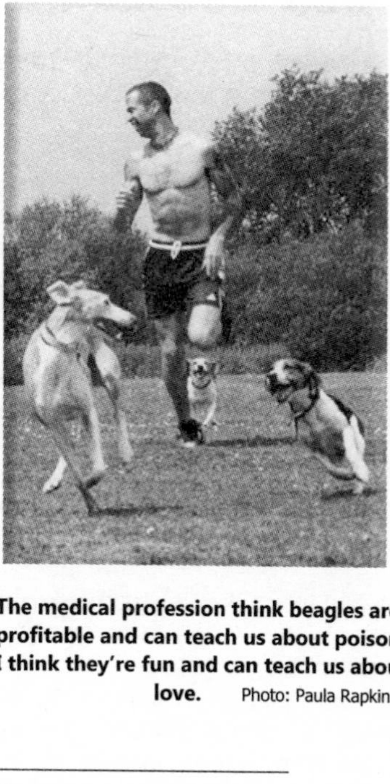

The medical profession think beagles are profitable and can teach us about poisons. I think they're fun and can teach us about love. Photo: Paula Rapkins

The beagle is the medical profession's canine gold standard, but they don't even work! Hundreds of millions put to a grim death to gather results that may be incompatible with others of their own species! The mind boggles. So what are we left with here? Business as usual! Whatever the stated intention, look at the outcome.

The outcome for our animals from all these products is not health but along the supply chain there is wealth. I'm not dissing all vets of course and I know good people who are vets but there's something seriously wrong with any group of people who participate in chemical experiments on live animals and inject cancer in our beloved companions.

[208] https://www.regulations.gov/document?D=EPA-HQ-OPP-2010-0229-0023

I have heard it said that animal vaccines must be safe because vets wouldn't harm animals. It is also suggested that they must be safe and effective, even if there are questions about some human vaccines because these have been tested on animals to save other animals and because animals are animals the results must be accurate. This cock-eyed logic doesn't sit with the infinite stream of vaccine-induced 'events' reported by owners. Events do sound rather benign, momentary, a weekend maybe? We are duly invited to attend as we might attend a social event or a charity event, for fun not danger. But the chemical events that these kind words belittle may turn out more like a terrorist outrage or an air disaster, albeit on a much wider scale and affecting many more lives.

Also there are no studies comparing the health and wellbeing of unvaccinated animals to vaccinated animals or to see if homeopathy is cheaper and more suited or if good nutrition is the best foundation for overall health. It's haphazard, harmful and doubtful of need. Yet still insurance companies often demand animals be vaccinated before they will provide insurance. So did the lab rats bring any gains for our cats or even our rats? An important consideration for one such as I. Seriously, so far there's not much to get cocky about in the miracle cure department. So who do you ask to help you decide if there's some value in these pet jabs and poisons?

Vets? Party line. Vaccine makers? Party line. Animal welfarists? Party line. Try it.

Me: The line they left out.

I looked to the rescue centres working hard to find good homes for the homeless and needy strays. These are the real warriors not just mopping up society's mess but dealing with the suffering of animals daily. Yet predominantly, as some kind of badge of honour these waifs are often offered to potential new homes as "up to date" or "fully vaccinated". And they repeat the party line about it all being necessary to save lives. They often mention the polio vaccination as some kind of proof, which of course it is! Other ill-informed animal lovers will demand the badgers be brought into this mess and be vaccinated in reaction to disease fears peddled by industry. They will repeat the words "protect", "conspiracy theory", "experts" and "polio". So what does this full compliance even mean for these rescued animals looking for safety from human ignorance, and according to whose advice and on what science are these lethal interventions based? I asked them all. Mantra. However it's dressed up what this means is fully vivisected and often paid for by voluntary public donations. With regard to the bigger cash generating animal rescue organisations, incredibly pharmaceutical sponsors can often be found supplying their vaccine products to help the poor strays.

One reward for the sponsors from our compliance with their vaccine schedules, aside the free advertising, is that our experimental puppy is highly likely to manifest any number of ailments that will 'sadly' need further veterinary treatments and more animal experiments. Or maybe a return to the rescue centre, messed up by the poisons and unmanageable in their new homes? Our ongoing participation in these experiments only further emboldens a greedy, relentless industry. And as for the next generation of animals born to today's DNA mutated mutts, we will only mourn.

But don't trust me, simply ask your medical expert for the relevant vaccine safety data, proof of necessity, the vaccine ingredients or the culture medium – that which grew the vaccine virus – and unless you get some satisfaction, which I am certain you won't, you may be left feeling it's time to leave. I asked and here's what I found. The good news is there are other ways. Remember, there is no luxury in ignorance except for the very people who are unable to prove the safety, effectiveness and necessity of these nifty little biological time bombs.

Medical science has broken the totality of natural laws in the human body to little pieces. It has studied and re-studied single processes and overestimated them. The symptoms of a disease became the main problem for research and clinical work. The medical theory of the old and middle ages to combine all parts in the body to a biological entity was pushed aside almost involuntarily, and finally became very far removed from our thinking. How such thinking of totality will help us to find the cause of cancer can best be seen in practical examples – not animal experiments – in the nutritional field of people who do not get cancer, and, on the other hand, of those who get it in greater or increasing amounts.

Dr Max Gerson.

Had one vaccine, had too many

No one in my lab wants to get vaccinated. This totally creeped us out. We weren't out there to pokes holes in vaccines. But all of a sudden, oh my God – we've got neuron death!

Professor Christopher Shaw [209]

I've looked hard and found the lack of evidence-based science that vaccine researchers talk about. But what about the increasing frequency we are invited to attend for boosters? Do annual injections make the vaccines somehow work better? By extension the pre-marketing proof of this is lacking, but it isn't really necessary now because these products have been extensively tested on the domestic population so we can see for ourselves what they are capable of.

A spokesman for Intervet, one of the world's largest veterinary drug manufacturers now owned by Merck, the world's largest drug company, told BBC Radio 4's Today programme in 2004: 'We base our recommendations on the science and the science we have tells us that **we don't know how long immunity lasts in any individual animal.**"

So, not got a clue or don't care to say? This 'don't really know' thing comes up a lot in the medical arena. They usually follow by inviting more research grants. This is money to play with, to invest in one's future research, to build upon. Few will use it to compromise the status and wealth of their donors or the status quo.

Is that basic information regarding the efficacy of their product really such a difficult thing to figure out? They don't know and didn't care to draw conclusions during development? They assure us the vaccines work but have no way of knowing if it's for one day or for life, so logically the best thing we can do is just keep buying those boosters and then it doesn't really matter, right? In gaga land! In reality too much of anything is usually harmful especially when it's delivered by needle and it is highly toxic.

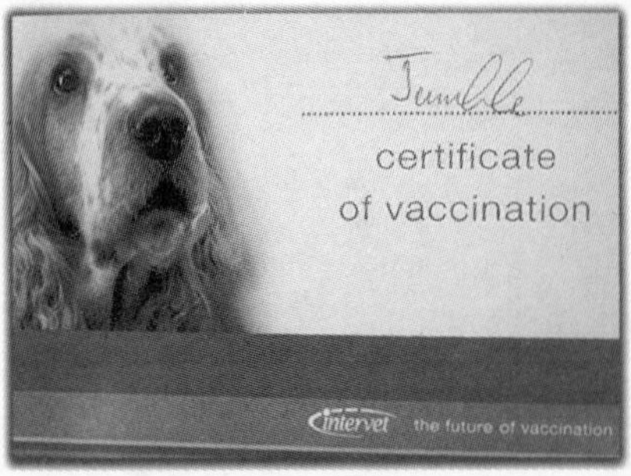

What does your animal's vaccine 'certificate' tell you? Check the crafty use of words to guide us their way. A certificate is a good thing right, something to be proud to possess. Does it say that your baby has been vaccinated repeatedly for things like distemper, hepatitis and parvovirus (DHP)?

Have these been given annually? This flies in the face of the vaccine manufacturer's guesstimates and the science; it is an unnecessary medical intervention and it is

209 http://whale.to/b/vaccine/shaw_h.html

dangerous. So your vet is either clueless or taking advantage. Either way your best friend is in harms way and you need to help him.

- *Routine vaccinations are probably the worst thing that we do for our animals. They cause all types of illnesses, but not directly to where we would relate them definitely to be caused by the vaccine.* Christina Chambreau, DVM
- *Above all, it must be remembered that even a 3-year license is a minimum DOI [Duration of Immunity] for core vaccines and for most core vaccines the true DOI is likely to be considerably longer,* ***if not lifelong,*** *for the majority of vaccine recipients.* [210]
- ***There is limited information available on the incidence and prevalence of canine diseases driving the use of core and non-core vaccines of companion animals. It is, however, recognised that there is an increasing body of scientific literature and opinion that suggests the DOIs of the core vaccines (as defined by the WSAVA Guidelines) for dogs may be considerably longer [9 years +] than the authorised claims for existing vaccines on the EU market.*** [211]

In a parvo outbreak in the UK in 2017 only two of the 12 cases reported had any substance attached, but in both cases the point was made clear that the dead dogs had had their protective jabs. So we could headline that 'In 100% of reported cases all dogs were fully vaccinated'. And this is the theme wherever you look.

- *One woman said that her eight-month-old puppy has had both sets of required injections (to guard against it) but she still died.*

- *Tracey Hand... from ... Gainsborough, lost her beloved dog Scooby to the virus on August 30 despite him being vaccinated against it.* [212]

- *My little Shih tzu got her booster yesterday then turned ill last night frothing and dribbling through the night got scoots... she is now on a drip in vets dehydrated so worried. Pray its only reaction to her booster... not Parvo virus.*

- *A family in our village has just lost two vaccinated dogs.*

- *A friends 8 month old puppy has caught parvo even though she has been vaccinated.*

---

210 https://onlinelibrary.wiley.com/doi/epdf/10.1111/jsap.2_12431

211 https://www.gov.uk/government/uploads/system/uploads/attachment_data/file/485325/Vaccines_VMDPositionPapaer.pdf

212 http://www.lincolnshirelive.co.uk/news/lincoln-news/fears-after-12-cases-deadly-402816

The Vets

Remember, the Order is most distinct to public vaccinators that it is only healthy children that are to be diseased.
Dr Walter Hadwen (1854 – 1932)

Taz had 7 of these parvo vaccinations in 7 years, for an infection which may affect puppies of a few months of age. He acted it but not for as long as we knew him was he a puppy.

Canine parvo is a mutated man-made virus that evolved from cats. It made its way into dogs in the late 1970's and spread so rapidly and simultaneously around the planet it appeared like it was being delivered by needle. The smart money says the original source of this virus was contaminated cat kidneys used for nourishing the distemper virus into life. Indeed, soon after its appearance parvo was classified as a mutation of the feline panleukopenia virus (FPV) and current taxonomy defines canine parvovirus and feline panleukopenia virus as a single entity which has returned home.

> *Since the emergence of Canine parvovirus (CPV-2) in the late 1970s, CPV-2 has evolved consecutively new antigenic types, CPV-2a and 2b. Although CPV-2 did not have a feline host range, CPV-2a and 2b appear to have gained the ability to replicate in cats.* [213]

Little in the vaccine department has been able to compete with the arrival of the parvo from a veterinary business perspective (aside from vaccine-induced vet visits), although new vaccines are being constantly produced to chase the endless viral mutations around and this must be very encouraging.

> *Parvovirus suppresses the immune system. Injecting the live virus, despite attenuation, can have serious implications for the animal's health and for simultaneous vaccination. Vaccine-induced immunosuppression has been well-documented following various vaccines, and it has been found that if the vaccine recipient is harbouring a sub clinical infection, or becomes exposed to a pathogen, clinical disease can occur.* **Catherine Diodatti MA - Vaccine Guide for Dogs & Cats.**

Taz had 8 lepto vaccinations each with a dose of mercury, yet mercury is toxic to dogs and causes grave harm, as it does to all the species it is tested on. Here's a thought: always was, always will be a deadly toxin. And, not that it changes this detail, but leptospirosis is so rare in the UK there are no records kept, and this is a theme too. Do vets mention the prevalence of each of these diseases when offering your baby a needle so you can weigh up the risk? They should. Who else will? Leptospirosis is being treated as a core vaccine and is recommended by a great many vets yet the science of necessity just does not demand it. So they are dishonest and/or ignorant and cannot be trusted? Let's have a look.

---

213 http://www.2ndchance.info/pankeuk-Ikeda2002.pdf

According to reports made to the Government's Veterinary Medicines Directorate (VMD) by pet owners, more than 120 dogs are feared to have died after receiving a dosage in the three years the product has been on the market.

In the last two years, regulators have received 2,000 reports of dogs having suspected adverse or fatal reactions. ***The regulator has however refused to reveal the total number of animals that had been affected*** *since the product came onto the market, prompting concern among dog owners that* ***the scale of problem is being kept hidden from the public.***

The VMD also declined to say whether it will consider taking the product off the market, because ***its researchers have so far failed to find enough evidence linking the vaccine to dog fatalities.***

In 2014 the European Medicines Agency advised the manufacturer to ***compare reactions to those recorded from the previous leptospirosis vaccine****. No conclusions have yet been reached and L4 remains on the market.* [214]

Vets are churning out **L**epto**4** vaccines regardless of everything. One internet forum with 14,000 members documented death number 78 recently. Titch, an 8 week old Jack Russell cross chihuahua puppy. He went blind and his kidneys failed just 2 days after vaccination. [215] Only in the hands of vets and vivisectors! And it isn't just the dead dogs is it; there are many more left injured, itching, irritable and allergic and harbouring mutations into the future.

Taz had 7 flu vaccinations in 7 years not to cure or prevent anything but to possibly "**reduce** clinical signs of canine para-influenza infection" and to "**reduce** viral shedding" for a period of time that "has not been demonstrated."

Its flu, it occurs most in kennels where there's overcrowding and stress, it's usually mild or inconvenient for the dog. They'll get over it.

The distemper virus in dogs is comparable to the human measles virus and the measles vaccine has been used in dogs to this end. We know all about the measles vaccine and this relative should be viewed with deep suspicion until we are shown proof otherwise. Encephalitis is a recognised complication of the live attenuated canine distemper vaccine.

Post vaccinal canine distemper encephalitis occurs in young animals, especially those less than six months of age. It has been recognised as a disease entity for a number of years, and is believed to be associated with

---

214 http://www.telegraph.co.uk/news/2016/07/02/dogs-dying-after-having-protective-vaccine-owners-claim/

215 https://www.facebook.com/groups/322967551247441/

vaccination using live virus. The pathogenesis of this disease is unclear, but may result from insufficient attenuation of the vaccine virus which causes subsequent infections of the CNS [central nervous system]; the triggering of a latent distemper infection by vaccination; other vaccine components; or an enhanced susceptibility of the animal (e.g., animals that are immunosuppressed). [216]

The distemper vaccine is considered effective in maintaining antibodies if given at the right time, but that as we know does not automatically equate with protection and we can find ample evidence of vaccinated dogs succumbing. But if antibodies are what we seek then the distemper vaccine is only needed once. Taz got it four times before we stepped in so three times he was subjected to unnecessary medical intervention with this one life-threatening product alone. The ingredients are little understood but it comes in a package of dangers which we underestimate at our peril.

1981: *Ten gray foxes seronegative for canine distemper virus were vaccinated with 1 of 3 commercial modified live-virus canine distemper vaccines. Of 5 foxes receiving vaccine A (chicken tissue culture origin), 4 developed significant titres (greater than or equal to 1:100) of neutralizing antibody to canine distemper virus and remained clinically normal after vaccination.* ***Two of 3 foxes vaccinated with vaccine B (canine cell line origin) and both foxes receiving vaccine C (canine cell line origin) died of vaccine-induced distemper. Five unvaccinated control foxes died of distemper after a known occasion for contact transmission of virus from a fox vaccinated with vaccine B. The results suggested that the chicken tissue culture origin modified live-virus canine distemper vaccine is probably safe for normal adult gray foxes, whereas the canine cell origin vaccines are hazardous. The results of this study tended to corroborate anecdotal experiences of veterinarians who have observed that gray foxes frequently die from distemper soon after vaccination with modified live-virus canine distemper vaccines.*** [217]

2017: Same vaccine, with added spin and ignoring the above:

There is ***a chance*** *a dog will have side effects from the canine distemper vaccine if a* ***live virus*** *is used. Side effects* ***may include*** *a low-grade fever, lack of energy and appetite, and irritation at the injection site. Not all dogs will have a negative reaction to the distemper vaccine. The slight chances of side effects from the vaccination outweigh the risks of a dog contracting the actual distemper virus.* [218]

Hepatitis is rare, puppies being the most vulnerable. The hepatitis virus in that component of the multi-dose vaccine is grown in the MDCK canine cell line, which

---

216 Braund's Clinical Neurology in Small Animals: Localization, Diagnosis and Treatment

217 https://www.ncbi.nlm.nih.gov/pubmed/7199036

218 https://www.vetinfo.com/canine-distemper-vaccine-explained.html

you may recall was originally harvested from the kidneys of a Cocker Spaniel in 1958. As we may deduce from the fox experiment, this may be a bit too much meddling for Mother Nature to tolerate. They can call it science but she ain't stupid. This was thought to be a female dog who they describe as "normal". What they have used her for in the decades since she died is anything but normal. Is this more than just a little bit weird? The growth medium, or compost, used to spark up this hepatitis virus also contains a foetal bovine serum. That's basically a baby cow's blood and dog kidney extract injected into my dog four times! You sick fcuks. [219]

> ***Bovine serum,*** *commonly used during vaccine production to provide several biological molecules and growth supporting factors for optimal cell growth,* ***has been the major source of contamination in veterinary vaccines.*** *The most prevalent bovine contaminants have been bovine viral diarrhoea pestivirus; parainfluenza virus type 3; bovine herpesvirus 1; bovine enterovirus type 4; bovine orbivirus (bluetongue); bovine polyomavirus and bovine parvoviruses.* [220]

Taz had two rabies vaccinations one to get him across borders and the other one a year later, yet he was never leaving the country again anyway so he didn't need two even by the rules made up by all these self-interest groups.

Dr Pitcairn's 'Complete Guide to Natural Health for Dogs and Cats' say

> *The most common disturbances following rabies vaccination are aggressiveness, suspicion, unfriendly behaviour, hysteria, destructiveness (of blankets, towels), fear of being alone and howling or barking at imaginary objects.*

The vaccine makers boast

> *Because Nobivac 1-Rabies vaccine is produced on an established cell line, it has safety advantages over inactivated brain-origin rabies vaccines.* ***Tissue-origin vaccines contain extraneous protein in addition to rabies antigen that can lead to autoimmune disease.*** [221]

Bless their little hearts. This is Merck, an empire built on evil trying to be kindly! In this new improved Nobivac Rabies vaccine promo they boast that the viral components are safer for our little piggy because they were sprouted in the established cell line of rabbit DNA over 100 years old, instead of fresher, allegedly more iffy brain or kidney material used in other vaccines. I think iffy is a given and safe is subjective. Who mentions that we are risking autoimmune disease with

---

219 http://www.sigmaaldrich.com/catalog/product/sigma/84121903?lang=en&region=GB

220 Human and animal vaccine contaminations: http://www.sciencedirect.com/science/article/pii/S1045105610000734?via%3Dihub

221 https://www.drugs.com/vet/nobivac-1-rabies.html

inactivated brain-origin rabies vaccines? And that the vaccine is only "an aid in preventing rabies." 221

Digging in we find our cat, dog or ferret will also be getting a shot of aluminium phosphate and mercury in their jab. Now, if you have been paying attention and have taken note of the health crisis the vaccinated human population is in, you may consider that injecting this highly neurotoxic nanoparticle cell mutating combo into our precious loved ones is probably not a good idea. And with each booster of course the burden accumulates and the body's ability to resist wanes.

> *Aluminium is extremely toxic, especially if you inject it. Mercury and aluminium are in Gardasil and Gardasil is an incredible vaccine. We looked at Gardasil and compared it to all the other vaccines... Gardasil was the worst thing we had ever seen in terms of the symptoms that were showing up. Gardasil has amazing list of reactions that stand out... and they include some very serious things. Coma... death... unconsciousness... suicide... Aluminium is strongly associated with depression. I think the vaccine makes them so incredibly depressed they can't cope.* [222]

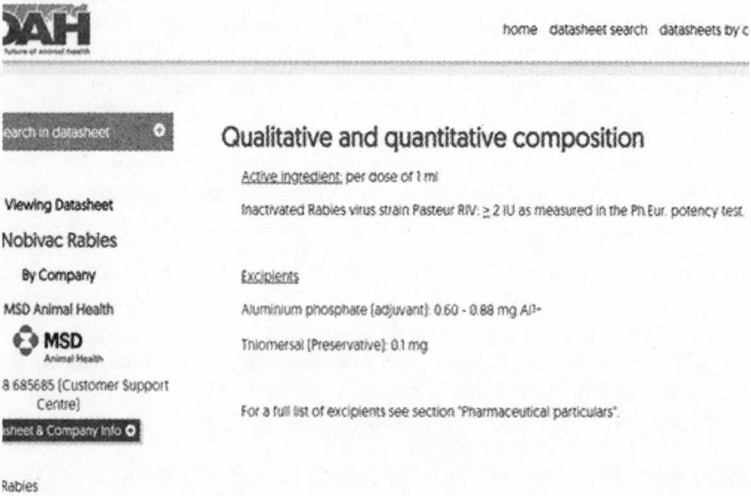
home datasheet search datasheets by c
earch in datasheet
Qualitative and quantitative composition
Active ingredient: per dose of 1 ml
Viewing Datasheet
Inactivated Rabies virus strain Pasteur RIV: ≥ 2 IU as measured in the Ph.Eur. potency test.
Nobivac Rabies
By Company
Excipients
MSD Animal Health
Aluminium phosphate (adjuvant): 0.60 - 0.88 mg Al3+
MSD
Animal Health
Thiomersal (Preservative): 0.1 mg
8 685685 (Customer Support Centre)
For a full list of excipients see section "Pharmaceutical particulars".
sheet & Company Info
Rabies

The makers of thiomersal, Eli Lilly, carried out a human trial on their mercury preservative in the 1930's and promptly observed the demise of 100% of their 22 already ailing victims, some the very same day, so concluded, since it was their trial and it was their product, that they died for other reasons and therefore there were no toxic effects to record. Simple science!

By 2007 we find mercury is still toxic in all its forms:

---

[222] Stephanie Seneff, Ph.D Senior Research Scientist, Massachusetts Institute of Technology

> *Eight of nine children examined in this study (a) had regressive autistic disorders, (b) had elevated levels of androgens, (c) excreted significant amounts of mercury post chelation challenge, (d) had biochemical evidence of decreased function in their glutathione pathways, (e) had no known significant mercury exposure except from Thimerosal in their vaccines/Rho(D)-immune globulin preparations, and (f) had extensive alternate causes for their regressive ASDs ruled out. It is clear from these data, and other emerging data that have been recently published, that additional autistic disorder research should be undertaken in the context of evaluating mercury-associated exposures, especially from Thimerosal-containing vaccines. Additionally, studies should also be undertaken to evaluate other databases/registries of patients to assess the compatibility of the present results with clinical observations for other children with autistic disorders. In light of the results of this present case series examining mercury exposure and its consistency with previous controlled studies of autistic children, the mercury factor should be considered in the differential diagnosis factors of regressive autistic disorders in children.* [223]

I see a pattern forming. If they'll do that to our children what hope do our animals have? Thousands of sickening experiments and hundreds of studies on this hazardous waste material in the years since that first indicator have replicated these findings yet they persist injecting it into everyone and everything they can get their bloody hands on.

> *Thimerosal used as a preservative in vaccines is likely related to the autism epidemic. This epidemic in all probability may have been prevented or curtailed had the FDA not been asleep at the switch regarding the lack of safety data regarding injecting Thimerosal and the sharp rise in infant exposure to this known neurotoxin.* [224]

This is getting silly. Necessity does not enter my mind. I'm not thinking science either. Animal welfare? Nah! A product to sell is what this is.

It's generally acknowledged and is always in the accompanying advice of vaccines that they should only be administered to "healthy" recipients, with a broad spectrum of exclusions. That's a big word, an important word and it's vital we consider it because all those complicated components in that needle are going to adversely affect health to one level or another.

Health may be compromised before the needle goes in if:

---

[223] https://www.researchgate.net/publication/6373722_A_Case_Series_of_Children_with_Apparent_Mercury_Toxic_Encephalopathies_Manifesting_with_Clinical_Symptoms_of_Regressive_Autistic_Disorders

[224] Mercury in Medicine - Taking Unnecessary Risks. A report prepared by the Staff of the Subcommittee on Human Rights and Wellness Committee on Government Reform United States House of Representatives. May 2003
https://vaccines.procon.org/sourcefiles/Burton_Report.pdf (page 15)

1. the animal is genetically defective
2. there is something wrong with the animal's diet
3. the animal is stressed at time of injection
4. the animal's immune system is not fully competent
5. the animal is exposed to a virus before or soon after vaccination
6. the animal is on other drugs or medication
7. the vet administers the vaccine inappropriately
8. the vet stores the vaccine inappropriately
9. the animal is incubating disease at the time of vaccination
10. the animal is pregnant
11. the animal has parasites
12. the animal is very young and has maternally-derived antibodies
13. a previous vaccine was contaminated
14. a previous vaccine was toxic and left a weakness
15. the animal has been recently challenged by pesticides
16. the animal is post surgery
17. the animal is post illness
18. the animal is allergic to any vaccine ingredients

What this all means is the immune defences are otherwise occupied and cannot adequately meet the extreme demands of the vaccine. This I equate to kicking someone in the head while he's lying unconscious on the ground - an image I have collected along the way of an action I cannot fathom which sickens me.

And when it does all go wrong we typically hear the medicine expert announce that the victim had a "bad reaction" to the vaccine, as though it were your baby's fault and nothing to do with the perpetrator. Seldom do we hear the experts announce that the victims of a bomb attack "reacted badly" to the bombs, but in the field of modern medicine things are not as they should be and there is no shame in the destruction of life.

Prof Peter Openshaw, a leading immunologist from Imperial College London, claims,

> *A lot of vaccine reactions are just inexplicable. It may be that someone had an infection before they got a jab, it may be something in their genetic make-up or sometimes there are allergic reactions. But vaccines are extraordinarily safe compared to the diseases they prevent.* [225]

Party line. Vets will seek to offload multiple vaccines and pesticide products during these brief appointments, not because of sound scientific research that says your baby needs them since the sound scientific research says the opposite. They are thinking more about themselves and about shifting stock. They know full well they may not get you through the door again for at least another year and of course many of us don't feel the need to go back for their idea of an MOT. And vaccines have a sell by date so they have to sell as much stuff to you when they have you in

[225] http://www.telegraph.co.uk/news/uknews/3336455/Secret-report-reveals-18-child-deaths-following-vaccinations.html

the shop as they can. It would be a very unusual business that operated any other way.

> *A good immune response is reliant on the reaction of an immunogenic agent and a fully competent immune system. Immunogenicity of the vaccine antigen will be reduced by poor storage or inappropriate administration. Immuno-competence of the animal may be compromised by a variety of factors including poor health, nutritional status, genetic factors, concurrent drug therapy and stress.* [226]

It's a fragile existence around these needles! Is it not a little bit obvious by now that it's not a variety of factors that make these vaccines dangerous but the vaccines themselves? What all this means with the waffle edited is that your dog may die or become ill if any of the above apply to him. And isn't it ironic that those with a robust immune system are the best equipped to fend off a virus and the very ones who don't need an artificial boost!

Do vets work through this list of potential life-threatening contraindications when customers attend for cancer causing vaccines? Do they themselves check off this list before the vaccine sale is agreed and the animal injected? I know the answer because I've been there. We may have an inclination our companion animals are struggling with an underlying health issue but they don't complain so how can we be sure? Perhaps your baby carries defective genes from a parent who suffered vaccine or pesticide-induced cell mutation? Does a vet know this is even possible? What is the right diet for a dog anyway? Do vets really know and based on what? Marketing of the food manufactures' products that the vets often sell? Manufactured food is at the root of many health issues in all captive species, especially humans, where it is often compounded by the expert's lack of understanding. 'Stress'? At the vets? Never! Do vets have any clue what's in the syringe? This information is scattered and not easy to come by. Common yet little understood effects of these vaccines are nervousness, anxiety and depression, linked to aluminium, so multiply that vet-induced anxiety each time the animal returns to be further immune compromised and there's another animal at serious risk of harm at the hands of experts with bills to pay.

> *In response to this [vaccine] violation, there have been increased autoimmune diseases (allergies being one component), epilepsy, neoplasia [tumours], as well as behavioural problems in small animals.* **Mike Kohn, DVM.**

Risking anyone's life by a deliberate intervention which is probably ineffective and probably dangerous to avoid an infection which will probably never occur and can probably be managed with much less risk is probably not a good idea.

We could gather from these vaccine risk warnings and from a rich human/animal experience that someone with a fully supported immune system, eating a clean

---

226 http://www.noahcompendium.co.uk/?id=-455536

nutrient dense diet appropriate to the individual would be best able to respond to a viral attack and not need a needle.

This very real harm mirrors that affecting the human population. We'd be fooling ourselves to assume otherwise. Of course the only credible side effect monitoring system can be a voluntary one not run by government or industry since these agents of deception cannot benefit from shoddy science coming under the spotlight and cannot be trusted with the lives of others. According to Merck, some of the effects of their products include "encephalitides... and many other less well defined viral infections".

Encephalitides is otherwise known as encephalomyelitis, encephalitis or the much easier understood: brain inflammation. Imagine how society would react to a serial killer on the rampage inflicting brain damage on children, even one, or a vivisector inflicting brain damage on some animals in his lab. Indeed we are soon up in arms, yet still we participate and passionately defend the very same crimes because we convince ourselves we are doing the right thing. Like philanthropists, doctors, psychopaths and serial killers.

> *Recent reports have raised concerns within the profession over the relationship between vaccination and delayed adverse events, specifically vaccine-associated fibrosarcoma in cats and immune-mediated disease in dogs.* ***Determining which vaccines pose a risk to which animals, and when, simply cannot be determined with the information available today.*** [227]

Oh yes it can. It's all of them.

I'm not picking on Merck or our vet by the way but they are up to their eyes in it. Other vaccines have mercury and aluminium mixed in them and that goes via vets into cats too. And ferrets. They all grow the virus the same way. One size fits all in gaga land and only there. Image that, we could have one government, same thoughts, one religion, one TV channel, a uniform, a set menu and the same colour car. Sounds mental! Like putting mercury into cats. Are we nuts? Maybe that's why they're often a little bit loopy! All the vaccines are swimming with poisons but the full ingredients are not readily available to the regular consumer. It's a trade secret don't you know! Commercial confidentiality is like national security. It's an excuse to cover up something dodgy. Logically they don't want you to know what they are up to because if you did you wouldn't give them your money and that matters more than anything.

Those human vaccines linked to so much physical harm contain 25mcg of thimerosal (50% ethylmercury) per shot. **The vaccines given to our companion animals have quadruple that amount @ 0.1mg of thimerosal in each injection.** So dogs aren't like people or are they? To the vaxers a Rottweiller's a Chihuahua - they're all the same. And this toxic data on thimerosal doesn't even consider the

[227] British Veterinary Association, in a letter to Catherine O' Driscoll (What Vets Don't Tel You About Vaccines)

hypodermic route, which we must remember bypasses most of our immune defences and takes the danger to another level altogether...

You couldn't even construct a study that shows Thimerosal is safe. It's just too darn toxic. If you inject Thimerosal into an animal, its brain will sicken. If you apply it to living tissue, the cells die. If you put in a Petri dish, the culture dies. Knowing these things, it would be shocking if one could inject it into an infant without causing damage.

Dr Boyd Haley PhD Dept of Chemistry, University of Kentucky

Section 11: Toxicological Information

Routes of Entry: Inhalation. Ingestion.

Toxicity to Animals: Acute oral toxicity (LD50): 75 mg/kg [Rat].

Chronic Effects on Humans:
MUTAGENIC EFFECTS: Mutagenic for mammalian somatic cells. May cause damage to the following organs: spleen, bone marrow, central nervous system (CNS).

Other Toxic Effects on Humans: Hazardous in case of skin contact (irritant), of ingestion, of inhalation.

Special Remarks on Toxicity to Animals: Not available.

Special Remarks on Chronic Effects on Humans:
May cause cancer based on animal data. No human data found. May cause adverse reproductive effects(fema
implanation mortality, fetotoxicity)and birth defects. May affect genetic material

Special Remarks on other Toxic Effects on Humans:
Acute Potential Health Effects: Skin: Causes skin irritation. Eyes: Causes eye irritation. May cause chemical co
inhalation: Causes respiratory tract irritation. May cause allergic respiratory tract irritation. Exposures to high cc
may produce unconsciousness with cyanosis(a bluish discoloration of the skin due to deficient oxygenation of t
and cold extremities and may also affect the cardiovascular system (rapid pulse). Acute exposure to high conce
of mercury vapors may also cause kidney damage and affect behavior/central nervous system, peripheral nerv
and autonomic nervous system, and liver and cause gastrointestinal effects (nausea, abdominal pain, vomiting
Harmful if swallowed. May cause gastrointestinal tract irritation with nausea, vomiting and diarrhea, headache.
high concentrations may affect respiration and cardiovascular system which may produce unconciousness with
cold extremities and rapid pulse. May also cause central nervous system effects and/or neurological effects, an
the urinary system (kidneys),and liver. Chronic Potential Health Effects: Skin: Prolonged or repeated skin conta
skin sensitization, an allergic reaction. Inhalation and Ingestion: Repeated or prolonged exposure may cause c
damage, and may affect the liver, and bone marrow. Chronic exposure to mercury vaporsbehavior/central nerv
peripheral nervous system (depression, irritability, nervousness, weakness, ataxia, fatigue, tremor, jerky gait, li
personality changes), metabolism (anorexia, weight loss) and cause gastrointestinal disturbances which is coll
to as "aesthenic-vegetative syndrome." Chronic ingestion may cause accumulation of mercury in body tissues
in salicylism which is characterized by nausea, vomiting, gastric ulcers, and hemorrhagic strokes.

Thimerosal Toxicity [228]

A field study conducted by Canine Health Concern during 1997, involving 4,000 vaccinated dogs, asked participants if their dog was ill, when did he become ill in relation to a vaccine.

68.2% of dogs in the survey with parvovirus contracted it within three months of being vaccinated; 55.6% of dogs with distemper contracted it within three months of vaccination; 63.6% with hepatitis got it within three months of vaccination; 50% with para-influenza contracted it within three months of vaccination, and every single dog with leptospirosis contracted it within that three-month time frame. 91% of Ataxia cases occurred within three months of a vaccine event; 81% of dogs who had tumours had them at their vaccine sites and first developed the tumours within three months of being vaccinated; 78.6% of dogs with encephalitis (inflammation of the brain) first developed the condition within three months of being vaccinated; 73.1% of epileptic dogs first became epileptic within three months of being vaccinated and 65.9% of dogs with colitis developed the condition within that first three months. 64.9% of dogs with behavioural problems started to be a problem within three months of vaccination; 61.5% of dogs that developed liver failure did so within three months of being vaccinated; 73.1% of the dogs who developed short

228 http://www.sciencelab.com/msds.php?msdsId=9925236

attention spans did so within three months of vaccination; and 72.5% of dogs that were considered by their owners to be nervous and of a worrying disposition first exhibited these traits within the three month post-vaccination period.[229]

The evidence is overwhelming.

The grim reapers at Merck comment almost in passing in their Nobivac Feline 2-FeLV product data that, "some reports suggest that in cats, the administration of certain veterinary biologicals may induce the development of injection-site fibrosarcomas". This is more spin and only undermines the considerable increase in risk of cancer posed by this vaccine.

Tumours comprising bone cells (osteosarcomas) muscle cells (rhabdomyosarcomas) cartilage cells (chondrosarcomas) and many other cell types are also showing up at the vaccination site.

This from the American Veterinary Medical Association (AVMA) in 2001:

> *Vaccine-associated feline sarcomas are a conundrum for the veterinary medical profession.* ***We do not understand the attributes of the feline immune system and genome that make cats susceptible to VAFS, yet we must continue to vaccinate cats against key infectious diseases. Vaccination was once considered an essential routine medical procedure with minimal risk. In the past decade, we have recognized that vaccination protocols must include assessment of the risk of sarcoma development.*** [230]

What a statement! This conundrum for the poor vets is really much more a conundrum for cats and their families caused by the vets. But it did give the prestigious AVMA an exciting opportunity. And it gives us special occasion to see how easily those we hold with high regard use the pain of others to prop themselves up. And we see how little they know. Take note they "do not understand" the feline immune system yet are injecting countless millions of cats with a liquid cosh meant to catapult this unknown entity into a state of emergency. So, with that we can see we are off to a very bad start with these people and should know not to expect too much.

With vigour and enthusiasm our cat heroes founded the Vaccine-Associated Feline Sarcoma Task Force (VAFS) and gathered together a whole mess of industrious fellows such as the American Association of Feline Practitioners (AAFP), American Animal Hospital Association (AAHA), American Veterinary Medical Association (AVMA) and the Veterinary Cancer Society (VCS), plus veterinary researchers and clinicians, the U.S. Department of Agriculture's Animal and Plant Health Inspection Service and the Animal Health Institute... blahdebladeblah.

---

229 https://chchealth.weebly.com/vaccine-survey.html

230 http://avmajournals.avma.org/doi/pdfplus/10.2460/javma.2001.218.697

They next constructed dozens of studies to, on the face of it, do something about the **hundreds of thousands** of cats that have developed terminal cancer at the vaccine injection sites, primarily after administration of rabies virus and FeLV (feline leukaemia virus) vaccines by their vets. Personally, I think the previous study that came up with these numbers should be able to reach a definitive conclusion, were that the true intention, but of course it wasn't. But it was going to be good for business.

This bold investigation by this top ranking group of vets into "the prevalence, causes, and treatment of VAFS", would surely, promptly uncover the cause and stop any more cats and their families from suffering. In gaga land! In the real world the establishment have learnt to never let a good crisis go to waste. And at times of crisis shortage it can be equally good for business to boost crisis production!

You would probably decide upon hearing of all these vaccine-induced cancers that pulling the vaccine until it was proven safe would be the best idea, as would I, but these people are not like us. These vets quickly scooped up $100,000 to help with this noble cause in donations from none other than a pile of vaccine manufacturers such as Pfizer, Intervet, Novartis and Bayer...

You think by now you probably know where this is going? Oh, you cannot imagine!

> *Vaccine-associated feline sarcomas are highly invasive and, often, rapidly growing neo-plasms* ***that require aggressive treatment, which may include a combination of surgery, radiation therapy, and chemotherapy. Task force-funded studies have shown the value of computed tomography and magnetic resonance imaging in determining the extent of these tumors before surgery or radiation therapy.*** [230]

Yes, they set to work spending these pharma funds on multiple studies to discover that medical CT and MRI scans are the most useful tools in cancer detection! This is a joke, right? Of course not, this is serious and it will naturally lead to more pharma treatments, which are seriously good for business too. Treatments that we all know will not make anything better for these cancer induced cats or any other cats. And as for the owners, gotta get them involved...

· ***When feasible, cats with histologically confirmed VAFSs should be imaged by computerized tomography CT or MRI. Advanced imaging data are very useful in determining the extent of surgery and/or the size of the radiation field that will be needed to maximize the chances for successful treatment.***

· ***Consult with an oncologist for current treatment options, which may include radiation, chemotherapy, surgery, or other modalities, prior to initiating therapy.***

· *Never "shell out" a sarcoma. Incomplete surgical removal of a sarcoma is the most common cause of treatment failure.* ***Employ oncologic surgical techniques to avoid seeding malignant cells. Remove at least a 2-cm margin in all***

planes, including the deep side. In some instances, this will involve reconstruction of the body wall, removal of bone, or other advanced surgical techniques.

· ***Submit the entire excised specimen for histopathology. Mark the excised mass with India ink or suture tags to provide an anatomical reference to facilitate subsequent treatment.*** 230

Eek! Didn't see all that coming when Tiddles got his elixir of life down at the vets!

Never mind you can pay in instalments, and life goes on.

Ahhh! About that...

> ***However, the addition of chemotherapy to radiation therapy and surgery has only modestly prolonged disease-free intervals. The unfortunate truth is that there are no good treatment options for cats with these tumors, further emphasizing the importance of tumor prevention.*** 230

They didn't know that chemo doesn't cure cancer before embarking on this venture? Perhaps they will go on to emphasise cancer prevention now they have discovered that as the best option? What do you think? This takes us back to my original hypothesis: the vaccines - focus on the vaccines...

Nah! They mention it in passing which tells us they are aware of the concept but there's no future for drug medicine in prevention. They decide instead it's best to ensure this feline gravy train just keeps right on rolling...

> ***Billions of dollars have been spent to understand the causes of and find cures for cancers in humans. In comparison, our efforts to understand and cure vaccine-associated sarcomas in cats are just beginning. There is still much to be done. Further research into the epidemiology, causes, treatment, and prevention of vaccine-associated sarcomas is essential to solving this problem.*** 230

And what do you know:

> ***Financial support of appropriate studies is expected to be a continuing need for the foreseeable future.*** 230

Do you think any of them blinked?

Just beginning, much to be done, more research, need more money... Sounds like our motive again. How about we work through the following paragraph and see if there isn't a key here to solving this grave mystery. I didn't compose it of course they did.

> ***Vaccine-associated*** *sarcomas in cats are most often fibrosarcomas, but many other types of sarcomas have also been reported. These sarcomas in cats are usually characterized by marked nuclear and cellular pleomorphism, high mitotic activity, and large central zones of necrosis, features consistent with an aggressive biological behavior. Often a peripheral inflammatory infiltrate consisting of lymphocytes and macrophages is seen.* ***Macrophages in these sarcomas often contain a bluish-gray foreign material identified*** *by electron probe x-ray microanalysis* ***to be aluminum and oxygen. Aluminum hydroxide is 1 of several adjuvants used in currently available feline vaccines. Similar inflammatory responses and foreign material have been described for inflammatory vaccination-site reactions in cats, dogs, and humans.*** 230

In that stunning announcement of the result of wide-scale animal experimentation on domestic cats we have solved the puzzle and can bring to a close the investigation into the prevalence, causes, and treatment of vaccine-associated feline sarcomas:

The cause is in the name and in the tumours; the rather unimaginative quest for a treatment is rapidly turned into a cure by addressing the cause - something almost unheard of in orthodox oncology; which in turn neatly resolves the question of prevalence. It's like medical Cluedo: the vet did it, in the surgery, with the needle.

So, no more vaccines, no more vaccine-associated feline sarcomas. Sorted! That was an easy one and it could have been done without a pile of self-interest business partners circulating money among themselves in order to promote their own cause and to discover things that should have been discovered during vaccine development if they were interested. However, it is always helpful to have more confirmation that aluminium and vaccines are linked to cancer. Devastating, for the uninitiated, but useful to know. How many doctors know this? How many vets? Tell them all. Tell everyone.

So, what did they do with these findings?

They press ahead regardless but do offer the following advice in order "to facilitate management of vaccine - associated sarcomas". Are you ready for this?

> *The task force has made initial vaccine-site recommendations in concert with the American Association of Feline Practitioners. In short, the task force recommends that vaccines containing rabies antigen be given as distally [far from the leg joint] as possible in the right rear limb, vaccines containing feline leukemia virus antigen (unless containing rabies antigen as well) be given as distally as possible in the left rear limb, and vaccines containing any other antigens except rabies or feline leukemia virus be given on the right shoulder, being careful to avoid the midline or interscapular space.* 230

I told you they aren't like us.

What this recognises is that digging out those vet-induced cancers from between the shoulder blades is no good for anyone, not least the cat, and of course the cat must come first. That cat is valuable. With the new improved science the vet can simply remove part of the affected limb when cancer appears and save the cat's life. A real live veterinary hero! So they get to vaccinate, amputate and you still have a cat with three limbs! A return customer. This is magic! Sadly (for some) an amputation commands a much higher price than the removal of a tumour but hey, we get to save a life and if in the event a second tumour appears where the other cancer causing vaccine was injected then a second leg amputation can be arranged. So the businessmen can cling on to that pussy for all it's worth.

Merck try to help too:

> *Surgical removal by a board-certified surgeon is considered the best treatment; however, complete removal is very difficult to achieve. When removing a fibrosarcoma, the veterinary surgeon will remove not only the tumor but also a wide and deep tissue margin around the tumor as well. Because it is difficult to determine the tumor's edges, recurrence is common. More than 70% recur within 1 year of the initial surgery.* ***The rate of recurrence is higher than 90% for injection-site sarcomas.*** *Even when surgical removal appears complete, recurrence is still the rule. Radiation treatment and chemotherapy are recommended to increase the tumor-free interval. Chemotherapy has been recommended for tumors that cannot be removed. Considering the invasive nature of these tumors, consultation with a veterinary oncologist (a specialist in the treatment of cancer) may be appropriate.* [231]

All that radiation scanning and surgical hacking and yet over 90% don't make one year before cancer is back. Meantime, in 2006 the AAFP and the (pharma sponsored) Academy of Feline Medicine Advisory Panel on Feline Vaccines "**stressed the importance of vaccinating the largest number of cats possible** within a population..."

Sick sick and sicker... The pharma loyalist at the AAFP later snuzzled up with Bayer on a further project seeking solutions to another problem they found with cats. Cats they figure don't like vets (worth considering) and according to the findings of this collaboration "cats represent one of the most significant missed opportunities for the veterinary profession." With a view to solving this problem of cats not needing vets and limited supplies of cats through the door, in 2013 the pussy pals produced a glossy brochure 'Ten Solutions to Increase Cat Visits' so to "provide practical tips for veterinary practice to implement in order to alleviate many of the obstacles to routine feline veterinary care." [232]

And they created a number of websites such as keepcatscomingback.com

---

231 https://www.msdvetmanual.com/cat-owners/skin-disorders-of-cats/tumors-of-the-skin-in-cats

232 https://www.catvets.com/public/PDFs/Education/Solutions/solutionsbrochure.pdf

As sick and twisted as all this is they may well have pulled it off.

After a sarcoma has been removed:

1. *Recheck by physical examination monthly for the first three months, then* ***at least every 3 months for one year****.*
2. ***Perform additional diagnostic procedures as appropriate for the abnormalities detected.*** [233]

Most don't make one year before the treatment fails and the cat is seriously ill again, yet every 3 months the vet will waste your time, freak out your cat and bill you.

Vaccines and vivisection are primitive and crude and deliver more misery than health, but they are very good for business.

That's all

I've thought about this a lot and asked around and I conclude that the single most important action we can each take to remove animals from harms way (aside not eating them) is to not subject them to experimental vaccines.

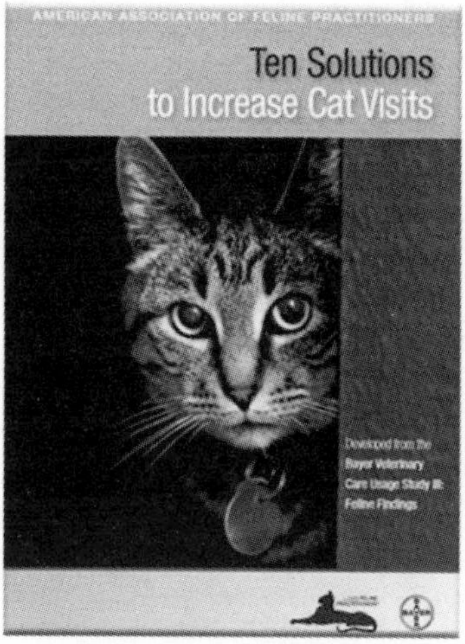

Problem, reaction, 10 solutions!

Animals don't get long enough here with us as it is and in the age of the cancer causing vaccines that brief experience is in many cases being spoiled by discomfort, disease and distress in order to satisfy the vested interests of people who have no interest in the happiness and wellbeing of humane beings and their loyal companions.

The fatal tendency of mankind to leave off thinking about a thing when it is no longer doubtful, is the cause of half their errors.
John Stuart Mill (1806 -1873)

[233] https://www.avma.org/About/AlliedOrganizations/Pages/tfguidelines99.aspx

Over to you

Unless we put medical freedom into the Constitution, the time will come when medicine will organize into an undercover dictatorship to restrict the art of healing to one class of Men and deny equal privileges to others; the Constitution of the Republic should make a Special privilege for medical freedoms as well as religious freedom.

Dr Benjamin Rush, Founding Father, noted physician, medical professor and an early surgeon general to all Continental armies.

The good news is that there are other ways to remove tumours and better yet to protect from tumours and to overcome viral infections without toxic jabs. We've looked at black salve. Simple nutrition, suckling, clean water (not from the tap) and love at the heart of our actions are the foundation for a robust immune system. Understanding the real risks posed by infections is important. Then we look to reducing the intake of toxins, particularly via needle via the skin and to increasing the use of natural solutions we can grow or source ourselves.

> *Cinnamon is recommended as an internal antiseptic by Dr C.G.Grant (British Med. Journal). When in Ceylon he discovered that persons working in cinnamon gardens seemed to be immune to malaria. On trial he found it valuable in gastroenteritis, recurrent boils and, he thinks, in typhoid fever. He was astonished by its wonderful influence in influenza, and earnestly recommends its free use by others.* [234]

Lemon, citronella, neem, bergamot, rosemary, eucalyptus, garlic, rosemary, cinnamon leaf and lemongrass oils can all be used to very effectively control insects.

Homeopathy is a healing art, one that doesn't damage the host or the foetus, as vaccines readily do. It's an art that vaccines try to mimic with a level of stupidity surpassing any other human endeavour. Homeopathy may not work for everyone, but what does? It undid 50 years of lurking vaccine damage for me and stands out the more I learn as the safest and surest virus intervention with application in both prevention and healing.

The core principle of homeopathy is that Like Cures Like. By giving a very small amount of the substance which contributes to your illness the intention is to spark the body to drive its own healing process and assist its innate tendency to self-regulate.

Some vets may suggest an antibody titre test if you express a desire to pull back on vaccinating. This test of antibody levels will give an indication of available immune defences against a given invader, and a measurable range is in fact the foundation of the vaccine immune theory and the typical end point of clinical trials seeking proof

[234] Cinnamon as an Internal Antiseptic Cincinnati Lancet-Clinic, July 1, 1889, p.352. from Dissolving Illusions - Suzanne Humphries MD Roman Bystrianyk.

of efficacy. But high antibodies are only suggestive of a superficial level of protection since immune defence is multifaceted and as such patients with high antibodies may still become infected while those with low or no detectable antibodies may be protected by a barely understood innate immunity. Regardless of vaccination animals are being exposed to wild viruses and naturally boosted with no physical symptoms, as are those of us who haven't been vaccinated against all this stuff they warn us to fear, and there is evidence that older dogs with no recent vaccination record have high antibody protection.

In 2017 following a wider trend the UK government announced banning prescription homeopathy. Herbal treatments are next in the firing line if we allow this to continue. Some vets are calling for homeopathy to be banned for animals too, arguing it to be unproven and by definition unsafe, bladeladeblah. The claim has typically been that homeopathy works in some people only because of the placebo effect. That doesn't wash in a community lacking true placebo, or in the animal model where proof of efficacy destroys the placebo theory, so here they just say it's unapproved by the medical authorities so it needs to be banned.

This vet and pharma babe in the UK claims in this Guardian newspaper piece that he only wants "evidence-based veterinary care" for the animals he treats. And don't we all, but his solution is not to find some instead he launches an attack on the increasingly popular non-pharma competition. "There are few things more heartbreaking than having to pick up the pieces after an animal has received inadequate care", he reckons. Indeed. But he isn't talking about cancer causing vaccines, pharmaceuticals, chemo, pesticides and greed. He is talking about unapproved "ineffective" homeopathy causing pets to die because of the ignorance of owners delaying the use of proven poisons such as vaccines, pharmaceuticals, chemo and pesticides by using the other.

He says we should trust him and all like him because his superior "medical knowledge is the result of years of study and training at formally accredited institutions, and based on sound research". I say after decades of the same collective repetitive behaviour from these self-important drug experts we can judge the relevance of these fine words by the outcome. Are they helping our animals stay healthy?

Demanding of the Royal College of Veterinary Medicine that they outlaw any hint of a safe alternative to the pharma poisons, the vet claiming the support of 1,000 others and some vet nurses and students, reckons "that a failure to end the prescription of homeopathic remedies in animal care is an endorsement of these treatments... also an implicit acceptance of vets who place animal welfare at risk by putting their personal beliefs ahead of evidence-based medicine and the body of knowledge our profession has accrued."

This is not science and animal welfare speaking; this creates division, isolates free thinkers and builds the monopoly of control. From this kind of public statement those vets who think outside the box experience isolation and accusations of incompetence and animal cruelty, they are being bullied, while the drugs keep flowing and the animals keep dying. It's the pattern we recognise!

I'd say by the same token any vets still in cahoots with the vaccine maniacs, knowing what we know, are well in the frame for the well documented harm this vile profession is doing through its reckless use of cancer causing poisons.

The case against homeopathy, he claims on behalf of the status quo **"has never been clearer, with every well controlled study showing that these remedies are no more effective than a sugar pill."** [235] The nerve of it! Would these be the same "controlled" sugar pill trials where the sugar pill has been replaced by a vaccine, drugs or some other unnamed substance? Same trials that say polio, lepto 4, Herceptin and the MMR are safe and effective?

In this 1997 meta-analysis of 89 placebo-controlled homoeopathy trials, the question was asked not can we improve something but can we disprove: 'Are the clinical effects of homeopathy placebo effects?' Nevertheless, from the negative came a positive...

> ***The results of our meta-analysis are not compatible with the hypothesis that the clinical effects of homeopathy are completely due to placebo****. However, we found insufficient evidence from these studies that homoeopathy is clearly efficacious for any single clinical condition.* ***Further research on homeopathy is warranted*** *provided it is rigorous and systematic.*
>
> ***We believe that a serious effort to research homoeopathy is clearly warranted despite its implausibility. Deciding to conduct research on homoeopathy recognises that this approach is a relevant social and medical phenomenon.*** [236]

One thing that I think the public tends not to know is that there's not a medical school in the United States that teaches nutrition.
Dr T. Colin Campbell, The China Study.

---

[235] https://www.theguardian.com/science/2016/jul/08/why-we-are-calling-for-a-ban-on-vets-offering-homeopathic-remedies

[236] https://www.ncbi.nlm.nih.gov/pubmed/9310601

Show & Tell

Numerous infectious diseases are described as idiopathic, meaning that "the cause is a complete mystery." For many idiopathic diseases, the causes become clear when certain techniques are applied to the patient's blood or other tissues.
Lida Mattman - Cell Wall Deficient Forms

You get by now they don't like other ideas and why this story of how we created a successful cancer treatment protocol will not be headline news. The managers of the media have kept the lid on this possibility for the benefit of a few who want to maintain control of the many. However unlikely it sounds that's exactly how it is because that's the intention.

Here you see the look of my neck after the first weeks of full adherence to the MannIcure. It doesn't look like the kind of state you would want to be in and in reality I am still riddled with tumours but they had stopped growing, some are shrinking and from my perspective this is just like a wild trip! (And I've done that too so I know what that's like). It was a clash of emotions but I had never felt so sure of myself. My mind was moving like the high speed time-lapse rise of a skyscraper as I was creating my future and it's coming on nice.

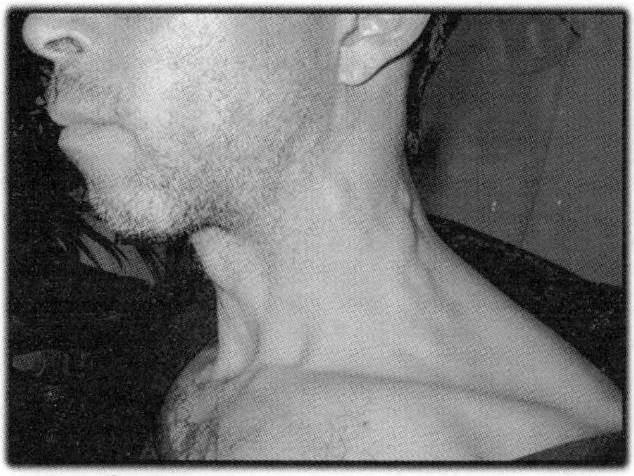

Shape shifting! This is what blood cancer looks like 10 months after chemo (in October 2016) and as cancer free as I was ever going to be according to the cancer treatment experts.

December 2016 I go back to the hospital for my monthly check up. I am now considered in such urgent need of more assistance they want me every few weeks but I space them out more. More chemo and a bone marrow transplant are top of the menu due to the speed of my chemo rebound and they want to re-evaluate and re-emphasise this urgency. You can see why from this image, this is one year after chemo and this cancer is all over me. It didn't work. But of course it was not my concern what anyone thought my destiny was to be because by now I was in a state of healing and I had my own plans. But thanks for your advice and opinions, I think it is wrong to send others to their death based on a stream of scientific fraud.

Hospital appointments are seldom fun. I mostly came away from mine with someone else's dire predictions regarding my future. It's understandable as this is the norm in that environment, and the expectations are low. We were bringing an odd balance to all this with our interpretation of what the future holds, to the evident curiosity of our hosts.

December 2016 I get this rookie right out of medical school. This was a little disappointing as we wanted to see how Dr Fear PhD responded to arguably the most significant moment in her career, me with less tumours than the last time we met but instead we got this kid half my age who we'd never met before and who was really out of her depth. They were all out of their depth now I think about it. She had on the one hand the previous commentary from her superiors regarding my status - disease progression all over the place, must repeat failed treatment and all that - and on the other she has some curious dude who is non-compliant and was not mentioned in her training.

She recorded the following on December 12 2016:

> *I met Mr Mann in Clinic today. He is feeling generally well in himself. He does suffer from night sweats but says these have not worsened in any way. His weight has remained stable. He has not suffered any infections recently although* ***on examination there were multiple enlarged lymph node in the neck bilaterally. There were also some lymph nodes palpable in the axillae as well... Mr Mann in himself thinks that his lymph nodes are regressing now but I think on examination there are still quite a lot which are palpable.***
>
> *We have offered Mr Mann a scan previously but he is not keen because of the risk factors of irradiation. I have discussed with him about having a scan done again but he does not want to go ahead with this at present. I have therefore given him another appointment in a few weeks' time and advised him that if he starts feeling unwell to contact us so that we can arrange to see him sooner.*

No one within the confines of the system had ever suggested anything other than that the cancer would progress and no one seemed to have any grasp of the possibility it could go in the other direction. Not a hint that I should think anything else possible. They don't mean it, the story has been ingrained though persistent programming and there are few who can imagine anything different. How terribly sad after all the research and all the sacrifices at the alter of the medical orthodox over generations, that few frontline representatives can encourage even the possibility of us self-inflicting less disease let alone no disease.

By the next appointment I attended two months later in February 2017 I had been able to turn up the dial full on my protocol and had reached such a point of transformation that there was no denying it. They often do though, but we had hit the jackpot with a top flight consultant haematologist who was genuinely interested in what we had done and was clearly thrilled. Doctors and assorted experts make up a collection of coincidence theories to explain what they don't understand, such as spontaneous remission (it just went away). It's a human condition and doctors are as prone to it as anyone, especially with the superiority complex many have about themselves. There was nothing spontaneous about this though, we had worked hard and invested heavily to bring this about and it can be repeated forever.

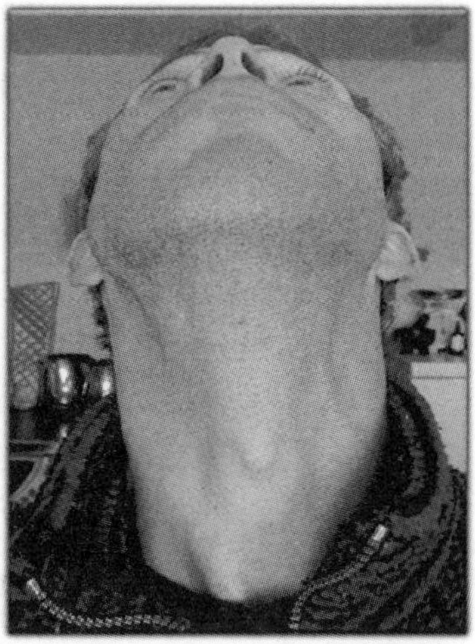

The MannIcure. Help yourself!
No sign of disease by January 2017.

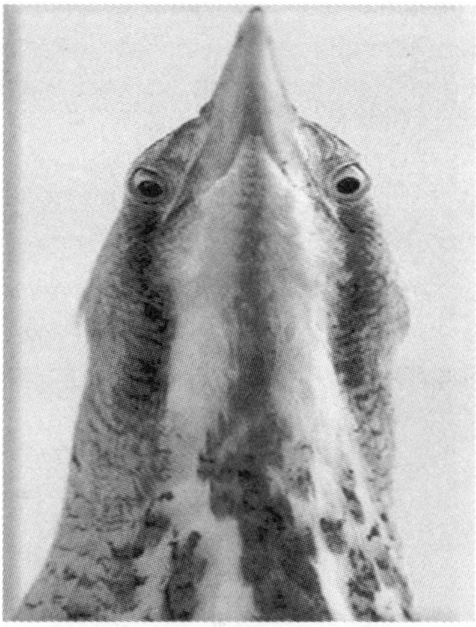

Photo: https://www.roeselienraimond.com/

Spontaneous regression or remission means the cancer gets smaller or disappears completely *outside the orthodox setting*. Pure chance! In hospital it's credited as the brave work of experts in medical science, outside the hospital it's the old coincidence theory that keeps things just as they are. One doctor of medicine responded to my story by blinking a lot, rocking slightly to the right before blurting "it's impossible" as he turned and left the conversation. He and I both knew he didn't want to say that, but he has been trained to respond in a particular way to what he sees. What I have done to restore my immune system is unknown within orthodox medical training and my reference to cancer microbes and blood cleaning and stimulating bile production is as baffling to the textbook trained mind as pharmaceutical drug names, vivisection and statistical analysis are to me. That said, a high percentage of doctors I have told of my journey have responded with warmth and encouragement and I think there is hope. My local GP surgery, for all the obstacles placed upon initiative and free thinking by the drug system that controls them, have been unwaveringly supportive and have never questioned or challenged my ideas. Of course they have seen my journey unfold.

The process of tumour fluctuations is also known to them as waxing and waning and is used to describe the uneven course of some lymphomas particularly of the slow growing (indolent) types. This may describe transient or short-term fluctuations in the size of lymph nodes that could be accounted for by inflammation or infection or other factors unrelated to the actual number of malignant cells. Waxing and waning has been likened to the daily fluctuations in the stock market, but ultimately it's of little significance what happens in the short-term, unless the cancer growth medium is changed.

No one ever asks but it might be worth considering whether that micro-environment in which the cancer thrives has been changed and caused the cancer to change. Does the cancer continue to grow when we do nothing to change the environment? Is it possible that the cancer might recede in line with an adjustment in lifestyle? By eck, I think we might be onto something! Microscopic experiments with the cancer microbe have proven this to be so and now we have a more scientific explanation than wishfully thinking it away. When the disease does die off for real there will be other indicators such as blood charts balanced, improved appetite and weight gain and observable improvements in how the patient feels and performs. The clinical signs and the patients are of far greater importance than charts and statistics and traumatised mice.

A study by Dr Harold Foster of recovered patients and this spontaneous remission mystery that so many ortho-docs refer to when confronted with healing showed some not surprising findings. Lifestyle and diet changes featured prominently with 79.5% cutting out sugar and meat. Dr Foster concluded that

> *'spontaneous'* cancer regression *tended to occur most frequently in vegetarian non smokers, who did not use table salt, white flour, or sugar and who avoided canned, smoked, or frozen foods... alcohol, tea, coffee and cocoa, but instead drank freshly pressed fruit and/or vegetable juices. Many took vitamin and mineral supplements together with various herbs.* [237]

Dr William Boyd studied this extensively and estimated in his book 'The Spontaneous Regression of Cancer' that just 1 in 100,000 cases appear to regress with no apparent cause.

> ***The wide fluctuations in the growth of tumors are due primarily to changes in the resistance of the organism (patient) and not to changes in the virulence of the tumor. It is the concept of control that is central to the phenomenon of spontaneous regression.*** 237

In 1950 Dr Engelburt Dunphy published four case histories and concluded:

> ***The occurrence of spontaneous regressions renders untenable the hypothesis that 'cancer is a progressive, lawless, autonomous growth'... Also, if there are factors that lead to progression of***

---

[237] Harold D. Foster, "Lifestyle Changes and the 'Spontaneous' Regression of Cancer: An Initial Computer Analysis," International Journal of Biosocial Research, vol. 10, no. 1, 1988, pp. 17-33. https://www.healmindbody.com/spontaneous-remission-of-cancer/

> ***tumors, then the alteration or withdrawal of these factors... can result in dissolution of the tumor.*** 237

Oncologist Dr WH Cole wrote that the term is an

> ... *erroneous classification because there must be cause of the regression.* 237

In 1933, Dr DeCourcy reviewed the literature on spontaneous remission and wrote:

> *There are no accidents in nature... I believe it is of the very first importance to give close study to cases of this kind with a view to gaining an insight... into Nature's methods of healing and to discover what can be done to make her work easier.* 237

Back at hospital February 2017, we'd filled our boots with all the likely debunking of our achievements by whatever doctor came in through the door and we were ready to do some debunking of our own. But there would be no need. We were all dressed up with nowhere to go but this appointment was worth the heavy weight of all of the last three years and we came away buzzing.

It's funny because I have no craving for the praise of others and I can take or leave the rambling of the debunkers but this was an exchange with a doctor to get excited about. The overall majority of our survivor testimonials refer to the peculiar reaction they get from their cancer expert when they show and tell of healing and that is what we anticipated, but we are in unchartered waters and like the first explorers this journey was intriguing at every turn.

Blood test done. Weighed. Waited. And we finally got to see my haematologist for the first time in over a year, he who had told me that I couldn't have responded better, and who would now have to face the fact I had! I had excelled! And all credit to him for coming to my party and bringing his joy! We exchanged pleasantries and bounced off each other. Alice says we're similar characters, although we don't meet on chemo. When we first met this dude we felt he was the right man for my journey and he has blended in nicely.

He asked the usual questions then went through my blood work while pointing to the numbers on his screen. "Red cell count: normal. White cell count: normal. Slightly elevated LDH but way down on the last count". He was really surprised by this as it had been rising for a year and we had been assured it couldn't be stopped without chemo.

Curious because my LDH had always been in range until Feb 2016 just after chemo finished and we saw the cancer growing again. LDH (a lymphoma marker) was now elevated to 682 and had risen to 814 that August. The range was 313 – 618. By the February of 2017 we had returned it with the MannIcure back to 580 (in the revised range of 240 – 480) which is where it was in the June of 2015, three months before chemo. By February of 2018 we had lowered it to 253, a significant achievement in itself. This shows the chemical intervention changed my disease negatively and that we changed my disease for the better.

Then he reads my haemoglobin which has risen back to normal too and causes him to observe with enthusiasm that this was actually "optimal for a young man". I was 50 at the time. Then I'm invited for my physical. Alice is my wife and she knows all about my physical. She's in her wheelchair. The room ain't large and there's a bed. There's the doctor and a nurse. Four of us. The physical does not require me to remove much clothing, only to allow the doctor access to my neck, armpits and groin. Nevertheless every time we go through this performance whereby this pointless paper thin curtain is pulled around the bed with three of us inside and Alice outside, to shield this process from her? She's seen my armpits. Of course I have to question why we do this but no one is really sure other than to observe this is how it is.

I don't mind in the slightest because I want to show and tell what I did. Alice knew.

I lie down.
He carefully examines my neck and observes: ***There's nothing there.***
He examines my armpits: ***There's nothing there...***
Then my groin with little expectation: ***And nothing there...***

What we do have is an air of puzzlement.

No one says another word for a couple of minutes as the curtain is pulled back to bring Alice back into view and the doctor goes to the sink to wash his hands. I tuck my t-shirt in and go back to my chair and exchange that covert wide eyed look with Alice. I can see through her excitement her urging me to "keep it shut!" I am reminded we are encouraging inquiry and not to spoil this precious moment with my questions. We want his! Anything! How does he explain this?

For what seemed like an age we were all quietly thinking. Alice and I are both chomping at the bit by now and we've waited a long time for this precious moment, eagerly awaiting that suggestion that this is somehow an accident or a coincidence. A misdiagnosis is obviously out of the question but what's left? The truth.

I can see him in the mirror as he towel dries his hands looking slightly puzzled, when he catches my eye. Struggling for the right words he eventually asked

What, err... Have you done something at home?

Well that threw me! Interesting since most true healers do so at home but no one ever asks how, yet this the most critical factor in making chemo look good.

"Why do you ask", I ask? There I go again, asking questions! In reply to a question, don't you know! Maybe I need to see someone about this. I could have told him at this moment what we did but we wanted to save the story for release in full context in due course.

Because your LDH has come down, he replied.

A big deal indeed! We did that and his admiration was palpable. And then there was the glaring absence of tumours for the first time in 4 years, arguably the biggest thing in cancer treatment! I swerved the question until we were ready to answer and would leave the explanation for the next appointment a year down the line when we would have had the time to advance my healing and lay it all out comprehensively, as you can see I now have. That was going to be another pleasurable experience for all of us. For my downer on the orthodox and the misguided nature of their approach to health I think this guy is a gem who genuinely wants to do the right thing for others.

As he concluded the appointment and shuffled my file back together and placed it to one side he observed curiously as much to himself as the rest of us:

Best left alone, I think.

I agree. He recorded later:

> ***I reviewed this gentleman in clinic today. He was entirely well and asymptomatic. I could detect no evidence of any palpable disease. His blood count was normal,*** *haemoglobin 166 g/l,* ***white count*** *5.8 x 10_9/l with a* ***normal*** *differential and platelets 286 x 10_9/l.* ***Biochemistry was normal,*** *his LDH minimally elevated at 580 U/L.*
>
> ***No intervention is required.*** *I will review him later in the year.*

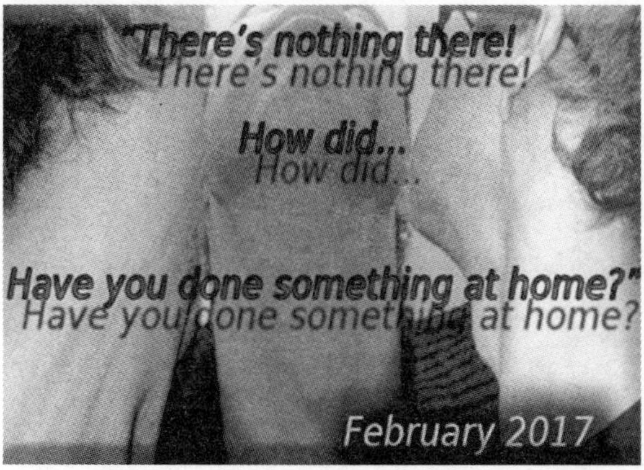

From an urgency just a few weeks earlier to see me every 4 weeks in preparation for heavy chemical intervention, these medical experts now **ask me** what I did to overcome cancer and when I would like to attend future appointments. I said I'll pop in once a year to show and tell. I think this says that collectively we have an opportunity to change the way we deal with disease, and we ought not let that pass.

Gerson himself viewed the blood cancers as more complex and difficult to treat than the solid tumours:

Their metabolisms are much deeper and more differently deranged than we see in other cancer types.

Yet still we have succeeded overcoming not just an inherently systemic, deranged cancer, decades in the making but chemotherapy and their mAbs too. A solid tumour presenting as a localised cancer will kill once it spreads through the blood to a second location. We were at the extreme end with cancer in the blood from the very beginning.

I will document each element of my protocol as fully as necessary to be clear the reason we included it. We are all significantly individual and we all present disease in a unique way but recovering the whole is a universal goal. There is no quick fix cure all but if you have the desire you'll find all you need within these pages. But for some minor tweaking, all that success requires is the will to live. I am not joking when I say that many of us have an unspoken, perhaps unconscious death wish and will resist all attempts at being persuaded to seek a long, healthy life.

It is said that it is much easier to kill someone than to save their life and so much easier to fool someone than to convince them they have been fooled and this experience with cancer has for me confirmed these truths gloriously. I was personally so excited to hear of the possibility I could save myself and I couldn't wait to get started. In fact I didn't wait, I changed my ways the moment I suspected something was seriously wrong. We had no idea how we were going to manage but we were determined and that is all you need to achieve anything. I am still watching people with cancer return time and again, encouraged by their peers and their doctor and the cancer charities, to be further traumatised, mutilated and poisoned by the toxic treatment on offer, while the cancer marches on regardless lunching away on the habits held dear.

Where I come from I'd hear the older people observe in their Northern twang how, "there's nowt funnier than folk". And how right they are! Here are some of the things people have said to me upon hearing of my treatment choice:

- *Oh, I couldn't be bothered with all them lettuce.*
- *Would the Gerson be able to make a treatment to suit me so I can get on with my life?*
- *It would be all on the news.*
- *I like my food too much.*
- *I need my toast.*
- *I trust my doctor.*
- *I'm just too lazy for all that.*
- *If it worked my doctor would have said something.*
- *I don't like juice.*
- *I'm not doing that! [coffee enemas]*
- *I've got the all clear.*
- *It'd be good if they could make it [lifestyle change] into a pill.*

- ***My** cancer's different, my cancer's incurable.*

And of course, straight from the front page of 'Every Idiots Guide to Killing Stray Thoughts':

- *You're just into conspiracy theories.*

We are a funny little creature. We can observe evolution and praise the wonder and even insist that's all there is, but heaven forbid we might have to get involved! One lady with cancer who introduced herself to me as "vegan animal rights", when faced with the notion of giving up eating out in restaurants, which was her passion "to spread the vegan message", said she would rather "thank the animals for their sacrifice" do the chemo and continue her protesting. And she did, proud to boast of her survival! Before the chemo they told her she had a curable cancer (5 years) and sure enough she made 5 years and was 'cured'. A chemo success story! And then it came back soon after and was no longer deemed curable so she would have to be maintained on mouse-made mAbs for the rest of her life. Watch that offer, as enticing as it sounds to pop a pill and get on with your life, your life will not be the same. Ask the question, just how long is that piece of string they have set on fire. I'm saying we don't have to sacrifice ourselves or the animals. You can if you want but you don't have to.

Healing the diseased human body with the application of a new way of thinking about food and medicine represents a paradigm shift in the way we live on this planet, but we are not a creature comfortable with change. I hear this kind of resistance right across the spectrum and gaze in awe at how few of us want that revolution when it comes down to doing something we would rather not be bothered with just this minute. And it's easy to see how and why the status quo simply gets on with its self-serving agenda. We do ask for it and seem to like to promote their cause!

I'm not judging by the way. Judging others is ugly and I am aware of the tendency the mind has to get us to judge others for not thinking like us. I am flawed and I'm working on it but I will respect all the earthlings and the extra terrestrials to be what they choose. I have plenty of time to play with now and appear to have undone the bodily damage so there's no reason why I can't achieve mind control. I'm also an observer, an inquisitive observer. Ooooh! Might just have to go back to the start of the book and award myself another title... Keith Mann **A**nimal**L**iberation**F**ront, **n**atural**H**ealer, **IO**. Why not!

Good luck to everyone trying to navigate this human experience at this time of great change, the choice is yours. Good health to those who desire it enough.

Let food be thy medicine, let medicine be thy food.
Hippocrates (460 -370 BC)

The MannIcure
- a functional work of art -

Non-Hodgkin's B-cell lymphomas account for approximately 70% of B-cell lymphomas. While its incidence is dramatically increasing worldwide, the disease is still associated with high morbidity due to ineffectiveness of conventional therapies, creating an urgent need for novel therapeutic approaches. [238]

Got one! For those who are curious, who want another perspective, something more than a hollow promise of a cancer cure just around the corner, here is the MannIcure. It is said that necessity is the mother of invention, well this is grandma. The protocol Alice and I devised to treat my cancer, restore my immune system and recover my health evolved at a point in time where all else we had tried had failed and cancer was sweeping like an unstoppable swarm through my body, aided by the toxic effects of chemo and rituximab. This protocol is incredibly powerful and cannot be understated. It did as requested, as rapidly as I desired. It saved my life. I am comfortable with words but struggle to express the significance of what we have here. To put this in some perspective I'll briefly outline my physical journey.

I had stage 4 non-Hodgkin's follicular lymphoma (NHL), one of the many subtypes of blood/lymphatic system cancers. The orthodox medical profession insist it is incurable. They are of course both right and wrong depending on our treatment choice. Orthodox pharmaceutical treatments do not cure and are not designed to do so.

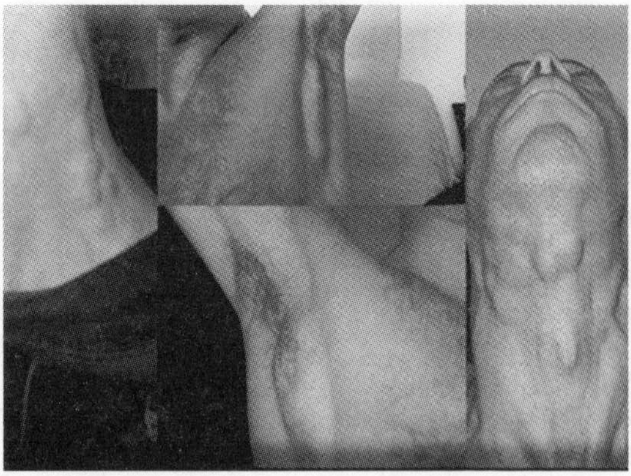

Gerson couldn't stop it. Chemo couldn't stop it. We stopped it.

My cancer had been reduced by chemo but rapidly rebounded and was growing again a few weeks later. I say again but I have no evidence it ever stopped. It hardly matters. I had a bone marrow biopsy and was told I had cancer "bubbling over" in my bone marrow. This rather unnerving finding, along with being refractory (the most significant marker), took additional time off my already poor prognosis. I startled myself and panicked when reflecting later that day on cancer 'bubbling over in my bone marrow', to the point of needing the toilet. I sat there wondering how anyone could realistically cure a cancer that was doing that in

238 https://www.ncbi.nlm.nih.gov/pmc/articles/PMC3248929/

the bone marrow. Our bone marrow actually produces our B cells as well as other blood cells but NHL is producing cancerous immune cells. You don't need that!

This all began in the summer of 2013. I began the Gerson Therapy immediately. Gerson holds an impressive track record with this and many other cancers and if you ask around you will find many satisfied customers no longer living in fear of cancer who testify to the incomparable results obtained by the immune system once restored to function. But Gerson doesn't work for everyone and couldn't catch my cancer, which was to become a refractory or relapsed cancer before we managed to stop it. That is like sitting on a time bomb. Or like having cancer twice! The new generation of cancer cells, the clones: are natural born killers, expert in surviving the Pharma's weapons of mass destruction. Traditionally we struggle in vain to outsmart the upstart cancer and the prognosis had traditionally always been grim.

But I'm still here and I'm in the clear. No sign of cancer.

We researched extensively to pull this thing together and continue to keep apace. Things are moving fast in the natural health arena. Not so much in the orthodox setting where cancer is as incurable as it was 70, 60, 50 years ago, but then why fix something that isn't broken? Alert to this uncomfortable truth we used our common sense and added in the wealth of information available in the alternative media where we find the natural healers and the testimonials and where the focus is on trusting not in a saviour out there but in the innate intelligence of the body to take care of itself at our behest. We set out not to suppress and contain in the short-term but to heal for good.

Doin OK.

The MannIcure is not a magic quick fix. We have worked hard under difficult circumstances to get where we are, and I have by necessity made it my life. I have tried to abbreviate to some essentials but nothing can substitute for ones own personal findings and understanding of the important role each element plays and just what it is we are aiming for. A critical factor in healing is to control what we put into our bodies. We must be our own doctors and be conscious of our undeniable right to decide our choice of medicine and not be bullied by anyone else.

We are rebuilding something amazing and corners cannot be cut. Think of yourself as a Grade 1 listed building rising from the ashes of serious destruction. You have to get it right from the foundations to the roof, but don't forget the wiring and the plumbing need to be in perfect working order too.

Sound advice has long been to not mix and match cancer protocols. They are what they are for a reason. There may be a tendency to pick and choose the favourable elements from various other protocols with little regard for necessity. It's critical to apply not what you want but what you need to heal and to adjust accordingly. There are many specifically designed cancer protocols that do restore health and they are designed as such for that reason, but they don't work for everyone. Nothing can beat common sense and instinct stemming from a broader understanding of the mechanism of the disease and the purpose of each of our ingredients in disrupting or correcting that mechanism.

The application of VEGA technology can assist in designing a protocol based on what your body needs, and you can be pretty certain that won't gel with any standardised therapy. VEGA can identify anomalies, and is a companion for you to share your remedies with.

So, let's take a brief look at how we believe we get cancer so we know what we need to deal with.

At the beginning of our time the sperm fertilises the egg and three essentials emerge: life, an immune system and the life-giving cancer-causing microbe. He is our friend, our dear, dear friend and without him we'd not be here. The job of the microbe is to cause the cell of the fertilised egg to divide and multiply rapidly until the embryo reaches full stage. At that time his job is finished. He will then return to the cells, harmless, helpful, and perhaps involved in cell repair.

Until the body becomes dominated by acidity as toxins build up quicker than we dump them, as we age, as we slow, we accumulate more and more. The blood loses its ability to move oxygen around the body, it darkens and the cells glue together and clog up the once pristine machine. The more we accumulate the worse the situation gets. All manner of subtleties may cascade, immune defences weaken, cells fail to function and devolve. Instead of breathing oxygen from a smooth running system the cells have to improvise and ferment to extract fuel. The microbes have to change their ways too in order to survive. And soon they thrive. These bugs are good and deserve our respect. These cancer microbes ultimately take over the lease by inserting themselves into the genetic machinery of the weakened host cells and replicate their own genetic code. And do they! And we call that cancer. This is a state caused by lifestyle. If we want we can change it or we can allow things to stay just as they are. Acidity, monitored via saliva on pH test strips at home, may be aggravated over the long-term by the usual offenders, the pharmaceutical drugs, vaccines, metals, chemicals, chronic stress, radiation, fake food, meat, alcohol, anger, resentment, envy and hate.

A cancerous cell has low ATP energy. Adenosine Triphosphate, the energy currency of the body. This is caused by the microbes inside of the cancer cells blocking the production of ATP through the interception of glucose. Glucose! Really? They want that, why?

Fuel! This is where the question of sugar feeding cancer comes to the forefront, as an unstoppable train sets in motion. Sugar should be removed in an instant, but cancer cells also now spew out lactic acid as a waste product of the inefficient, unnatural fuel manufacturing process we are entangled in and this needs fixing just as urgently. This is then recycled through the liver and returned to the blood as glucose which of course these cancer cells gobble up, gain strength from and in return spew out more lactic acid. And on it goes. All the time the body advances deeper into acidity fed by these by-products, which provides the perfect environment for cancer to ferment away uncontrollably.

The microbe is still our friend though, whatever we might think about cancer. He may now start to present signs that something is wrong in his natural environment that he needs help addressing, physical symptoms such as weight loss in the host, fatigue, abnormal blood readings, or the traditional lump we love to hate. This is our wake-up call, like the alarm we love to hate.

This is our chance to change direction before our habits cause these microbes to reach that critical mass. The body makes tumours and the body unmakes tumours. We can draw parallels with the science of vaccine virus replication. Each virus requires a very specific medium in which to grow and if it isn't right the virus can't grow. The medium is critical to the mass. The better suited the growth medium our lifestyle creates the better able the cancer virus are to multiply, the more acidity there will be, the more cancer cells, the more cancer microbes, the more tumours, starvation and death. It's a slow process, often taking many years to manifest, but less so as our internal and external environments get all the more toxic, as we might observe from the numbers of children now with cancer. We are speeding things up with the crap we consume daily!

For cleaning up the environment we applied the principle of nutrition and detoxification for health restoration based on Dr Max Gerson's findings, with updates. He provides by far the best foundation and his research is the best documented, it has been practiced and proven by the more outward looking, open-minded health practitioners of our time to the benefit of many.

We applied the pleomorphic cancer microbe principle which has been espoused by many unrecognised and persecuted researchers for hundreds of years and is being increasingly utilised for the restoration of health. In this, disease causing pathogens will shape-shift to suit their environment, for their own survival. We applied the electrical energy principle. This requires the cleaning and maintenance of the cells so they can resonate, vibrate, communicate and sing their song as they must for optimum performance. We see ourselves conducting an orchestra, finely tuning each precious instrument from the triangle to the hobo, daring not to ignore those wonderful musicians without whom there would be only silence.

We aren't aiming to just kill cancer cells but to heal. We kill cancer microbes inside the cells. We approach whole body healing from many angles. We change the overall internal environment with clean nutrition, magnetic pulsing and electrically stimulated blood cleaning and boost immunity by first removing the burdens. We are re-oxygenating the oxygen deficient cells with ozone and organic vegetable juices and healing flax oil. We are reactivating our natural killer cells and other immune system agents with modified rice bran NK Cell Activator, Agaricus Blazei mushrooms and beta glucans. We get into cancer cells with organic sulphur or DMSO and send in vitamin C and colloidal silver to kill microbes, while our finely tuned electrical pulses energise. Sulphur calms down the lactic acid cycle. We clean up all this debris with ozone water, saunas and coffee enemas. Wrapped around a positive attitude this provides a sound foundation for healing.

We think we did pretty good.

This is alien speak to the bulk of the human population not least to those managing the mainstream media and orthodox medicine, but of course they cannot heal and are not trying to. Thinking differently means we do things differently and achieve different results.

Too easy, eh? It isn't easy, it takes will power - think giving up drinking, smoking, eating packaged food, doing normal things normal people do. Nightmare! But it is entirely possible. And not so terrible as leaving behind the ones who love us.

We're better off not expecting scientists to prove this works. Scientific research as we know it has a way of proving and disproving everything depending on who is paying for the results and it's fair to say there has been no investment made in proving the worth of any natural protocol. We based our findings on science and on instinct and common sense. And on the work of independent researchers and those who have healed before, always bearing in mind that the cure is in the cause, not the chemist.

With love.

Man is the only species clever enough to make his own food... and stupid enough to eat it.

Dr Zoe Harcombe PhD

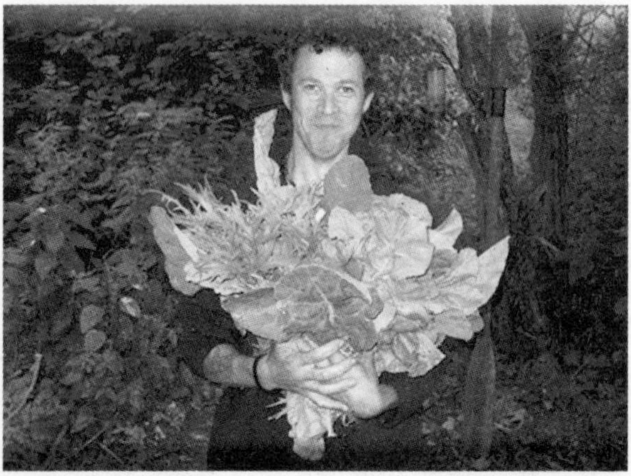

Food Fortification

After more than 25 years of cancer work I can draw the following conclusion:

Cancer is not a local but general disease, caused chiefly by the poisoning of foodstuffs prepared by modern farming and food industry. Medicine must be able to adapt its therapeutic methods to the damages of the processes of modern civilisation.

Dr Max Gerson 1958

The principle of biological totality is the essence of the MannIcure. To replace replenish and restore. The foundation of this is our nutrition, or if you prefer it's the all-in-one immunisation. The jury of six men and six women who healed came back with a unanimous verdict: nutritional deficiency leads to a diseased state that can be reversed. This comes from the daily consumption of nutritionally depleted, microwaved; genetically engineered, chemical coated, salt laden food-like-products soaked in preservatives, dyes, artificial flavours and sweetened. This is just one processed meal by the way. Repeatedly every day, til death do us part.

Scurvy is cured with vitamin C (ascorbic acid), which by definition prevents scurvy. Whooping Cough doesn't like high dose vitamin C nor does diphtheria and a great many other conditions. What do we do when our arteries become clogged or when we are diagnosed with type 2 diabetes? We change our diets. Pellagra is cured and prevented with niacin, B3. B12 and folic acid cures and therefore prevents pernicious anaemia; rickets, viruses and cancers don't like vitamin D, and night blindness invites vitamin A and so do measles. Beri beri is a B1 deficiency. And so on.

> *The importance of vitamin A in reducing the morbidity and mortality caused by measles and other infectious illnesses has now re-emerged. The potential importance of correcting vitamin A deficiency, as a practical and inexpensive public health strategy to reduce childhood mortality in the Third World, is being tested in many locations.* William R. Beisel MD, FACP Historical Overview of Nutrition and Immunity, with Emphasis on Vitamin A.

While the established order won't admit it, if we care to look at human populations with high intake of B17 from apricot seeds, such as the Hunza, high in the Himalayas, where there is no incidence of cancer and take notes from people closer to home who use the nutrient to kill cancer and utilise the whole range of vitamins and micronutrients in food to recover and maintain health, we see a common theme developing.

Were it not for the discovery that nutrients prevent and cure, the Great would probably never have stuck with Britain. Only the addition of citrus fruit to sailing crew supplies when Britannia was crossing the seven seas and seeking empire status saved that day and many more lives than the drugs we have today! Scurvy was wiping out entire sailing crews and stalling all efforts to take over the world until the lowly lime was introduced, and from that point onward Great Britain ruled the waves and could pillage at will. That simple fruit cure had been ignored for over 250 years because the medical experts of the time considered such a simple solution to be too outrageous for brilliant minds to contemplate. Dismissed as the fanciful imaginings of witch doctors, the search went on for mystery bugs hiding in the port holes and piss pots of those doomed voyages as two million sailors perished.

How many missed opportunities to save lives before we figure out who the real experts are?

This total nutritional approach is the bedrock on which we will rebuild our temples and reclaim our land from the ravages of toxicity. What will our grandchildren be growing their food in if we don't stop poisoning the soil? We can all do this one purchase at a time but for healing it's necessary to detoxify entirely. I urge readers who are serious about creating a cancer friendly nutritional foundation to study the Gerson books for a fuller understanding of the principles and the finer details as I do not have the space to lay out all of Max Gerson's findings here. That said we have slightly evolved the MannIcure from the Gerson dietary rules, like the measurements of the juices and adding extra flax oil, protein (butter beans, chick peas, kidney beans) and soft seasonal fruit such as raspberries and blackberries which are considered too aromatic for the Gerson Therapy. Nevertheless, there are key elements which should not be changed and which we must address.

Always Organic

Potato fields are sterilized before planting with a soil fumigant that kills all of the soil microbes and nematodes. When the potato "eyes" are planted, a systemic insecticide is sprayed over the fields to kill any bugs that may eat the sprouts. A month or so after that, the first herbicide is applied to kill any weeds hardy enough to grow. Because most of the soil nutrients have been eliminated, synthetic fertilizers are dripped into the potato rows every week, like an IV drip of chemical nutrients. Mid growth, many potato fields are sprayed yet again with the highly toxic organophosphate Monitor to kill aphids, potato beetles and other insects. Finally, to control blight before harvest, potato plants receive successive sprayings of a fungicide containing mefenoxam and clorothalonil, both acute toxins. Given this chemically intensive growth cycle, it's not surprising that a majority of potatoes, especially Russets, test positive for multiple pesticide residues.

Cindy Burke - To Buy or Not To Buy Organic

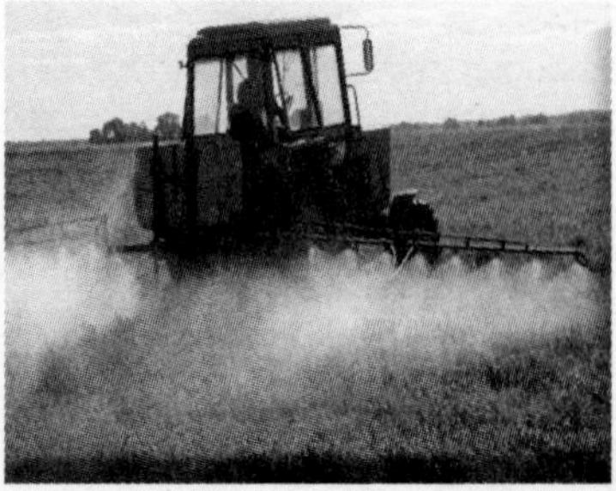

Aim for everything organic. Synthetic pesticides kill. They are poisons. Pesticides are known to be carcinogenic, neurotoxic and cause hormone disruption, developmental or reproductive disruption and cancer! That thing we are trying to get rid of. Pesticides don't contribute to healing and they do not provide nutrients to the plants covered in them. You may be able to find some toxicity studies on some animals for some pesticides - and even they provide little comfort - but try and locate any that assess the accumulation of this crap inside humans. No can do. Has anyone with letters after their name encouraging you to eat pesticides ever mentioned the studies linking pesticides to Parkinson's disease?

We found that for every 1.0 µg/L of pesticide in groundwater, the risk of PD increases by 3%. [239]

A sick body like a sick society needs to remove its toxic burden in order to heal. Then the daily fuel intake shifts from dirty to clean, harmful to helpful.

The average number of these chemicals applied to a potato crop has risen from around 5 in the 1970's to an excess of 30 today. Wheat chemicals have multiplied from 1 or 2 in the early 70's to over 20 today, onions and leeks are up to 30. [240]

The agricultural soil is damaged and depleted after generations of poisoning, overwork and under-nourishing, so depleted and yet the standard artificial fertiliser only contains three basic mineral substitutes of nitrogen, phosphorus and potassium (NPK). This is a poor substitute for that which we deplete from the earth that utilises over 50 known minerals such as iron, manganese, magnesium, zinc, calcium, sulphur, iodine and copper to grow healthy crops. I know from my experience getting my hands dirty just how important it is to generously feed the soil in order to keep it, the plants and the consumers healthy. The soil is our external metabolism.

We are now encouraged, by government no less, to eat at least five portions of fruit or vegetables each day and this would be a good thing except for the pesticides we are also encouraged to eat and 5 being a measly, random, unscientific amount. Medical and scientific evidence shows that a diet rich in fruit and vegetables helps to combat cancer and other diseases and none have established this as a fact more than the Gerson Institute. We can quite easily find a whole heap of animal toxicity studies that show just how deadly these poisons are.

We are advised to include this token gesture of healthy plant food into our 'staple of fake' in order to provide some nutrition. I am not a big fan of government advice on anything but I do take notes. 'Organic' stands out in this government advice, for its absence. We should use plant foods as medicine in order to flood the body with alkaline nutrition, not as a sticking plaster to make government look like they're trying.

Salvestrols (a type of phytonutrient) are important anti-pathogenic substances produced by plants to protect themselves from pests and disease in a similar way that mammals have evolved to use them. However, the use of so many chemical pesticides means that plants which are not organically grown will not produce high concentrations of salvestrols because they are no longer exposed to the attacks which caused the plant to produce what they needed in defence of themselves. It's estimated we have lost 90% of this supply since we started applying synthetic

239 https://www.ncbi.nlm.nih.gov/pubmed/25939349

240 http://www4.dr-rath-foundation.org/Newsletter/articles/shocking-new-data-on-pesticides-in-food-presented-at-london-conference.html

poisons to our crops in order to intensify production and a similar pattern will naturally follow for the many other trace elements we are slowly discovering.

These plant-derived compounds are essential for our well-being and cannot be made in the body and must therefore be supplied through our diet. Salvestrols, from that Latin word *salve*, (to save) are converted in the body by an enzyme reaction into a form that is toxic to malfunctioning cells, but because this enzyme is only present in sick cells salvestrols protect healthy cells.

The cancer diet takes us back to basics. We think we are highly evolved beings but even as mature adults we are only just beginning to learn how to eat! Or more accurately we are relearning how to eat for life in place of that habit of living to eat to which we have become addicted. Salads can be made delicious when we use some imagination instead of the traditional loveless salad cobbled together with cucumber, tomato and an iceberg lettuce leaf or two. We have evolved way beyond that to mixing rocket, oak leaf lettuce, mizuna if you like em sharp, purslane, red salad bowl, mustard leaves, flower heads, flashy butter oak, baby leaf salad, sprouted lentils and cherry tomatoes, grated beetroot, carrot, peppers and courgettes of all colours. A blend of flax oil, lemon, cider vinegar, garlic, herbs make a tasty drizzle for a proper salad.

The principle of unprocessed raw or lightly cooked organic food is to keep the nutrients while creating as little work for the digestive and elimination organs as possible. We are using our energy efficiently. It's green and sustainable! Poisons into the soil are not. A sick metabolism requires all the help we can give it. Those packets of unreadable ingredients force the body to invest a lot of energy unravelling them for very little nutritional reward. It's a poor use of our resources. On top of that the popular processed brands are not organic and not really food. More food-like products. This applies equally whether it says 'vegan' on the packet or not. This is not living food and there is no evidence to back up the belief that nutrient depleted chemical concoctions do no harm. Conventional wisdom says eat and all will be fine, but we are not fine and this lazy approach has proven ineffective at either maintaining health or recovering the health of people crippled with rising chronic diseases.

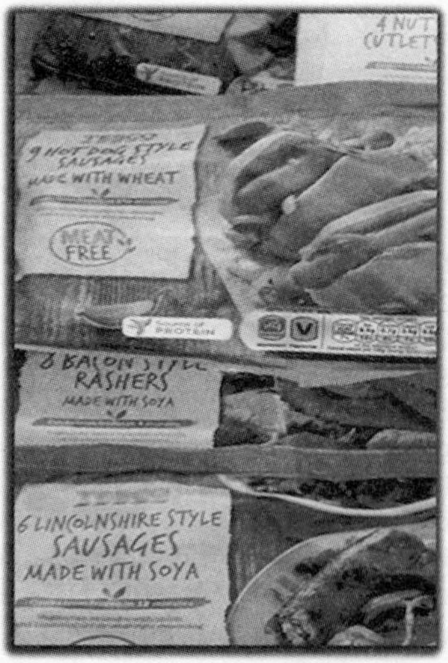

Alternatives to fresh food are linked with degenerative disease.

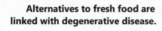

Aside all that, pesticides are the antipathy of vegan, food, health and life! It's inconvenient to avoid and it isn't sexy but prevention is better than cure and organic is the first gesture we can make to prevent disease setting in and perhaps the biggest favour we can do for the environment.

Most studies on non-Hodgkin lymphoma and leukemia showed positive associations with pesticide exposure. Some showed dose-response relationships, and a few were able to identify specific pesticides. Children's and pregnant women's exposure to pesticides was positively associated with the cancers studied in some studies, as was parents' exposure to pesticides at work. Many studies showed positive associations between pesticide exposure and solid tumours. The most consistent associations were found for brain and prostate cancer. An association was also found between kidney cancer in children and their parents' exposure to pesticides at work. These associations were most consistent for high and prolonged exposures. Specific weaknesses and inherent limitations in epidemiologic studies were noted, particularly around ascertaining whether and how much exposure had taken place. [241]

Encouraging the next generation away from consuming animal bits, pieces and body parts and the heavy energy our incessant destruction of the other earthlings creates, is a step forward in the development of our consciousness. But teasing that generation into the norms of processed junk food and pesticides instead and the associated health issues, and death drug treatments that inevitably follow only moves us sideways at best.

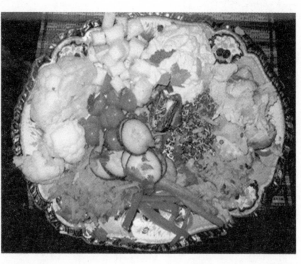

Protein is another question that inevitably comes up. The ability of animal protein to turn cancer on and off in experiments is dramatic. The China Study is a good book to learn how this works. Professor T Colin Campbell was every bit the enemy. Brought up a dairy farmer and hooked on milk he graduated into vivisection so he could mould his passion for destroying animals into greater and greater profits. Campbell wanted to be remembered for discovering how to make sheep and cows grow faster. Instead, along the way he discovered that children who ate high protein diets were the most likely to develop liver cancer. From this hidden fact would mushroom the most important study into the role of cancer and nutrition ever undertaken. And from its findings, flying in the face of official wisdom, another successful career was derailed.

Animal protein intake was convincingly associated in the China Study with the prevalence of cancer... this association is an impressive and significant

241 https://www.ncbi.nlm.nih.gov/pmc/articles/PMC2231435/

> *observation, considering the unusually low intake of animal protein. Diet and disease factors such as animal protein consumption or breast cancer incidence lead to changes in the concentrations of certain chemicals in our blood. These chemicals are called biomarkers. We measured six blood biomarkers that are associated with animal protein intake. Do they confirm the finding that animal protein intake is associated with cancer in families? Absolutely. Every single animal protein blood biomarker is significantly associated with cancer in families. These experiments also demonstrated that the body could "remember" early carcinogen insults, even though they might then lie dormant with low protein intake. That is, exposure [to a carcinogen] left a genetic "imprint" that remained dormant with 5% dietary protein until nine weeks later when this imprint reawakened... with 20% dietary protein. In simple terms, the body holds a grudge.* **T. Colin Campbell, Thomas M. Campbell: The China Study**

I limited my vegetable protein intake in the first few weeks of cancer kill but increased after that time to a balance.

No animal protein.

I load up on organic gluten free porridge oats and all the fruit I can get my hands on and soak and sprout organic pulses. Everything should be fresh and not from a packet or bottle, tin or jar. No mushrooms. No drinking tea or coffee. Turn chick peas into humous, butter bean mash and kidney beans mashed with sweet potatoes, squash, peppers and herbs made into oven cooked burgers. Rice or quinoa wrapped in cabbage leaves. Herbs of all sort. Fat chips done in the oven without oil. Flax oil infused with dried herbs added when they cool. Garlic potatoes with tenderstem broccoli, grilled spring onions and cherry tomatoes, roast parsnips with pea and mint gravy. Cook onions in water, not hot oil. Smoothies are easy and raw and each tastes different depending on what's in the fridge! Excluding fruit, which can be eaten by the barrow load but not juiced.

Potatoes are a staple. Dr Gerson had been in the thick of WW1 and saw how the German army was sustained on potatoes, the centre piece of every meal. This advice is standard Gerson Therapy. Bubble & squeak, potato cakes with garlic, herbs peppers, tomatoes and celery; oven chips, whole onion and parsnips drizzled in a flax oil, garlic chopped coriander vinaigrette. That's me living on the edge. I love food and I'm eating to live.

Sprouted pulses, it should be noted, start to attract mould after a few days even in the fridge. Smart arse here didn't notice this and would at times store them for a couple of weeks. Eating mould is not an ideal with or without cancer. If in doubt get the magnifier out and check these little bundles of goodness for any furry piggyback riders or simply don't keep them for 2 weeks!

Oven cooked root veg dipped in home-made tomato soup. Pea soup, carrot and coriander and tomato and basil. Watercress. One or two ingredients, slowly cooked and simply delicious. We need to lose the salt, the stock cubes and bouillon powder and retrain our taste buds. Once my salt addiction was gone this became easy and once the cancer was in retreat an absolute must. I relish in the recovery of new found friends once written off by their drug experts alive for the sake of simple lifestyle changes.

Oil & Fats

Getting this right is critical.

Max Gerson recounts an early clinical experience in 'A Cancer Therapy - Results of Fifty Cases' with a patient in Paris in the 1940's, while experimenting *with* humans.

> *This was a very interesting case. I had to work against the whole family, and I had plenty of trouble. There were many physicians in the family. But anyway, I came through in that case. She had cancer of the breast which regrew. Every time the family insisted that she was "so much down". She weighed only 78 pounds. She was skin and bones and they wanted me to give her egg yolks. I gave her small amounts of egg yolks - the cancer regrew. Then they insisted that I give her meat, raw chopped meat. I gave her this and the cancer regrew. The third time, they wanted me to give her some oil. I gave her this and the cancer regrew. But anyway I could eliminate the cancer and cure. And still I had no idea what cancer was.*

I avoided all oils while healing other than uncooked organic cold pressed flax (linseed) oil. I use the flax oil on salads, houmous, potatoes, lentil pate. Avocados are considered too fatty for the Gerson Therapy and I did lay off for those two years but I reintroduced them occasionally once my healing was well under way and I felt it was right. See how I went from terrorist to moderate rebel!

Additional healthy fat was a big instinctive draw for me and so was an increase in protein, something I had restricted to one tablespoon daily on Gerson. I upped my intake of flax oil greatly and in doing so my body continued to restore at an impressive rate. Fat is a very grey area and not least in lymphoma. I needed and thrived with more oil than anticipated. The good oil is cold pressed and organic and comes in amber glass bottles for protection from the light. Flax Farm in the UK deliver it freshly pressed chilled, to your door. The light alone breaks down the oil molecules but heating sends them crazy and alters the fatty acid chains turning the oil harmful. All the oils we use when heated become rancid and detrimental to healing.

I have detected particles in oils treated with steam... which are highly toxic for man.
Dr Johanna Budwig (1908 – 2003)

Dr Johanna Budwig PhD was the senior expert researcher for pharmaceuticals and fats in the German Federal Health Office in the 1950's and she made some groundbreaking discoveries which ultimately brought her into conflict with the establishment and set her on a path to resolving the problem of cancer using the Budwig diet.

A common observation of modern nutrition is a deficiency in omega-3. Dr Budwig established that essential polyunsaturated fatty acids, linoleic acid (LA - omega-6 fatty acid) and alpha-linolenic acid (ALA - omega-3 fatty acid) are key elements of cell membranes. Without a properly functioning membrane cells lose the ability to protect themselves from opportunist microbes, to perform vital life processes such as the dividing, forming new cells and communicating. Udo Erasmus PhD states, in 'Fats That Heal Fats That Kill':

> *Frying and deep frying are completely prohibited if optimum health is what you are after or if you are attempting to reverse cancer or any other degenerative condition using natural means. Safe frying is a contradiction in terms. The 60g (2oz) of margarine and shortenings we consume each day contains more than twice as many toxic food additives' than are found in the other food that [we] consume each day.*

There is a clear recurring theme in research into the heating and consumption of oils which suggests that the oil we disrupt with heat disrupts our electrical potential when absorbed. Oils when heated lose their electrical spark and their nutrient content making them not only dead food but toxic and dangerous too. Cold pressed oil, specifically flax/linseed oil, serves to hold oxygen in the cells it nourishes and acts as a barrier to invaders. This also serves as a kind of electrical transmission facilitator delivering signals along cell membranes and throughout the body.

Frying food in hot oil rearranges molecules, and as we might imagine if we were to burn the electrical cables of an appliance or pour fat into the circuit we would create serious disruption in the communication of the power supply and risk serious consequences. Such crude analogies may be easy to comprehend and it is worth considering that oils also become corrupted when exposed to light and oxygen (air), such is their sensitivity.

The Cancer Tutor:

> *Without the proper metabolism of fats in our bodies, every vital function and every organ is affected. This includes the generation of new life and new cells. Our bodies produce over 500 million new cells daily. Dr Budwig points out that in growing new cells, there is a polarity between the electrically positive nucleus and the electrically negative cell membrane with its high unsaturated fatty acids.*
>
> *During cell division, the cell, and new daughter cell must contain enough electron-rich fatty acids in the cell's surface area to divide off completely from the old cell. When this process is interrupted the body begins to die.* ***In essence, these commercially processed fats and oils are shutting down the electrical field of the cells allowing chronic and terminal diseases to take hold of our bodies.*** [242]

[242] https://www.cancertutor.com/scleroderma/

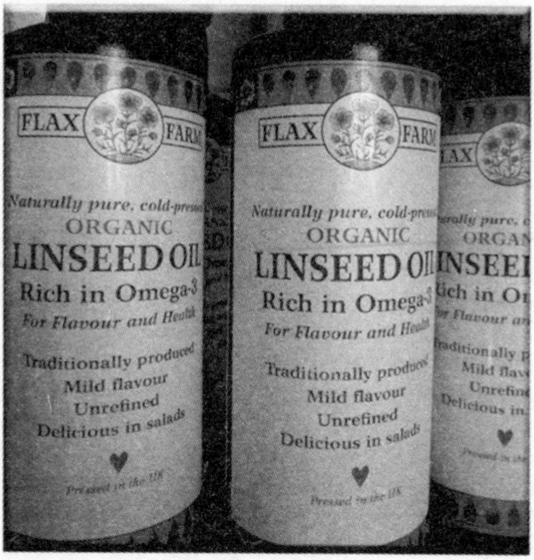

We are seeking to deliver maximum nourishment to the cells consistently so we remove that which hinders and replace with that which helps. This means no more cooked oils. Eliminating heated oil in itself removes a significant body of food from the standard menu. No pasties or pies, no processed, packaged food-like products, no margarines; nothing fried; no biscuits, crisps or take-aways. We are not good at harmonising oil once its composition has been compromised by heat and often times repeatedly. We only have to look at the kitchen sink after a meal to see how incompatible the oil is and that's just the aspect we can see, so it shouldn't come as any surprise when the healing science suggests that getting this junk out of our system might help it run more smoothly. We are literally eating ourselves to death and if we want to heal we need to stop.

We use only flax oil while overcoming cancer *and never heated*. Flax oil has a predominance of omega 3 which is anti-inflammatory, a balance we are seeking to restore and considered to be essential in resolving many modern health conditions. Modern diets tend to include 20 times more omega 6 than omega 3, which can promote inflammation. There is evidence long-term consumption of flax oil alone could result in an uncommon deficiency in omega 6. I therefore introduced a small amount of hemp seed oil after one year N.E.D. However during the protocol I did not risk any other oil other than the proven flax seed oil.

Refined Sugar

If you've ever made wine, you'll know that fermentation requires sugar. Stagnant swamps ferment. Cancer cells ferment. Refined sugar doesn't really need an introduction. It has no physical health benefits and does not serve any helpful role in curing anything other than cravings. Sugar makes tasteless or gross food-like products taste like something you need to eat. It encourages us to fill up on junk food in place of health food. It's addictive. Sugar feeds candida. Yeast, fungus and mould all fall into this category of cancer nourishment and as in kids, sugar makes the cancer microbes more active. Ortho-docs will tell you that there's no evidence that sugar feeds the cancer (while using a sugar to light up cancer for their scans) and that all cells need sugar to survive and that cutting out refined sugars could instead be dangerous. We have a choice and theirs is more fun and less bothersome, but remember their advice to load up on processed sugar and fat doesn't contribute to healing.

Sugars contribute significantly to acidity and inflammation and cancer cells depend on steady glucose availability in the blood for their energy. Refined sugar, refined grains and anything else refined will contribute to the cancer cells energy supply. As the body works to balance the pH in the face of a rise in acidity, it will use up available minerals even leaching them from bones causing further imbalance.

Cancers can use fructose just as readily as glucose to fuel their growth. The modern diet contains a lot of refined sugar including fructose and it's a hidden danger implicated in a lot of modern diseases, such as obesity, diabetes and fatty liver.

Dr Anthony Heaney of UCLA's Jonsson Cancer Center

The metabolism or use of energy by cancer cells and the tumours they form is much less efficient than the evolutionary perfection of normal cells. Normal cells use oxygen, aerobically, a process which is significantly more efficient. Fermenting cancer cells perhaps in a reflection of our lifestyles and preferred treatment choices have devolved to a primitive state where they are generating energy from inferior raw materials, requiring much more to get by. We may observe that malnutrition is commonly recognised as one of the main causes of death for cancer patients, who literally starve in deference to the opportunist microbes that our food choices have provided a home for. The irony doesn't stop there of course because next we opt to pile in a mess of toxic chemicals to deal with this problem, *knowing* deep down if we are honest that this is unlikely to happen.

Sugar feeds cancer, increases cholesterol, can weaken eyesight, cause drowsiness and decreased activity in children, can interfere with the absorption of protein, causes food allergies, contributes to diabetes, can decrease growth hormone, can contribute to eczema in children, can cause cardiovascular disease, can impair the structure of DNA, can cause hyperactivity, anxiety, difficulty concentrating, and crankiness in children, contributes to the reduction in defence against bacterial infection (infectious diseases), greatly assists the uncontrolled growth of Candida Albicans (yeast infections) and contributes to osteoporosis. **Nancy Appleton, PhD, clinical nutritionist, Lick the Sugar Habit**

Dairy

From our extensive research, one idea seemed to be clear: lower protein intake dramatically decreased tumor initiation.

T. Colin Campbell, Thomas M. Campbell: The China Study

Out of sugar? Good. What's the next best thing for keeping cancer content? Dairy! Dump that too. Or, mix em up in a cake with some margarine and you got yourself the making of a cancer charity fundraiser and a bumper harvest for cancer cells! There are a couple of exceptions to this dairy rule in natural cancer therapies notably the Budwig diet in which the casein (the whey) is drained from organic milk/yoghurt which is then fast blended with organic electrically charged, cold pressed flax oil making a cottage cheese, a readily absorbable sulfur rich protein.

For a general overview of dairy, as is generally consumed without any such consideration, we call on the findings of The China Study. In the first large comparison between the regular Western diet and the Chinese plant-based diet, rats and mice confirmed beyond doubt that the sacred protein of cow's milk, casein, causes cancer, in rats and mice. In controlled experiments the researchers were able to switch cancer on and off by adjusting the amount of animal protein in the diet of their test subjects. Not much good on its own, but with cancer growth seen initiated at between 10-20% dietary protein intake in rodents and in humans and further accelerating with increase, this is stunning information.

> ***Casein affects the way cells interact with carcinogens, the way DNA reacts with carcinogens, the way cancerous cells grow.***
>
> *The initiation stage [of cancer] is far less important than the promotion stage. This is because we are very likely "dosed" with a certain amount of carcinogens in our everyday lives, but whether they lead to full tumors depends on their promotion, or lack thereof.*
>
> **T. Colin Campbell, Thomas M. Campbell: The China Study**

It is clear, says Campbell, an accidental whistleblower and fully converted plant nutrition advocate, **"we should not have our children consume diets high in animal-based foods"**. Again it borders on the comical that these cancer growth factors can be controlled in the home and when taken out of the equation have the clear potential to improve survival and limit human cancer incidence and death rates. This alone is superior to the treatment 'response' on which the almighty orthodox cancer industry depends on for its survival and of course the ortho-docs are keeping it quiet! Worse still they encourage us to feed our cancer with these very antagonists.

Wheat and gluten

Gluten has no nutritional value. It is a protein found in **b**arley (the grain, not the young leaves), **r**ye, some **o**ats, **w**heat and **s**pelt (BROWS) and we don't need it. Gluten can cause ill-health and allergies and gluten sensitivity is increasingly common so no, not going to help healing and at best it will be a waste of space! Quinoa, buckwheat (a pseudo grain somehow related to rhubarb) and millet are alternatives.

Meat

> *The rule of thumb: If it contains something that came from an animal, it is forbidden.*
>
> **Webster Kehr. Independent Cancer Research Foundation**

Meat represents death. We are returning our hearts and souls to living foods and working to harmonise with the world we live in. Violence doesn't belong as a normal daily event. Meat is acidic and typically awash with adrenaline (road kill maybe not so much) and animal protein feeds the cancer process. Farmed organic animals do not die peacefully of old age. They die as babies usually before their first birthday in awful circumstances just like the rest of the edible animal kingdom, so if it isn't necessary then it causes unnecessary suffering and accordingly that's a crime.

Again consulting The China Study, we find a firm indicator on meat:

Pancreatic enzymes can be destroyed by contact with acids. Also, a diet comprised mostly of refined foods and meats may result in an acidic body chemistry that depletes these enzymes. Cancer cells metabolize foods very inefficiently and generate acidic wastes. This extra acidity can further compound an already bad environment for pancreatic enzymes. The excess acidity also enables the cancer to spread by using acid dissolved normal cells as its food source.
I think this strongly acidic environment, especially local to the cancer, is the primary reason that cancer does not normally heal on its own.
T. Colin Campbell, Thomas M. Campbell: The China Study

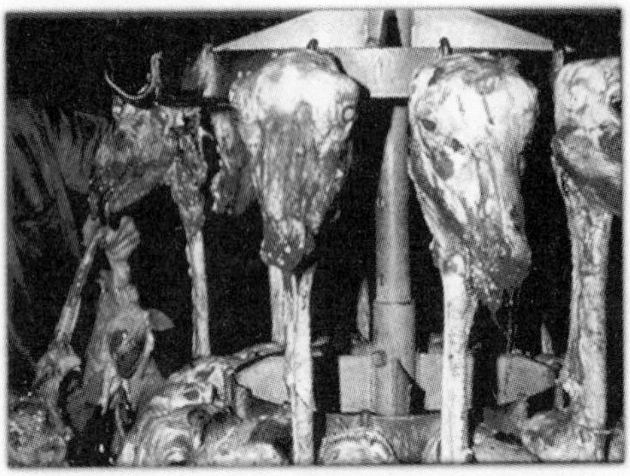

All meat was excluded by Gerson from the Gerson Therapy. So too fish and other animal protein also nuts, seeds, soya and protein powders due to their high fat/protein content and sluggish digestion. Meat doesn't break down easily and is known to use up excess pancreatic enzymes in this process. These enzymes are known for their ability to dissolve the protein coating typical of cancer cells and are essential in fighting cancer. Processed meat is known to go one step further and to cause cancer and as most animal feed is now genetically modified and loaded with antibiotics and growth promoters who knows what else it might brew up.

Soya

The jury is still out on soya generally and it's heresy on the vegan scene to deny this stuff but I'm not a believer in the product commonly consumed. I've had no need or desire to experiment with processed soya anything in my healing and I don't see any benefit. I think soya has been turned from a harmless potentially helpful bean into a suspect. Extracts of the bean itself in its raw unprocessed organic form may hold potential in treating some cancer but we've been taken to a place far far away from there and you will struggle to find a credible cancer therapy that recommends eating it.

Soya milk is processed and most soya milk products have really undesirable ingredients added as flavours, such as MSG, and fillers and even the organic additive free options should be avoided when healing from cancer, if you ask me. I like soya milk but won't be drinking it again, understanding as I do of its potential for aggravating cancer. I haven't used it to heal and do not consider it beneficial in restoring health.

Home made soya milk would of course be a better option but still not for cancer patients. Vegans are being tempted back into the box from which we have started to emerge with these enticing new product ranges that food manufactures have created to keep their customers. Been there done that and I get it, but it's slow kill poison not health food. And yes folks vegans do get cancer. The last thing they want is for the burgeoning mass of lifestyle vegans to lead the way by moving society back to the simple things where we grow our own food in clean healthy soil and set a healthy example. We set out on the right path to whole food veganism but we took the junk diversion when it hit the shelves and are now being misled. We can now see this if we open our eyes. We know enough now to get back on track. Right now vegans appear no less ailing than the rest of society and are no example of a healthier way. The revenue of the big corporations we love to hate are the big losers in our food revolution. And revolt we must.

We get these unseen extras when processing food into flavoured products. The biggest GM crop is soya/soy which by volume adds up to around half of all GM crops grown worldwide. Ninety-three percent of soya beans grown for the world market are genetically modified **herbicide-tolerant freaks** and as far from organic as plastic. Most go into animal feed but the by-products are used as lecithin, emulsifiers and hydrogenated oils for processed ready meals and biscuits. Funny how our animals once ate our food waste and now we get fed theirs! Soya oil also goes to make DL - alpha-tocopherol, the synthetic vitamin E food supplement found in vaccines. Resourceful but insane. But then who doesn't like a bit of creativity in recycling!

Plants in this genetically altered state can tolerate any amount of Monsanto's Roundup while all around wither and die. But they pay a price and so do we. Glyphosate is an organophosphorus compound sold as Roundup broad-spectrum systemic herbicide and crop desiccant which allows farmers to shower their fields to kill weeds easily, but it's absorbed through the roots and foliage and may not slot so readily into the wonderful web of life. The Monsanto Roundup Ready soybean was the first off the production line but lots of plants have been disrupted in this way since, and redesigned to withstand potent herbicides such as glyphosate and supply is increasing at a dangerous rate. [243] Of course the emergence of glyphosate resistant weed species is becoming a costly problem, probably requiring new more devastating poisons. Or better still a few old ideas. But where in our goal for health does this stuff belong?

---

[243] https://www.ers.usda.gov/data-products/adoption-of-genetically-engineered-crops-in-the-us/recent-trends-in-ge-adoption.aspx

Soya also contains phytic acid which inhibits absorption of other nutrients, and phytoestrogens, which when taken in excess could potentially create their own problems. VEGA told me no to tofu and other soya products and I suspect that will be the case for most cancer patients. Processed soya for sure, oestrogen driven breast, uterus and ovarian cancer in older women for sure. Soya has a higher content of phytoestrogens than just about any other food. Phytoestrogens are plant-based oestrogens that mimic oestrogen in the body and there are still uncertainties on the effect. The better human research gives the thumbs up to soya, but not as we know it in the West. There is a place for the Eastern tradition of fermenting foods such cabbage and tempeh (cultured soya) once healed. A supplement containing fermented soya extract can be used in cancer treatment and is tested as a potential agent in the RGCC blood test but evidence for its worth is scant. If in doubt leave it out.

> *After a long fermentation process, the phytate and 'anti-nutrient' levels of soybeans are reduced and their beneficial properties become available to the digestive system.* **Weston Price Foundation**

Genetically **M**odified **O**rganisms

Wreckless scientists have interwoven toxic plant and insect genes into crops to kill insects and worms and an awful lot of papers written about animal experiments using GMOs confirm the dangers yet for the majority of these products there are simply no safety studies to refer to.

Under globalist moves for narrowing control of everything into a few hands, their 'food code' as dictated through Codex Alimentarius* backs nations and manufacturers into a corner on choice. In the EU now, **at least 85% (around 107 million tonnes) of the compound farm animal feed is genetically modified or GM-derived**. Of 148 GMOs licenced in the EU, 7 varieties are soya bean, one a sugar beet, two are micro-organisms, and there are 27 varieties of maize and 3 varieties of rapeseed.[244]

The European Food Safety Authority is as lazy with the science and as reckless with safety and health as the drug makers in scattering around this lethal material. Compare the GM language with the vaccine loyalists' cover-up of their contamination:

> *The recombinant sequence is present in the GM plant only as a single or low copy number, which makes the* ***potential absorption a rare event and therefore difficult to detect... when more studies are carried out with more sensitive detection methods, such recombinant DNA fragments may be more frequently found in the future.***
>
> ***It is therefore possible that DNA fragments derived from GM plant materials may occasionally be detected in animal tissues, in the***

244 http://www4.dr-rath-foundation.org/PHARMACEUTICAL_BUSINESS/health_movement_against_codex/index.htm*

same way that DNA fragments derived from non-GM plant materials can be detected in these same tissues.

No technique is currently available to enable a valid and reliable tracing of animal products (meat, milk, eggs) when the producer animals have been fed a diet incorporating GM plants.

***There is no reason to suppose** that GM feed presents any more risk to farmed livestock than conventional feed. GM feed, which **is very unlikely** to contain viable GMOs, is digested by animals in the same way as conventional feed. Food from animals fed on authorised GM crops **is considered to be** as safe as food from animals fed on non-GM crops.* [245]

Mono**S**odium **G**lutamate

If you are vegan then you will probably be drawn to the booming range of cheating meats, the soya cheeses and the sausages and pies as they advance along the aisles. And you may feel positively smug about it, as I did. These concoctions can taste good, as is the purpose of all processed meals loaded with flavour enhancers, and there is a draw to a cruelty-free meal that makes us look normal, because junk food is what everyone eats.

But there's a little secret, hidden away in the endless list of barely pronounceable ingredients on these packaged products, and it's this that gives flavour to the devitalised end product. One of the most likely flavour additions to all the processed packet foods after sugar is MSG, aka agent E621. MSG is a non-essential amino acid and a very effective and addictive flavour enhancing salt that is produced by fermentation of wheat starch, sugar beets or molasses. This sounds like it should be pretty harmless, but regular consumption of MSG is associated with neurological conditions such as MS, with cancer, reproductive disorders, obesity, eye damage, fatigue and disorientation, depression, rapid heartbeat, tingling, numbness and migraine headaches. MSG has dire consequences for lab rats too.

Researchers fed rats MSG and destroyed the retinal cells that allow vision. A decade later neuroscientists using this method of destroying eyesight to study visual pathways to the brain found that MSG not only destroyed retinal vision cells but also parts of the brain. This was caused as neurons became overexcited and burnt out. This is what's known as excitotoxicity, and that has led researchers to describe MSG as an excitotoxin that can set in motion radical hormone fluctuations and nervous disorders. While the naturally occurring glutamates in food aren't dangerous, processed free glutamic acids like MSG are.

The Arizona Center for Advanced Medicine believes this product increases the growth of cancer cells in the body and other research separate of industry concludes that MSG acts like an excitotoxin slowly poisoning cells and potentially affecting brain

---

[245] https://www.food.gov.uk/science/novel/gm/gmanimal

activity to the point of causing learning difficulties. MSG is a neurotoxin, able to penetrate the blood brain barrier.

However it's packaged MSG is an unbalanced compound that simply does not belong in the human body especially at the levels we are building and it is certainly not health giving. The deceptive labelling is every bit the cover up of a crime. MSG has attracted a bad reputation and its pushers know it and have taken to subterfuge to keep it flowing.

I was a Marmite/yeast extract fan and was mortified to discover that it and just about all else processed and tasty was only thus largely because of this hidden ingredient. MSG or its main component glutamic acid can be found in textured vegetable protein, glutamate, hydrolysed vegetable protein, yeast extract/nutrient, sodium/calcium caseinate, hydrolysed yeast/protein, autolyzed yeast and the ever delightful multi-use gelatine which is a gooey tasteless substance made from boiled down animal by-products such as ligaments, tendons, bones and associated matter which is often mixed with sugar and flavourings and some E numbers to pack out sweets, or candy for children. Yumeeee. And of course vaccines!

Whey protein, bouillon/vegetable broth, malt extract/flavourings, soy protein, seasonings, soy sauce, maltodextrin and vegetable gum, corn starch, chicken, beef or pork smoke and natural flavouring are other potential daily sources. Commercial pet food is of course much the same.

Home-grown healing! You couldn't eat all that but when juiced it's easy.

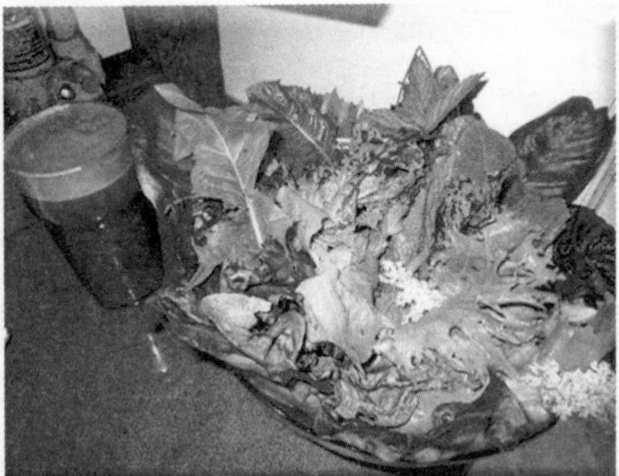

Whoa! Slow down soldier! I get it - this is a lot of stuff to avoid. And the first question is what's left? Curiously it used to be just those on the standard meat and two veg diet that would ask me this question, but as an indicator of how dramatically human society has been misled about what food is, even vegans who were not long ago reasonably savvy about what food is now ask me what we can eat if processed food is avoided. Vegans are still human and humans want more. In this case more food choices. While I have mentioned a few of the veggies I eat there is so much more. It seems silly to list a pile of fruits and vegetables, pulses and grains but seeing as all this food is becoming rare in our convenient society I'm gonna. Besides which, this is it folks and it ain't all bad with a will to live and some imagination. We start from basic ingredients and cook with consideration to the precious life-giving nutrients on a low heat, slowly. No artificial anything processed into a packet, no heated oil, no salt, no sugar, no MSG.

It's over to you to make like Adam and Eve, and to make a new world that works in the interest of healthy families.

Apples, red, green, yellow peppers, cauliflower, leek, purple carrots, broccoli, onions, potatoes, parsnip, peas, fennel, celeriac, spinach, sweetcorn, pumpkin, sweet potatoes, beetroot, green beans, runner beans, kidney beans, butter beans, broad beans, squash, radish, cabbage, beetroot, lettuce, chick peas, courgette, mango, pineapple, celery, pears, plums, artichoke, kale, lemon, lime, Brussels sprouts, cucumber, garlic, bananas, peas, tomatoes, melons, dates (in moderation), ginger, aubergine, green, brown, red, French lentils, dried fruit (in moderation), yam, rice (with consideration to current widespread arsenic contamination of crops), quinoa, millet, buckwheat, bok choi, turnip, pumpkin, swede, gluten free oatmeal, watercress...

With no end of colours, varieties and endless fresh herbs to choose from and with a little imagination you can do a lot more than just heal with plant food and remember this is just the beginning of a new way of looking at food and disease control and yes, we need to think about pest control and not get stressed about odd shaped carrots and a cabbage leaf with a hole in it.

Juicing

Many cancer patients struggle to eat and have digestive issues, juicing to the rescue!

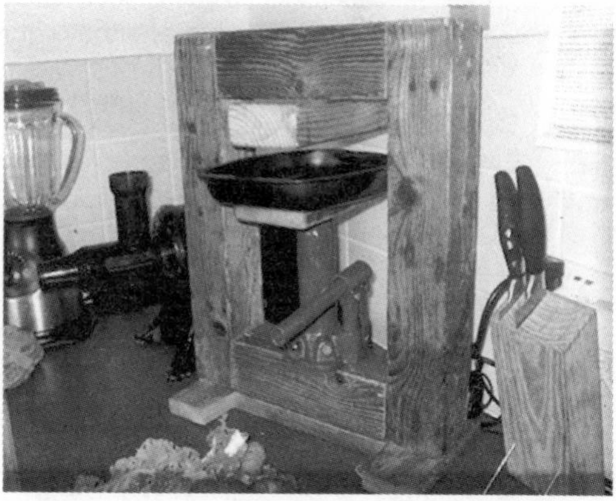

With a view to delivering the greatest concentration of micronutrients and phytonutrients into our body as efficiently as possible juicing is the most potent delivery system we know of. Max Gerson went to great lengths to measure the nutrient content of the ingredients he used to cure terminal cancer patients and with a whisper of the technology and resources we have available today, and with no cancer training he achieved remarkable success. His findings in many areas have stood the test of time and have proven he was way ahead of his time. It's important to use the correct juicer that doesn't over heat the produce and one that will extract the most nutrients. A two stage masticating juicer with a pulp press is the ideal and the most expensive. **Pure** Juicers offer the best machine and excellent aftercare.

We later used a Norwalk but started with a Champion and a homemade pulp press which works out a great deal cheaper. That's our press on the previous page. Cost around £30 for parts.

Everything juiced must be organic, of course, or we risk condensing poisons and adding to the problem. And no, pesticides cannot be washed away. I used to think this was a solution but it isn't that simple. The chemical residue can be reduced of course but because pesticides are sprayed over entire fields they poison the soil. Systemic pesticides migrate up inside a plant following absorption to await unsuspecting insects and end up in the pollen and nectar. Washing them away is not an answer.

Carrots are particularly efficient at absorbing from the soil and are used at times to detoxify the soil, so it's not hard to see how they might offer more health properties if grown in living soil with all the micronutrients, compost and humus that has evolved there forever, rather than more and more barren nutrient deficient dirt, exhausted from years of intensive growth and so much chemical spraying that the farmers fall ill. As we can see from exploring lymphoma studies there is a distinct pattern of agricultural links to blood cancers. Farmers, the canary in this coal mine get it more concentrated than the typical trickle feed the rest of us get but we know it builds up and we know the role these poisons play in cellular disruption.

Gerson have a set prescription of 4 green juices, 3 carrot juices, 5 carrot and sour apple juices plus one grapefruit/orange juice per day. 13 x 8oz each. They are this way for a reason and if you do the Gerson Therapy that's the recommendation and this is sound advice generally. We eventually adapted the juices mixing carrots with whatever lettuce leaves we could grow or source and making 5 x 16oz per day with over 20 varieties of lettuce in each juice through the summer months. These are deep green and deeply nutritious.

Carrots are surprisingly low on the glycaemic index and are loaded with calcium and a heap of other minerals and vitamins and alongside the equally nutrient dense lettuce provide a powerful punch of nutrients.

I often wondered why half the number of juices @ 16oz wouldn't work the same way and save a lot of time and effort. I answered my own question by doing just that - less juices same juice - but only after religious compliance for 2 years to the Gerson 8oz rules had failed me. It matters that the juiced pulp is crushed during the juicing process to extract the maximum and the finest nutrition. It does well to remember that Max Gerson was so far ahead of his time that most still haven't caught up. Variation in juice material once healed is a treat in itself.

Green juices are my preference and the greener the better. Lettuce seeds, as an example, cost £1.40 for 200 Cos (Romaine) from organic suppliers. It's not so easy to grow the amount of produce needed all year round but the possibilities would be endless with a wider community working together on cleaning up our diet, our health and the environment. Add red cabbage, watercress, green pepper, Swiss chard and the good old sour apple, ground and pulped into a Green Guinness. Fill your boots! The widening consensus seems to be that, as Gerson said, fruit itself is not a cancer feeder but juicing removes the fibre and condenses the fruit sugars delivering them to cells easier so we are cautious with what we juice and when healing stick with what we know works. Our adaptations worked incredibly well.

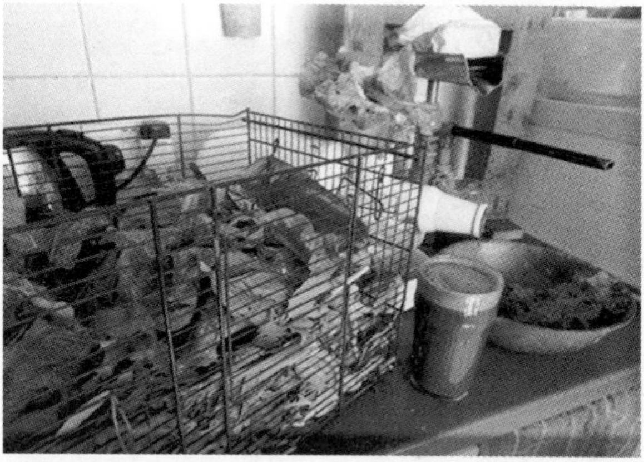

The juices are used as a powerful detoxifying tool and help to balance electrolytes when used alongside coffee enemas. Good advice is to swill with water after a juice or brush teeth to stop your teeth from rotting.

The juicing of cabbage and kale is not recommended as this family contain goitrogens known to block the synthesis of thyroid hormones and interfere with iodine metabolism and suppress thyroid function particularly when raw and condensed in juice.

Having established the MannIcure and watching its incredible success I was able to fit in growing my own food around the rest of the protocol. Being able to heal while soaking in the bath and sweating in the sauna gave me time to rest and doubling up on juice quantities released some time from the pressure of the Gerson protocol, the principle of which was always at our foundation. I did a deal with the guys at the local recycle centre where they would set aside the old rodent cages for me and these I would use to protect my seedlings and then to collect and carry my leaves and the trays make great beds for growing seedlings. This not only took these cages out of circulation so no more rodents would be held captive in them but also enabled a protected crop of leaves and let me shake off any lingering insects before they reached the kitchen. Simple things maketh this Mann.

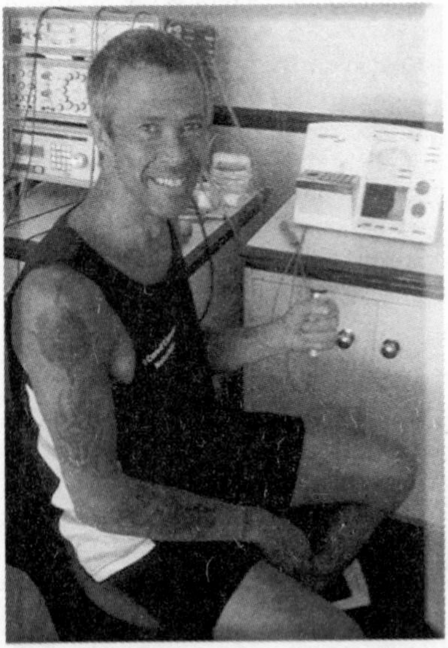

VEGA Bioresonance Diagnostic System

I can't speak highly enough of this bit of kit. This is the fast track big-clue diagnostic tool we've been waiting for. Actually it has been waiting for us! Shop around and compare practitioners – quacks are everywhere. This futuristic medical system can perform a deep non-invasive whole body physiological investigation and taught me everything I needed to know to fill any gaps and deficiencies to bring together my healing. VEGA brought home to me in less than 30 minutes a link between my cancer and the contaminated polio vaccine from over 50 years earlier, a far more common occurrence than you might at first think if you are new to the subject. In the right hands there is very little the VEGA Expert cannot diagnose. Tumours, if present, can be classified as benign, pre-malignant or cancerous. This German ingenuity can narrow down and even identify the cause of a cancer, it will find imbalances, deficiencies of hormones, enzymes, minerals and vitamins like a librarian can find a book, it can read tooth decay and the presence of a virus. It will even diagnose depression and can do all this in a hair sample, human or animal. This is an extremely powerful tool that only personal experience can confirm but I cannot stress the importance of finding a practitioner you can trust.

VEGA could transform our medical system and the health of the population overnight with its ability to magnify the subtle electrical currents that flow between every cell in the body, diagnosing with ease and even predicting disease. It is able to signal the presence of toxic metals and other pollutants and it can measure how well an organ is functioning. We regularly tested all my supplements in my 'circuit' and adjusted accordingly, removing what my body clearly did not want and adding what it did. We tested our water supply and found confidence in reverse osmosis and distilled water but not tap water. It is important to realise that VEGA cannot think ahead and doesn't know what your goal is. While we are advised to maintain our cancer therapy long past there being no sign of disease VEGA simply sees no sign in the now, but your goal is to ensure no sign in the future. There may therefore be no obvious need for supplements at the point of no evidence of disease but we are seeking to drown this cancer out and restore our body defences to the full so we maintain the presence we established to get rid of all of the cancer and leave no room for a recurrence.

The ideal would be to obtain your own machine and learn how to use it. More realistic in the short-term is to find a suitable practitioner who will work with you.

Using VEGA to prescribe remedies is also possible. If a body system is out of sync a good practitioner can place homeopathic, herbal or other medication onto the electrical accessory table of the VEGA device in order to observe the changes in the electrical readout. The medication then becomes part of the energetic circuit. The remedy's subtle motion patterns are conducted through the computer, similar to the invisible flow of electricity. A true placebo placed there for example would give a negative or neutral reading whereas a true remedy tested for potential efficacy will equal the frequency of the energetic imbalance of the patient and bingo! Comparing pharma poisons against herbs for example may prove incredibly enlightening! And at the end of a half hour scan you have a clear choice of treatment. Take it or leave it.

But, shhhh! Don't tell your doctor. This is the end of their monopoly and they will be obliged to warn you that this system (not that most will have ever even heard of it) has not been approved by their authorities. Of course they don't approve! Unapproved is like something unclimbed or unexplored - it's an opportunity. VEGA practitioners are not meant to divulge cancer findings to patients even though this information is revealed and is incredibly accurate and could be used to save lives. EAV Assessment and Screening or electrodermal screening and Sensitiv Imago are similar bioresonance systems to VEGA and there are numerous others.

Thermography or thermal imaging has been around for many years and the technology is way in advance of the radiation dose MRI and CT scanners for detecting abnormal cancer activity. It's non-invasive and non-toxic which is a good start and should inspire doctors who are taught to first do no harm, but of course that's not going to happen any time soon because habits are habits and doing harm seems to be a side effect the industry is happy with. Thermograhy uses super sensitive state-of-the-art infrared cameras and sophisticated computers to measure thermal emissions emitted from abnormal tissue. Cancer cells are more ravenous than normal so put out more heat energy. This technology can detect abnormalities before the onset of a tumour. It's as simple as it's effective and not quite VEGA but a step up from the radiation technology.

While much less useful in my view and a great deal more expensive an RGCC blood test (see pages 417-418) can indicate the best options for treating cancer, based on test tube analysis of circulating cancer cells.

Cancer Microbe Killers:

The Trojan Horse

This is a cool idea. Three ingredients make up our delivery system but there is room for flexibility. We utilise several cancer microbe killing elements in the protocol but getting them into cells can be tricky so we use a couple of tricks to target delivery. There are more than a dozen treatments that are known to kill the microbes inside the cancer cells. Chemo isn't one of them. Chemo kills the cells the microbes live in; the microbes quickly move into newly damage cells (thanks in no small part to the chemo) and carry on as normal. We want to target the microbes while repairing the cells and their environment. Here are some options. We could use bicarbonate of soda, B17, turmeric, cinnamon, colloidal silver or vitamin C. The Trojan horse, coming up next, infiltrates these microbe killing substances directly into the cancer cells to do their work.

1. Organic sulphur - MSM

(Methylsulphonylmethane)

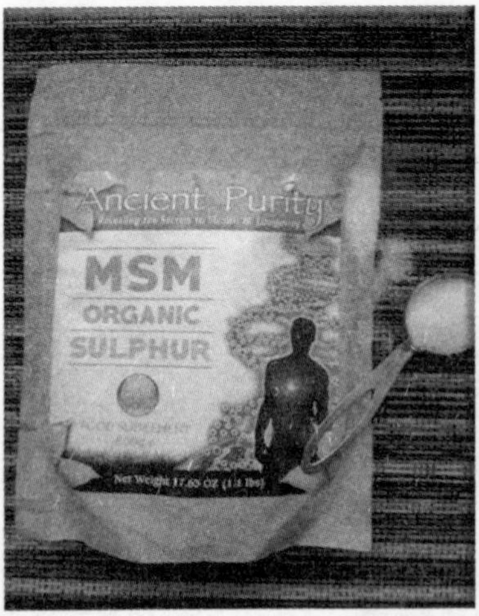

- Opens port to cancer cells to allow in cancer microbe killing agents
- Blocks the lactic acid cycle
- Regenerates cells
- Transports oxygen around the body
- Transports waste out of the body

We prop open the cancer cells with sulphur.

True organic sulphur grabs the oxygen from the water and transports it across cell membranes into the oxygen staved cells weakening the microbes and enabling the start of cellular regeneration. This process is of course dependent on the general environment being compatible with restoration, which takes us back to the nutritional foundation of the cancer protocol.

Sulphur is one of those essential elements which is depleted from our food supply due to modern farming methods. Sulphur also helpfully mops up lactic acid in the bloodstream which the cancer cells are creating and is being recycled to glucose providing them with fuel. This is a self-perpetuating cycle strengthened by the consumption of refined sugars, but our daily sulphur dose disrupts this cycle (aka the cachexia cycle) depriving cancer cells of a key supply line.

This element is an important consideration for alternative practitioners and patients particularly in advanced cases where this cycle will be in full swing. It is entirely possible that this missing element alone could account for why some of the more established cancer therapies such as Gerson and Budwig are experiencing less success today with cancer patients, as stand alone protocols, and is taking even longer than was the case when the soil and therefore the food supply contained greater amounts of sulphur (and less poisons).

> *Since 1954, rates of disease in the U.S. have gone up approximately 4,000 percent. And in 1954, chemical fertilizers were mandated by our government. Fertilizers such as ammonium nitrates and sulfates, which lack bioavailability, appear to have broken the sulfur cycle. A study of the periodic table of elements shows sulfur, selenium, and tellurium as being the only three oxygen transport minerals. Further study shows that chlorine and fluorine are detrimental to such oxygen transport, yet these elements have*

been added to make our teeth "healthier" and our water "more pure" or free from bacterial infestation. These elements are poisonous at higher concentrations, and they block the uptake of both oxygen and sulfur. Drinking city tap water is discouraged in the Study for this reason. [246]

Ancient Purity's crystals are derived from the pine lignans of marine pine trees. We do not use MSM/sulphur tablets or powder. The organic crystals from a quality source are our gold standard. MSM tablets often contain additives which block the bioavailability of the sulphur. Many powder and tablet versions have been heat treated and processed which taints and weakens the sulphur. If the purification process uses crystallisation there can be toxic waste in the end product. The most desirable process is through distillation.

The sulphur tastes pretty benign and is made by dissolving 1 tablespoon in a glass with 2 or 3oz of distilled or reverse osmosis water, not tap water as the chlorine it contains will neutralise the sulphur. It is necessary to guarantee you are not consuming any chlorine. This means we don't shower without a chlorine shower filter (£16.99 cytodoc.co.uk). If you can't fit one or don't have a filter it is advisable to shower many hours away from drinking the sulphur. Humans don't store sulphur and it's no longer adequate in the food supply and only stays in body for around 12 hours. Therefore we take at least one tablespoon every 12 hours introducing steadily. Upon initiating the cancer protocol in order to load up on my stores and for the next 18 months I took 1 tablespoon 3 x daily. I included it in 3 Trojan horse shots each day to use it to its full potential. After one year of being N.E.D I reduced to 1tbsp MSM twice a day (approximately 12 hours apart) including 3x a week within the Trojan horse (colloidal silver + DMSO).

Available from: Ancient Purity in UK [247]

2. DMSO

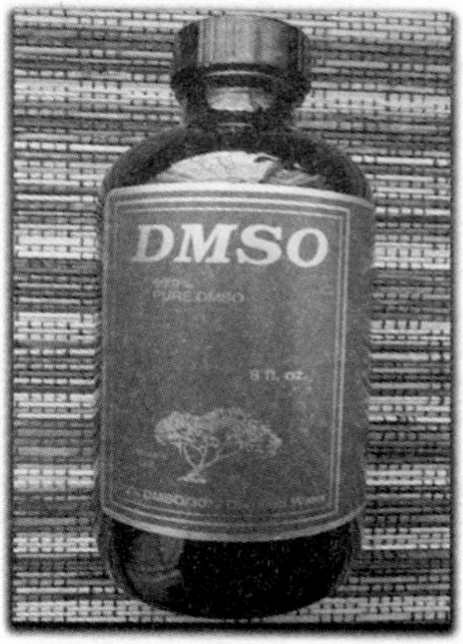

Dimethyl Sulfoxide is a wood solvent, a natural product from the wood industry and one of our most powerful multi-functional anti-cancer agents.

DMSO is well known for its ability to pass through the cell membrane as has been verified by many researchers and therapists for over 50 years. DMSO has been used in the medical setting for all manner of conditions and traumas; it reduces inflammation, increases delivery of oxygen and reduces blood platelet stickiness. And it is one of, if not the most potent free

246 http://www.naturodoc.com/sulfurstudy.htm

247 https://www.ancientpurity.com/msmsulphur

radical scavenger. Tens of thousands of papers have been written and published on the implications of DMSO but of course being a natural product, it isn't a favourite of our dear friends down at Big Pharma Boulevard.

But it doesn't stop there. Since DMSO opens the window to cancer cells very efficiently this allows us to carry in microbe killing substances. DMSO is also important for delivering treatments which are destroyed by the digestive tract since DMSO readily carries medications transdermally, through the skin, such as black salve, therefore avoiding dilution by stomach acids.

It should be noted that DMSO will carry with it all the ingredients we mix it with which is one reason we limit our intake to the purest ingredients. Always! No fillers add-ons or hidden ingredients in anything. Avoid what it touches. No plastics, rubber or latex. Alternative microbe killing agents may be used interchangeably in this seek and destroy process we just follow the same principles, either following on 15-30 minutes after MSM or mixed with DMSO.

DMSO can cause a severe body odour, the worst side effect! From October 2016 I was taking 15ml DMSO once a day in the evening just before bed mixed with 2oz of colloidal silver, 15 minutes after taking sulphur. To fully utilise this window I took a teaspoon of bicarbonate of soda soon after and as the last thing of the day. There is some research showing potential for MSM and DMSO mixed together.

I maintained my daily dose for 1 year beyond N.E.D (no evidence of disease) and have reduced to 3 x per week.

Also available: [248]

3. Colloidal Silver

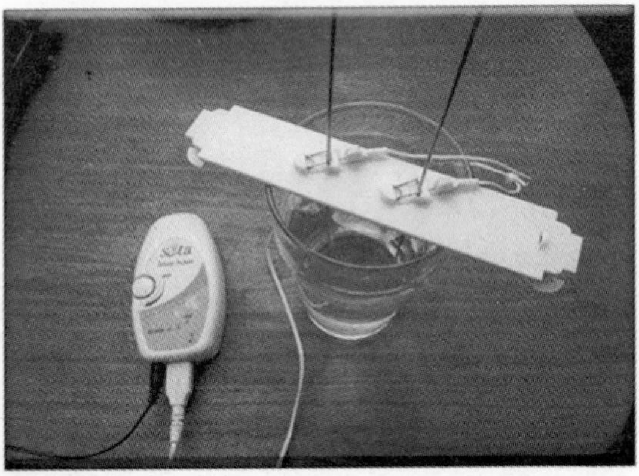

[248] https://www.luckyvitamin.com/p-15429-nature-s-gift-dmso-liquid-unfragranced-8-oz
http://cancercompassalternateroute.com/therapies/dmso/#

Another of those once popular antibiotics, until the 1930s. Then came the Pharma. But we're back! Colloidal silver is less destructive, it consists of silver atoms suspended in distilled ion-less water, small enough to penetrate cells and poison the pathogens within and has been used successfully to combat even antibiotic resistant MRSA infections. The quality is superior when it's homemade in a clean dust free glass and our Silver Pulser doubles up to make the ionic silver colloids as required. This is a pretty tasteless clear liquid. A 500ml glass takes 2 hours to make and provides a supply for a few days which we take 15 – 30 minutes after organic sulphur and/or with DMSO to carry the silver into the cancer cells. We would set aside a day to make up a batch to last a couple of weeks, stored in 500ml amber bottles. Discard if it goes dark.

I took 2oz 3 times a day until 1 year past N.E.D and then reduced gradually to 3x a week within the Trojan horse.

Detoxification:

1. Coffee Enemas

We can continue to wait for the dodgy clinical trials and animal experiments to study the role of coffee enemas, the science of the coffee bean and the workings of a rat's arse or we can just get on with healing in spite of the ignorance of the medicine men.

Detoxification is an absolute priority. There are of course numerous elimination pathways and coffee enemas provide us with a superb stimulus for one of them. Breaking down disease deliberately must be accompanied by the organised elimination of these surprisingly powerful toxins from the body so they don't circulate and do further damage. Coffee enemas are not colonics. We're focussing on stimulating the liver. The liver is a large organ with hundreds of functions and is central to the recovery of our health. The liver is always struggling badly in a cancer patient and needs support and this is what we are here to do. Luckily it has an amazing capacity for regeneration of itself when given assistance.

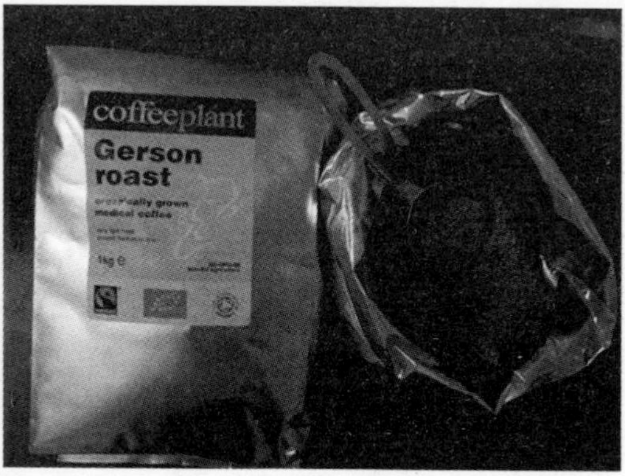

Enemas have been utilised for many years by human cultures much smarter than ours and coffee enemas are increasingly used by alternative practitioners and patients in naturally treating cancer and other ills. Lessening the toxic burden we all accumulate is the beginning of healing. Enemas have been priceless for me. They provide a relaxing downtime in a hectic schedule as the caffeine reacts in the opposite way to oral consumption and they relieve pain too. The coffee stimulates the production of glutathione, a key antioxidant for targeting free radicals. The caffeine enhances liver function and in turn stimulates the processing and excretion of metabolic wastes from the gall bladder. Gerson recommend them every four hours early in the Gerson Therapy and more when necessary. I found 3 or 4 a day ideal during the heavy detox of my protocol initiation, but one year later I utilise them as I feel is necessary, typically two a day. The body heals best when in sleep and a coffee clearout is a good way to start a day.

Listening to what my body is saying has been much more useful than listening to what other people have told me. The doctor I spoke to who told me my healing was impossible also insisted that coffee enemas were dangerous, so I asked how he knew that they were dangerous and he said "There have been studies". And with that simple belief, false as it is, he dismissed decades of practical use, clinical proof and arguably the best thing he could ever offer his patients.

> *The enzyme-intensifying ability of the coffee enema is unique among choletics because it does not allow the re-absorption of toxic bile by the liver across the gut wall, it is an entirely effective means of detoxifying the bloodstream through existing enzyme systems in both the liver and the small intestines. The blood serum and its many components are detoxified as this vital fluid passes through the individual's caffeinated liver.*
>
> **Charlotte Gerson, Morton Walker - The Gerson Therapy**

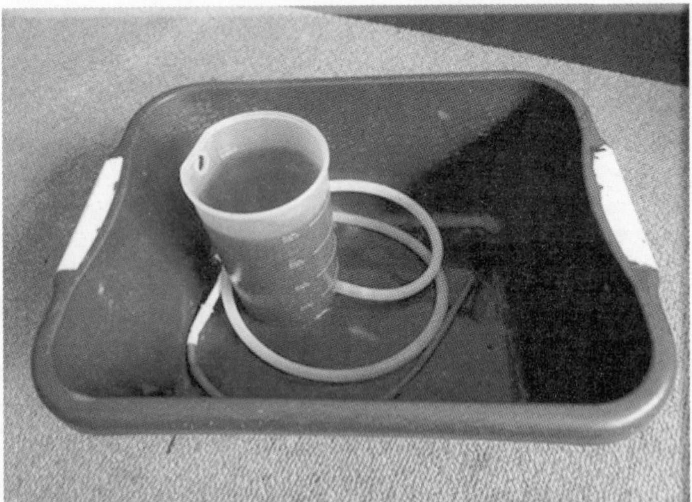

I tell you, when you have subterranean smells, human waste products and large parasites being propelled from your arse like a rocket engine, along with the coffee you have been holding there to flush it out, it doesn't matter what anyone else thinks. This is not any old coffee, and no: no sugar, no milk. We use Coffee Plants

Gerson roast organic medical grade coffee [249] and prepare the prescription according to the experts on the frontline. The preparation is important. I make a bigger batch and fridge it. Coffee Plant recommends not keeping it for more than one day but we find 2 or 3 works fine. Get the biggest pan you can find that isn't aluminium and add 27 heaped tablespoons of organic coffee to 2700ml of distilled water and boil uncovered for 5 minutes then simmer for 15 minutes with the lid on. Strain off the granules through a sieve and discard them; top the liquid back up to 2700ml with more pure water. Cool it put it in the fridge and you have coffee concentrate for a couple of days and are ready to go tease your innards. To dilute this for one enema mix 300ml of the coffee concentrate in a jug (shaken first) with 300ml boiled distilled/reverse osmosis water and 300ml cold water making it the right temperature. [250]

I began as most users do by setting up a comfy spot on the bathroom floor: pillow, enema mat, disposable gloves, towel & book. Seriously you need to be close to the toilet if a) you are new to this or b) you have excess toxic issues because once this healing process begins you are going to know all about it. I set up my stall on the comfort of the sofa once I got a feel for things and have never missed the toilet yet! Yeah I'm boasting. Healing is art. Now I hook to the wall, slip in the tube (it's very thin and it doesn't hurt even up six inches) turn the tap - fill me up, pull it out, read my book. We hold it for 12 - 15 minutes, each 3 minute cycle all of the blood passes through the liver so we effectively get 5 washes per enema. Any longer than 15 minutes and toxins get reabsorbed. This is a unique, creative, relaxing and painlessly effective way to stimulate the overburdened liver to dump stored waste.

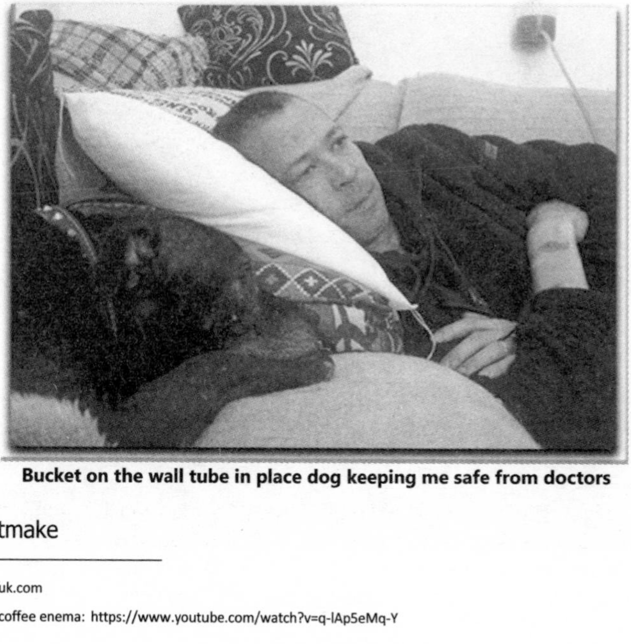

Bucket on the wall tube in place dog keeping me safe from doctors

Upcouldntitmake

249 www.coffee.uk.com

250 How to do a coffee enema: https://www.youtube.com/watch?v=q-lAp5eMq-Y

Curious eh, how it is considered perfectly rational to drink coffee but you are seen as a little bit bonkers if you want to shove it up your arse. But who decides and on what basis? Orally, caffeine serves to switch on the sympathetic nervous system and send the body into a fight or flight state, which in turn compromises digestion and the liver's detoxification mechanisms and all else that isn't needed while it focuses on dealing with the perceived on-rushing threat. Perhaps understandably taking it rectally has the opposite effect and switches on the parasympathetic nervous system, which in turn stimulates nerves in the lower bowels which triggers the liver to release stored toxins. It's kinda neat. And best of all we now have a choice. You don't have to do this, but you can.

One consideration with enemas is the possibility of causing an electrolyte imbalance. But we already solved that as the juices maintain the equilibrium, providing a great deal of nourishment to a battered body. We take in at least 24oz juices to each coffee enema to keep the balance.

2. Ozone

In all serious disease states we find a concomitant low oxygen state. Low oxygen in the body tissues is a sure indicator for disease... Hypoxia, or lack of oxygen in the tissues, is the fundamental cause for all degenerative disease. Oxygen is the source of life to all cells.

Dr Stephen Levin, renowned molecular biologist and geneticist, author: Oxygen Deficiency: A Concomitant to All Degenerative Illness

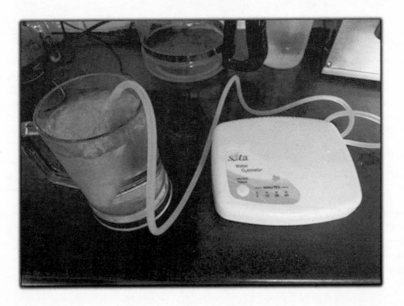

Dr Albert Wahl said:

> *Simply put, disease is due to a deficiency in the oxidation process of the body, leading to an accumulation of toxins. These toxins would ordinarily be burned in normal metabolic functioning. Ozone's effect on damaged cells is quite specific. It attacks the pathogenic materials that don't have a protective coating; it assaults diseased cells that don't have the all important protection of cell wall enzymes.*

Oxygen and ozone are not home to viruses. Viruses are anaerobic so treatment with a high concentration of oxygen and ozone can be very effective in killing them. We are only interested in ozone for the purpose of this protocol. Healthy cells emit a balanced electrical charge and have a strong enzymatic barrier making them effectively invisible. Ozone carries an extra atom of oxygen and is unbalanced electrically. Free radicals are also unstable molecules with a missing electron. Ozone has a spare, helpfully, and that is donated to bring balance.

All diseased cells, including cancer cells – as well as viruses, harmful bacteria, and other pathogens – are also similarly electrically imbalanced. Because of the imbalance that ozone shares with diseased cells, they're attracted to each other. It's a fatal attraction, a dance of death between the diseased cells and remedy.

Included in the essential three piece Sota package is an ozone water generator. One of the simplest and least expensive ways to flood the body with ozone on a consistent basis is to ozonate cold distilled, reverse osmosis or spring water at home. **No tap water**. The colder the water is the more ozone it can hold and the longer it can hold it. And it's more refreshing but more of an aggravant for the stomach to which some patients will be more sensitive. In such cases less cold water and smaller measurements may be advisable. I like to start the day with two cold pints. Also effective against fungi including systemic candida, athlete's foot, moulds, mildews and yeasts. Ozone has the ability to clear blockages in vessels; it oxidizes and breaks down the plaque allowing for better tissue oxygenation in deficient organs. A steady, regular supply helps to gradually adjust the internal body environment.

I took off with three pints a day or more if I could squeeze them in. It takes some juggling to fit the ozone water in away from food and supplements, so not to reduce absorption but this is a healthy habit to hone.

Ozone water is an oxidant and vitamin C is an antioxidant and so we want to take them away from each other. This applies to other antioxidants such as CoQ10. Vitamin C has an active life of about 4 hours and taking R-Alpha-Lipoic Acid in conjunction increases vitamin C's active longevity in the body. Ozone an hour before vitamin C is therefore preferable to an hour after vitamin C.

> *The production of harmful free radicals comes from the existence of toxic compounds and waste products stored in the cell... Ozone/oxygen mixtures create the good free radical oxygen forms that seek out and destroy all these incomplete*

toxic compounds by binding with them. We call this process oxidation and it is a normal function of the human body that has been suppressed due to a lack of sufficient oxygen.
Ed McCabe, author of O2xygen Therapies

3. Sauna

Wrapped in my sauna blanket, sweating healing.

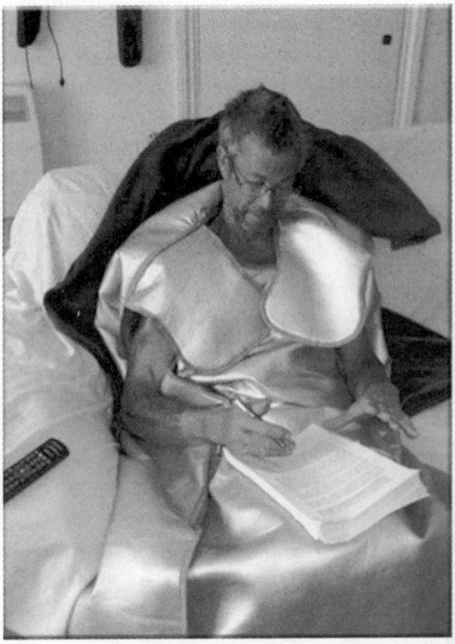

Sweating opens up another detoxification pathway little utilised by many of us. The infrared sauna is a simple addition to any serious healing protocol. Infrared saunas boost fluid circulation and force the stagnant junk toward the body surface and out through the pores of the skin. An incredible amount of fluid is flushed out in these blankets including heavy metals, chemicals and beneficial elements such as potassium, magnesium and sodium. Saunas come in other designs but we want infrared and this blanket version is ideal and emits low EMF. Firzone supply: [251] Thinking this thing through you will have noticed our protocol replaces the good stuff we lose in the sauna via our bathing and juices.

Hyperthermia or heating the body is a well-known and underused method of killing cancer cells which are weaker than normal cells and more susceptible to damage from heat. Disease does well in a body with a low temperature and cancer patients often have a low body temperature and raising it is one of our long-term goals. Cancer often grows in toxic tissues with poor circulation and oxygenation. Infrared saunas help cleanse from the inside.

Organ Support:

1. Liver

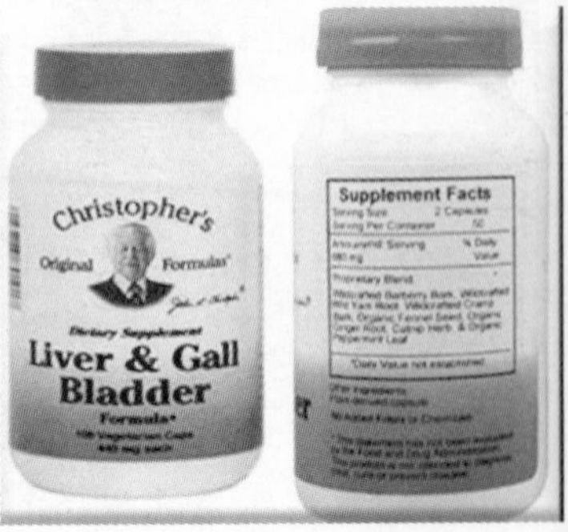

Cancer patients will always have a poorly functioning liver at diagnosis and the pressure will mount as the body heals, but the liver responds well to encouragement and has an impressive ability to repair itself.

[251] https://www.firzone.co.uk/shop/3-zone-infrared-sauna-blanket.html

Max Gerson figured in the 1950's:

> *In more advanced cases it takes a long time, about one to one and a half years, to restore the liver to as near as possible to normal. For the first few weeks or months the liver has to be considered as weak and unable to resume its normal functions especially that of detoxification... for that reason it is necessary to help the liver.* [252]

First we remove the burden of alcohol and pharmaceuticals. Magnetic pulsing of the liver, Christopher's Liver Formula (3 capsules x2 daily away from food until 1 year NED then gradually reduced to 2 capsules daily), homeopathy and coffee enemas served me very well in liver restoration.

2. Kidney

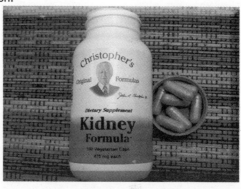

It was a concept that was difficult for me to grasp until I lived it, but once the cancer starts dying off the elimination organs can become overwhelmed with the amount of toxic waste they have to process if it isn't managed carefully. I had a lot of the stuff to dump and it all happened considerably quickly and I did feel an ache in my kidneys for weeks. This was reflected in VEGA readings. At one point during my big healing that pathway got quite blocked so I pulled back a little on magnetic pulsing and blood pulsing, reduced the Trojan horse delivery to twice daily and increased saunas, enemas and body scrubbing to help free me up. I'd say this strategy worked wonders and enabled me to return to my full protocol after a month. I took 2 of these capsules twice a day for 18 months as I felt the requirement and I am now down to half that as maintenance.

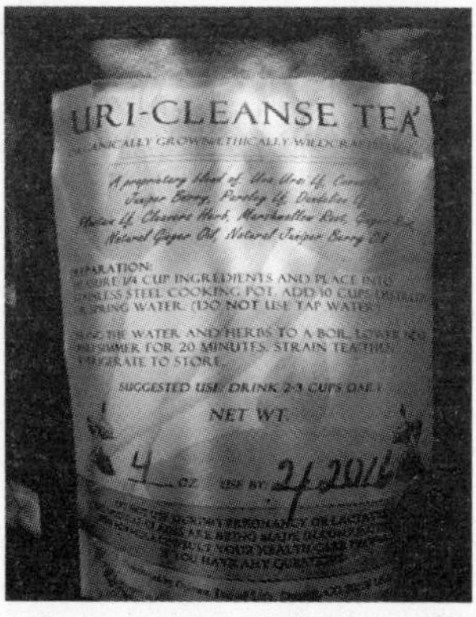

Hippocrates soup, created by Hippocrates himself and adopted by Gerson is a staple of the Gerson Therapy and designed to help cleanse the kidneys. A recipe of celeriac (or celery), parsley, tomatoes, onions, garlic and potatoes, cooked slowly like all good food and milled to remove the fibre.

Homeopathy has great potential and served my kidneys well through my healing.

I have taken herbal supplements throughout my journey Christopher's Kidney Formula served me well: wildcrafted juniper berry, parsley root, marshmallow root,

---

[252] Dr Max Gerson. A Cancer Therapy - Results of Fifty Cases.

goldenseal root, uva ursi leaf, lobella herb and organic ginger root. Uri-Cleanse tea, another herbal formula that has helped my kidneys in challenging times.

To help the flow of my lymphatic fluid at home I rebound on a small trampoline for 10 minutes twice a day. Well that's not strictly true, I try to do it twice but I don't think I managed twice very often, since half the day I have food or juice or a pint of ozone water in my belly or I am otherwise engaged. Me failing to meet that goal notwithstanding, the weightless effect of this bouncing motion plays a very important role in activating an otherwise sluggish waste disposal organ that relies on our physical movement to keep it dumping our waste, in my case harbouring long lost evidence of the work they have had to do on my behalf. First of all tattoo ink showed up in the middle of a surgically excised lymph node in 2013, my last tattoo was 13 years prior yet I was always physically very active in the meantime. In tracking back my disease using much more advanced technology we discovered that my lymph system was suppressed by the carcinogenic polio vaccine.

Immune Support:

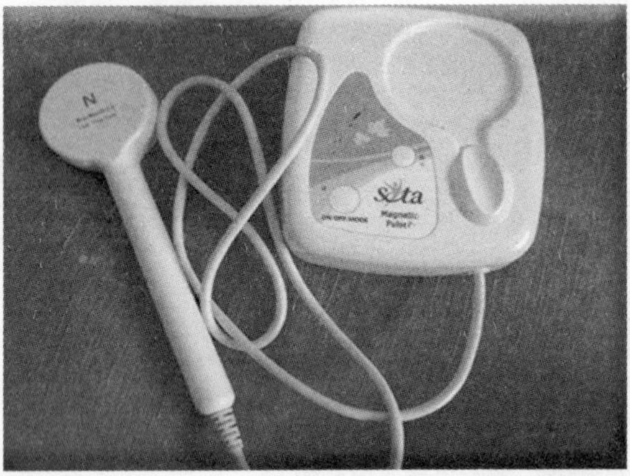

1. Magnetic Pulser

This is part two of the three piece Sota support package. In total they cost close to £900 and I can't think of money better spent.

This device emits a pulsed magnetic field aimed at the tissues and organs. Again this element of our protocol serves multiple purposes. First it creates an energetic vibration that the cancer microbes simply cannot handle. You know when you feel a bad vibe from someone you meet? Welcome to the world of the once indestructible cancer microbe, the incurable cancer you hear so much about. These microbes, according to independent researchers who study them, do not die via the standard methods used to kill viruses, bacteria and fungi and can withstand boiling, radiation and poisons in massive doses, such as chemo and fungicides. They seem to like the less hospitable environments and the little blighters just keep on growing.

Or did. The world is rapidly changing folks and it ain't all bad. In fact it is something as simple as what we have compiled here that could be good for everyone.

This Bob Beck/Sota Magnetic Pulser penetrates deep to reach the organs. The pulsed magnetic field helps to stimulate the natural flow of electrical voltage of cells and thus the recovery of the immune system and kill the bugs that are hiding away in tissues where they don't belong. With this support package the white cells will then gather again to mount a defence of the host and the red cells will realise their role and spread out as intended to transport oxygen freely. We are being gently sparked back to life with electrons by these bio-electric devices, electrons which are known to be highly potent antioxidants.

The Magnetic Pulser has many other applications than cancer, such as the control of bleeding, healing of wounds, breaking up fat, reducing pain and inflammation and calming nerves. The envelope of high energy from the magnetic pulsing and the blood cleaning, the immune boost and the detox I'd describe as forcing the cancer tumours into a meltdown, as might be the fate of a sceptic, bigot or debunker in the face of too many big ideas such as this!

We had beavered away for weeks identifying and understanding this one element trying to figure out the difference between Hz and microcurrents, gauss and carrier waves... back and forth pressing product suppliers for specifications and their research, and researchers for their opinions on immune stimulation versus immune modulation... This mattered greatly with my over stimulated immune cancer and we didn't want be winding that up any more!

It goes without saying that the equipment must be fit for purpose. We sniffed around the internet and found integrity and good intent in our eventual supplier. What you don't get are bold claims of anti-cancer activity from equipment suppliers, such as ours at Cytodoc/Sota. There are rules and those rules state that only industry approved products can be sold to treat cancer; and of this product they do not approve. They cannot afford to! And suppliers of products that do have true healing potential have to be careful not to be too honest about that in the face of threats, intimidation and assassination.

We came to understand that what we were looking for needed to carry the correct pulse of energy through the skin. And into lymph nodes. Viruses hide in lymph nodes and organs and since I had all that going on in my cancer riddled lymphatic system, we were overexcited at finding something readily accessible with the ability to assist that very organ and strengthen my immunity. Alice had by now become expert in how to cut through false claims and questionable interpretations of specific pulse waves; through the principles and practical application in the destruction of cancer and through a confusion of scientific bluster, like my life depended on it. This kind of support is essential for anyone serious about healing; someone to rely upon to do research. With due attention to detail and reading between the lines we ended up with a firm understanding of what we were looking for to square the circle on my protocol and we knew where to source it. That and an understanding of the cause and the mechanism of the disease enabled us to bring cancer to heel.

Take note. We can maybe save you some time, once I finish talking!

We ticked all boxes on the Monday ordered the equipment on the Tuesday got it on the Wednesday, as promised, and started on the Saturday. I started with the blood pulser, introducing gradually, along with making our own colloidal silver and then slowly introducing the Trojan horse. Next I introduced the Magnetic Pulser, shortly followed by drinking ozone water and soaking in magnesium + bicarb baths. I introduced gradually in order to manage the detox and die off of cancer cells. We knew what we wanted and by now fully expected, but you never know for sure until you try.

I began by doing 10 seconds with the pulser in each tumour region then moved around. Kind of a general clean up. The magnet in the paddle gets warm after 20 minutes use and switches off. If you are keen and able you can keep switching it back on and keep going all day long. I did push it to the limit but not for a whole day! We are aiming to work up to two hours minimum every day. It took a matter of weeks for my tumours to begin to soften, change shape, shrink and then over coming months and some longer to steadily dissolve and revert. All it takes is a small sign you are on the right track and you realise your life is in your hands and it doesn't matter how long it takes. It will take as long as it takes. There are no rules. We are making up the rules as we go along, learning and sharing. **We use the 'N' side of the paddle, the north. The South side may have the opposite effect and actually stimulate growth.**

In a situation with just one cancer lump to deal with, we are still seeking to clean out the whole body so are well advised to move this paddle around the body and not just the lump. The body will deal with the lump when the whole protocol is in synergy. And that is such a big deal and I hope you are paying attention because we have nothing to lose from exploring this brave new world, and everything to lose if we don't. I found a map of the human body a good purchase for reminding me where my organs and lymph nodes are located.

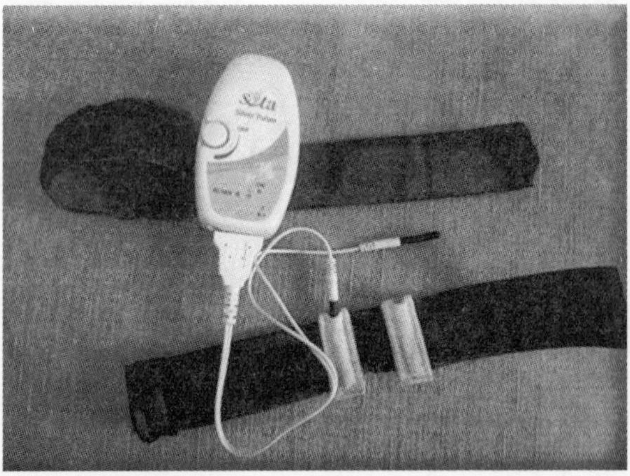

2. Blood Cleaner/ Silver Pulser

This Silver Pulser is made by SOTA, it uses an alternating current to better penetrate the skin. This brilliantly simple medical breakthrough puts out 27- 31 volts and is multi-functional. It pulses very subtle energetic vibrations that kill foreign bodies passing through the veins via the wrist worn electrodes and it's priceless.

The mainstream media reduce such wonders to an adolescent state, headlining not hope but something about Nut Quack Sonic Death Ray Claims. This level of education subjects many MSM followers to death by drugs. But what other people say only matters if we allow them to control our actions.

My blood has physically changed and now actually looks like it should as can be viewed with a Darkfield microscope. And I have no cancer. Is there a connection? When my Silver Pulser isn't zapping microbes and viruses swimming through my life blood, it's making colloidal silver. We are trained to think it smart to own a smart phone and no doubt it can be a life-saving device but it is also dangerous and intrusive and can't compete with the simple brilliance of this little health giving gem.

The Silver Pulser was like a domino at the front of the line that set off an amazing healing cascade, the likes of which you only experience once in a lifetime. I couldn't have managed my self-imposed detox without the whole MannIcure package. But just as noteworthy is the speed, effectiveness and pure simplicity of this arguably one of the most important medical devices of our time. For someone with a life-threatening heart condition a pacemaker would of course be their preferred invention but for someone with a degenerative disease, a bacterial infection, a viral infection or a need for a clear out then this has got to be worth a try. This is what you buy for that friend who has everything.

Or, if you have the wherewithal you can make one for yourself one. Make everybody one! That's all Sota did. There's no patent to be had on an electrical current so if you have some idea how to construct a circuit board the instructions are laid out @ iamkeithmann.com. Do consider not all Bob Beck/silver pulsers/Rife devices on the market are equal and may not generate the correct frequency. Sota are proven. Cytodoc.com is our trusted supplier of this equipment in the UK and Canada. It's important. Use the code Mann11 at Cytodoc and you may get a discount. Again the aim is for a minimum of two hours pulsing each day, with the cotton sleeves of the wristband housing the electrodes placed directly over the pulse of the wrist approximately in line with the little finger and the thumb. We are all unique and for example the placement of Alice's electrodes is much too close together for me to use the same wristband. It is important to feel the pulse in the fingers and to keep the cotton sleeves wet.

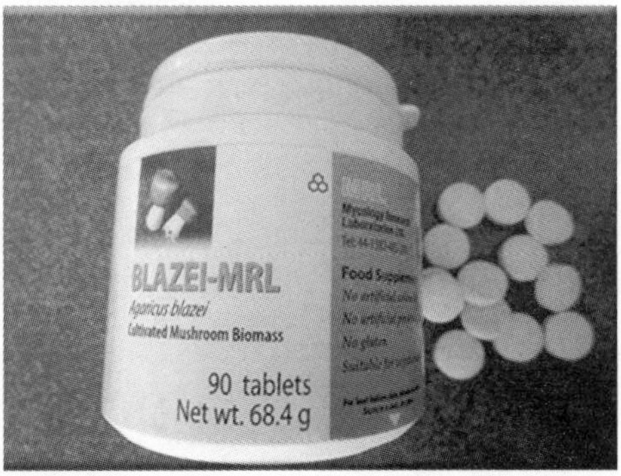

3. Agaricus Blazei
(the miracle mushroom)

Mushrooms get a bad press. They are from that fungal family whose compost is mouldy and moist and not really associated with health. But it's not that simple.

According to the International Journal of Medicinal Mushrooms, Agaricus Blazei "shows anti tumour activity & immunological enhancement." My 2015 RGCC blood test scored 25% cytotoxic potential, after artesin at 40% and ascorbic acid/vit C at 35%. David Hoffmann says in 'Medical Herbalism: The Science and Practice of Herbal Medicine'

Based upon in vitro, in vivo, and some human studies, the mycopolysaccharides found in medicinal fungi usually simply called ß-glucans, appear to have immunomodulatory, antitumor, antimicrobial, lipid-lowering, and glucose-regulating properties.

My instinct said take the mushrooms. Not to feed my belly but to kill cancer. The RGCC blood test said they'd do that. So we did some reading and we found they support immunity as well as kill cancer, so like collectors of rare antiques we went foraging and isolated the best quality assured supply of Agaricus Blazei mushroom then asked our electronic expert VEGA what she thought. She gave a very clear confirmation too, which is good enough for me.

The only doubt that remained was how much of what kind of support it would give me. It is a minefield where a product is promoted for its support of immunity, as this may hang over a vague interpretation of boosting, modulating, regulating, stimulating and so on. Ever vigilant about aggravating my immune stimulated cancer as opposed to working with it, we had to narrow this down to the exact detail as best we could with a week of emails and calls to suppliers to establish the best modulator of my individual needs. Our supply came from Mycology Research Laboratories Ltd and supplied by revital.co.uk

In for a penny in for a pound, I took 6x daily (@ 500mg each, two per meal) and continued for a year after being N.E.D. I then reduced gradually to a maintenance dose of two a day. It seems to have done me no harm! I'm a fan of the mushrooms.

4. NK Cell Activator™(Biobran)

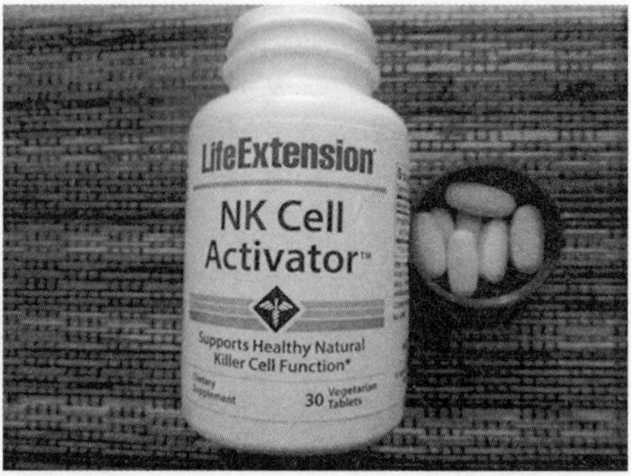

Natural Killer cells are crucial components of our innate immune system and our first responders. Mine seem to have been asleep but they are up now and are back on duty with the help of NK Cell Activator™. Ultimately our level of immune activity depends upon the quality and quantity of nutrients in our diets and the amount of toxins we eliminate.

- *Clinical significance of natural killing activity in patients with advanced lymphoma.*

  We recently determined that patients with spontaneous lymphoma regression had elevated natural killing activity prior to regression. *To clarify the clinical significance of natural killing activity in patients with advanced lymphoma, a prospective study was performed at a single institution in 43 untreated patients. Survival was analyzed to detect prognostic variables.* ***In patients with advanced lymphoma, natural killing activity is a valuable prognostic factor and may also predict the response to chemotherapy.*** [253]

- *Natural killer (NK) cells are important components of the innate immune response with crucial roles in eliminating viruses, regulating dendritic cells, and killing malignant cells.* The Blood Cancer Journal

- *The highly cytotoxic NK cell line... seems to be an attractive alternative for use in adoptive immunotherapy, because it was shown to exhibit substantial antitumor activity against a wide range of malignancies in vitro... which make them unique among the few established NK and T cell-like cell lines.* [254]

- *In one clinical study, scientists documented a three-fold increase of natural killer cell activity in healthy individuals within three to four weeks of receiving 500mg daily of the rice bran compound found in NK Cell Activator™.* [255]

NK Cell Activator™ (effectively the same as Biobran) contains modified rice bran shown to be a powerful immune 'modulator'. NK Cell Activator doesn't increase the actual number of NK cells, instead it strengthens existing NK cells and they in turn activate T cells:

- *Biobran... is able to increase NK cell activity by as much as 300% in just a couple of weeks, whilst T and B cell activity are increased by 200 and 150% respectively. Research has also shown that it can help significantly boost natural antibody production, as well as other parameters of the immune system.* [256]

I began taking 3000mg (6 tablets, 2 each meal) NK Cell Activator™ in September 2016 and maintained the dose for 8 weeks reducing to three a day (1500mg). After 2 months the optimum immune modulation is reached. Pulling back too soon can cause immune function to fall back. This is a simple product and not over rated but you don't get a lot for your money and at 6 a day they don't last long. One bottle of 30 lasts 5 days at around £22 a bottle buying in bulk. At the peak of cancer growth to the end of 2016 my killer cells clearly needed that help, by January 2017 I was down to two a day, by May 2017 as we anticipated VEGA saw no need. Thinking for

---

253 https://www.ncbi.nlm.nih.gov/pubmed/9533657?dopt=Abstract

254 https://www.ncbi.nlm.nih.gov/pubmed/11522236

255 https://www.ncbi.nlm.nih.gov/pmc/articles/PMC5795547/

256 https://www.biobran.org/benefits

myself I continued a maintenance dose of two a day for a year after being N.E.D then finally reducing to one a day. Every 12 months I shall do another round of 3000mg for 4 – 8 weeks.

5. Vitamin D3

Vitamin D3 is the sunshine vitamin. We say cancer is a microbe and that the sun is a friend not an enemy and should not be shielded from the body with chemicals. Many of us are now deficient in vitamin D which is compounded by sun screening and atmospheric spraying.

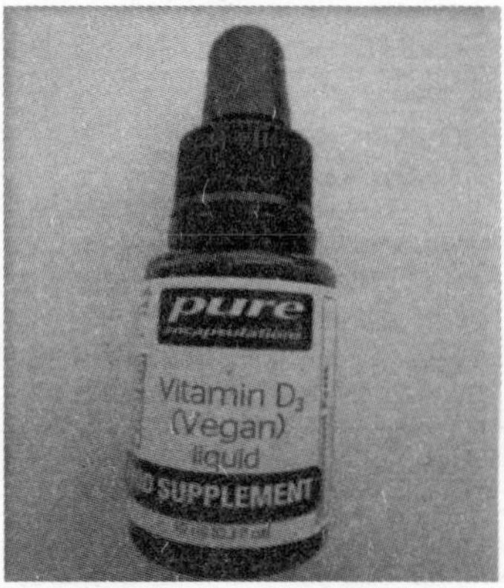

> *Worldwide, an estimated 1 billion people have inadequate levels of vitamin D in their blood, and deficiencies can be found in all ethnicities and age groups. Indeed, in industrialized countries, doctors are even seeing the resurgence of rickets, the bone-weakening disease that had been largely eradicated through vitamin D fortification.*
>
> *Why are these widespread vitamin D deficiencies of such great concern? Because research conducted over the past decade suggests that vitamin D plays a much broader disease-fighting role than once thought.*
>
> *Being "D-ficient" may increase the risk of a host of chronic diseases, such as osteoporosis, heart disease, some cancers, and multiple sclerosis, as well as infectious diseases, such as tuberculosis and even the seasonal flu.* [257]

There is no substitute for the sun, but this little bottle of juice is a good second best it is chemically indistinguishable from the vitamin D form produced in the body and this detail matters. It also matters to load up on more of this nutrient while seeking to heal than we would be able to get from the sun.

The synthetic form, D2, called 'pre-vitamin D' which they add to cereals and drinks as a kind of gesture only makes the makers look kindly, fortifying us by replacing some of the nutrients removed through farming practices and almost entirely extracted during processing. This is not the same and is not as easy to absorb. For many reasons we don't get enough sunlight on our skin and in our eyes and this is becoming increasingly recognised as a medical issue, so much so that doctors

---

[257] https://www.hsph.harvard.edu/nutritionsource/vitamin-d/

prescribe supplementation, pharmaceutical of course, but in the form of D2 which probably contains peanut oil (arachis) or soybean oil, alpha tocopherol, and calcium.

> *Quite simply, vitamin D3 is approximately 87% more potent in raising and maintaining serum 25(OH)D concentrations and produces 2- to 3-fold greater storage of vitamin D than does an equimolar amount of D2.* [258]

Studies published in the Journal of the National Cancer Institute in 2005 reached the conclusion that "**solar radiation may have a beneficial influence in both the incidence and outcome of cancer**". How is it we need reminding the sun is our friend? Sun worship is what we do! Or did! Currently we seem to prefer liars, paedophiles and parasites.

Headlines warn of self-inflicted toxic vitamin D overdosing, of uneducated people buying on the internet, dreaming of healing. This is a lead into more regulation of all high quality nutritional supplements, a process that has been under way for years. Perhaps next they'll limit our access to the sun, maybe sell us 'sun permits' to protect us from overdoing it. Some genetic epidemiology professor at a posh college said in a 'toxic health warning' piece in the Independent newspaper in 2017:

> *The usual prescribed dose in most countries is 800 to 1,000 units per day (so 24,000-30,000 units per month). However, two randomised trials found that at around 40,000 to 60,000 units per month* ***Vitamin D effectively became a dangerous substance.***

Did it? After just two of those fake placebo trials? If you keep your wits about you you'll hear quacks quack.

> *Until now we have believed that taking vitamin supplements is 'natural' and my patients would often take these while refusing conventional 'non-natural' drugs. Our body may not view supplements in the same misguided way. Vitamin D mainly comes from UV sunlight converted slowly in our skin to increase blood levels or is slowly metabolised from our food. In contrast, taking a large amount of the chemical by mouth or as an injection could cause a very different and unpredictable metabolic reaction.* [259]

Sure it could. For the first 6 months I took 15,000 IU a day, that's 450,000 a month. Cancer burden greatly reduced, according to my VEGA as of January 2017 I should continue to take 11 drops per day, 11,000 IU (international units), way beyond the meagre recommendations of the know-sod-all-about-health sickness industry who float around the 500 IU a day mark like they float around the idea that 5 pieces of pesticide seasoned fruit and veg a day is enough to prevent disease and that toxic symptom treatment is better than a whole body cure. My blood tests revealed low

---

258 http://www.gssiweb.org/en/sports-science-exchange/article/sse-147-vitamin-d-measurement-supplementation-what-when-why-how-

259 http://www.independent.co.uk/news/uk/home-news/health-warning-over-toxic-levels-of-vitamin-d-sold-in-supplements-a7625331.html

vitamin D early in diagnosis and consistently elevated at 120+ after supplementation, yet still I appeared to need much more. This is another big consideration for anyone serious about restoring balance. My note to self was not to rely on the blood test or the drug expert. On through the summer I continued on 7,000 IU a day and have no sign of cancer and my willy didn't drop off.

A year on I'm doing pretty good on 180,000 IU a month, six drops daily as my maintenance less than half of what I was on for the first six months of my protocol. While looking for the frightening vitamin D trials which this quack failed to reference, and which I couldn't find, I found some trials that make vitamin D overdosing appear less scary.

- *The single 300,000 IM dose of vitamin D is regarded as an effective and safe to* (sic) *promptly improve vitamin D status in GDM [gestational diabetes mellitus]* [260]
- *The U.S. IOM has also set the 'no observed adverse effect limit' (NOAEL) of vitamin D supplementation at 10,000 IU/day. "If extremely high doses are ingested above the NOAEL this may cause vitamin D toxicity, although reports of this are rare."* [261]
- And this trial on mrha.gov found 50,000 IU monthly, or 16,000 IU daily for one year *did not produce toxicity.* [262]

Now there's a thing. Through the obsession with trying to disprove everything they often reveal the truth.

For cancer patients in particular vitamin D is a must. And the level needs to be maintained high. Bill Henderson says in 'Cancer Frèe', "to heal cancer, you have to elevate the Vitamin D level in your blood and **keep it there forever".** Ideally, he suggests, at 70 ("adequate for most people" in the orthodox range) or higher. I'm floating higher (September 2018 after a long hot summer I'm at 224 in the 50-200 range and now at 6,000IU daily. 75-200 is described as "optimal" in the orthodox range) and I am healthy. I'm keeping mine higher than they advise.

> *Low Vitamin D Linked to Worse Prognosis in Type of Non-Hodgkin Lymphoma*
>
> *Vitamin D's connection to cancer is an active research topic. Prior studies have shown a survival benefit among patients with higher vitamin D levels for diffuse large B-cell lymphoma and chronic lymphocytic leukemia. In addition, earlier peer-reviewed research at Wilmot showed that low vitamin D levels among women with breast cancer correlated with more aggressive tumors and poorer prognosis; and that vitamin D deficiency among African Americans might help to explain higher death rates from colorectal cancer.*

Wilmot's director concluded:

---

260 https://www.ncbi.nlm.nih.gov/pmc/articles/PMC3470091/

261 http://www.gssiweb.org/en/sports-science-exchange/article/sse-147-vitamin-d-measurement-supplementation-what-when-why-how-

262 http://www.mhra.gov.uk/home/groups/par/documents/websiteresources/con137942.pdf

Our data, replicated internationally, supports other published observations linking Vitamin D deficiency with inferior cancer outcomes. [263]

The cells of the human body are teaming with vitamin D receptors. Vitamin D helps to modulate the immune system, to reduce inflammation and control infections. Winter sets in - get no sun - flu sets in. Vitamin D helps to ensure that the body absorbs and retains calcium and phosphorus, both critical for building bone. The ultra-violet radiation of the sun is a source of energy which is clearly undervalued.

Available here [264]

6. Vitamin C (liposomal)

There is overwhelming evidence of the protective effect of Vitamin C and other antioxidants against cancer of the breast.

Gladys Block, PhD. University of California following review of 90 studies on the relationship between vitamin C and cancer.

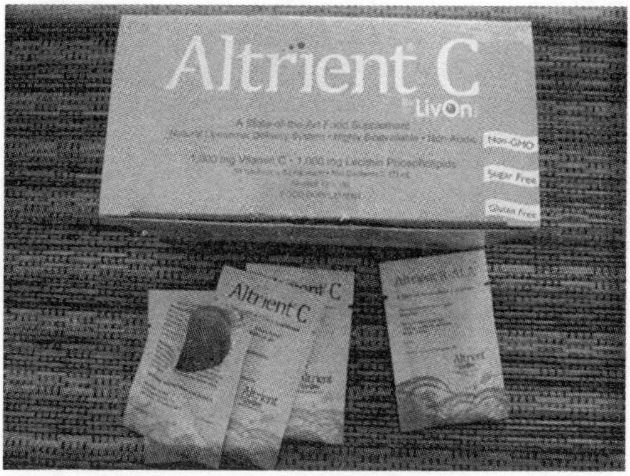

- *Most animals synthesize their own vitamin C*
- *Although defective, humans carry the gene that would provide the ability to synthesize vitamin C*
- *C-synthesizing animals produce vastly more vitamin C than the 90 mg government RDA*
- *C-producing animals radically increase production when faced with severe health challenges*
- *Non-C-producing animals are much more susceptible to disease than animals in the wild*

livonlabs

263 https://www.urmc.rochester.edu/news/story/4283/low-vitamin-d-linked-to-worse-prognosis-in-type-of-non-hodgkin-lymphoma.aspx

264 https://www.purebio.co.uk/shop/index.php?route=common/home

Vitamin C is one of the best recognised and most utilised natural cancer therapy ingredients. It is typically used intravenously in extremely high doses. Doses that freak out most programmed orthodox adherents, but then they aren't permitted by the drug companies to use it and wouldn't know how. Dr Linus Pauling won the Nobel Prize twice. He is recognised for his work with vitamin C and healed himself of kidney disease with a low protein, salt free diet and vitamin supplements. He discovered in his research that a daily intake of up to 10g of the vitamin aids anti-cancer activity within the body. The actual discovery of vitamin C is credited to Dr Albert Szent-Gyorgi who was also awarded the Nobel Prize in 1937. Some practitioners infuse 100+ grams when targeting cancer, which when administered in such doses by intravenous infusions readily kills cancer cells and only cancer cells. The National Institute of Health and many others have proven the anti-cancer effect of high blood levels of vitamin C as well as improved patient well-being, decreased inflammation and decreased tumour growth.

6a. R-Alpha-Lipoic Acid

I took 15,000mg of this liposomal product daily orally at initiation, reducing steadily to 2,000mg maintenance over 1 year. As cancer reduced so did my need. VEGA 3 months later indicated I could reduce to 11,000mg, by 6 months I was down to 5,000mg and so it has continued in line with decreasing cancer and health restoration to the point where I was at 3,000mg in May 2017 and I'm now sticking with 1,000mg daily.

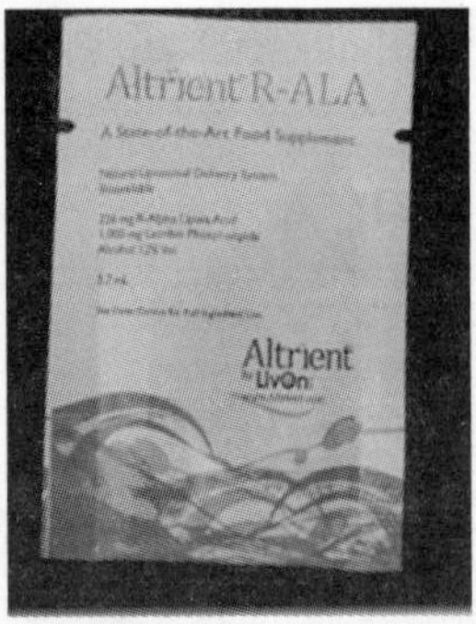

6b. Extra C

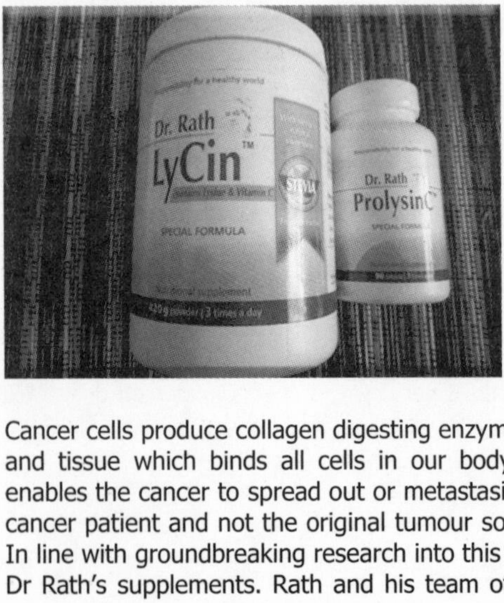

R-ALA is optional. We added the antioxidant liposomal R-ALA at initiation primarily for extending the active life of the vitamin C in the body but ALA is also a potent antioxidant and has anti-cancer credentials. One a day with liposomal vitamin C. Lacking funds we ran out of supplies after a few weeks of use but noticed no slow down in my healing so never added them back in.

Cancer cells produce collagen digesting enzymes to eat into the surrounding collagen and tissue which binds all cells in our body and it is this hole in de-fence that enables the cancer to spread out or metastasise. It is this process that usually kills a cancer patient and not the original tumour so stopping the spread is half the battle. In line with groundbreaking research into this specific pathological process we added Dr Rath's supplements. Rath and his team of researchers at the Dr Rath Research

Institute specifically formulated these products to neutralise this collagen digesting enzyme and rebuild surrounding collagen. They tell us:

> *Our extensive research conducted on more than two dozen cancer cell types has shown that this nutrient combination is effective in controlling cancer in multiple ways: stopping its growth, spread, the formation of new blood vessels in tumors (angiogenesis), and inducing natural cancer cell death (apoptosis).* [265]

A few months prior to protocol initiation I begun taking three synergistic products we tested. **Altrient C** (liposomal) "goo" (phospholipids+sodium ascorbate) x 15,000 mg, **LyCin** powder (L-lysine+ascorbic acid, calcium ascorbate, magnesium ascorbate), **ProlysinC** tablets (L-lysine, L-proline) all of which are also high in vitamin C. The Rath products I took at the doses recommended on the bottles.

This specific combination of natural vitamins, amino acids, polyphenols and other micronutrients work in biological synergy to help control critical aspects of malignancy. Alone they weren't enough but once my cancer had been significantly controlled by the full protocol, according to VEGA, I appeared to have no more need for the latter two of these supplements, the ones used specifically to repair collagen and stop the spread of the cancer. We'd check again months later and get the same feedback but ignored this detail as VEGA is in the moment and we were thinking ahead so maintained my dose for one year past N.E.D, removing all but LyCin and liposomal thereafter, which I continue to take at 1 dose daily. Goo, by the way, is not the scientific term, it's mine. It properly represents the texture of liposomal C.

Liposomes, or Liposome Encapsulation Technology has been used by pharmaceutical companies and researchers for nearly 50 years. Only more recently has it been adopted by healers for delivering nutrients to heal at home. Traditionally high dose IV in a clinical setting has been the only viable option for those wanting to use vitamin C therapeutically. This is not an alternative but it does remove the injections and the need to attend clinic and it can provide a huge benefit at less cost over an extended period.

As we learn more of their potential for targeted delivery, high absorption and bioavailability we will see this technology increase exponentially for sending nutrients, medication and supplements where they are needed. Unlike standard oral doses which have to bypass the well recognised destructive behaviour of the gastric juices and are therefore watered down somewhat if not eliminated outright, liposomes sneak the good stuff past this obstacle. Additionally this delivery system does not create laxative complications as other sources might do at high doses. Put simply the vitamin C is encapsulated within phospholipids, the oily goo, enabling it to be very efficiently delivered to the cells and tissues. Or if you prefer the technical chatter it's a "microscopic artificial vesicle consisting of an aqueous core enclosed in phospholipids molecules, used to convey vaccines, drugs, or other substances to target tissues".

---

[265] https://shop.dr-rath.com/en-us/contentlanding/homepage/home

7. Homeopathy

What can I say? Try it, for everything. Homeopathy is a stand-alone treatment for many ailments. Who would expect to find organ damage caused by a cancer causing vaccine yet there it was! So what do you do with that information? Go back to the machine that found it and design the appropriate restorative homeopathic remedy, of course! Homeopathy helped erase this scar on my soul.

I continue to take homeopathy for liver, lymph, kidney and immune support.

Homeopathy has a significant role to play in infection management for humans and animals and is a safer more effective option than toxic vaccinations.

8. Beta 1,3D Glucan

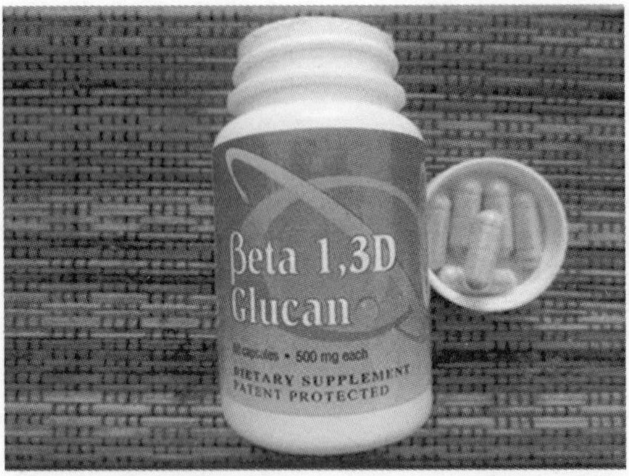

This is another immune support supplement to give us a rounded package. This is what's known as a biological response modifier. Beta Glucans have been tested by researchers for 50 years with 140,000 papers published and are used in many areas of the world to good effect.

The world leading researcher on Beta Glucans, Vaclav Vetvicka PhD says in 'Beta Glucan: Nature's Secret':

> *There are other agents that stimulate the immune system. However, glucans are in a class apart, because those other agents can push the immune system to overstimulation. This means they can make matters worse in the case of auto-immune illnesses such as lupus, multiple sclerosis, rheumatoid arthritis,*

allergies and yeast functions. Glucans, however, do stimulate the immune system, but never to the point where it becomes overactive. In addition, glucan is one of the few natural immunomodulators for which we know not only the composition but also the mechanism of action.

Beta Glucans activate immune cells including T-cells, natural killer cells, macrophages, cytokines and interleukin. It is important to source a proven brand. We chose the one with the best research and word of mouth in support of its effectiveness: Transfer Point. Dose according to body weight (1x 500mg capsule per 50lbs). Taken in the morning at least 30 minutes before food. Beta Glucans are most often purified from baker's yeast but also mushrooms, grains or seaweed, this is foodstuff we are not typically consuming when removing cancer, but the purification process makes them safe and beneficial. I took these for almost a year prior to initiating the MannIcure, partially inspired by mainstream science which suggested they may enhance the effect of rituximab. They didn't appear to help rituximab, or maybe they did and it's even more useless than we have given credit for! I aim, with time, to reduce to a maintenance dose of 1 capsule a day.

Cancer Killers:

1. Curcumin

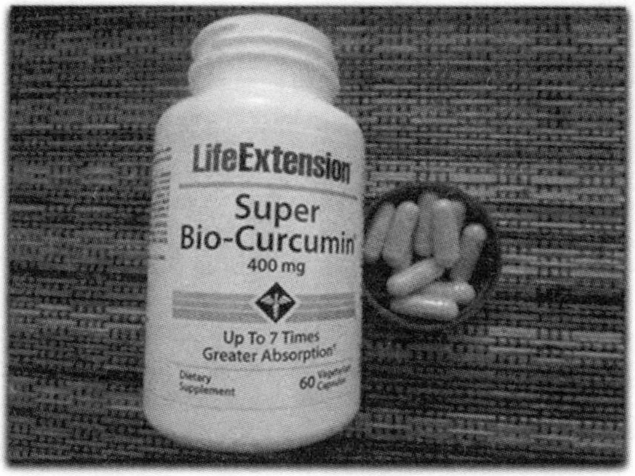

Curcumin is widely recognised as anti-inflammatory and anti cancer and my RGCC blood test recorded that my malignant cells had a sensitivity for it. Genistein and quercetin were other options for me in this class of cancer growth inhibitors. I didn't get to test everything in my list of options due to limited funds and not really any need.

From TheTruthAboutCancer.com (don't miss this series of documentaries with those at the cutting edge of the natural ways to heal):

Turmeric's active ingredient is an extracted compound called curcumin. Studies have shown that curcumin helps prevent several forms of cancer including breast, lung, stomach, liver, and colon because of its anti-inflammatory and antioxidant properties. It stops the development of cancer by interfering with the cellular signaling aspects of the chronic disease.

Curcumin's nearly miraculous "smart kill" properties work to inhibit the growth of tumors and the spread of cancer in fundamental ways at the cellular level. It has the laboratory-proven capability to inhibit a particular cancer-promoting enzyme (COX-2), impede blood supply to cancer cells, induce tumor-suppressing genes, stop metastasis (the spread of cancer throughout the body's organs), kill lymphoma cells and prevent the regrowth of cancer stem cells.

The ability to target cancer stem cells is one of curcumin's most powerful anti-cancer properties, as a recent study revealed.

It is important to source a good quality curcumin supplement. Cheap is not cheerful and not always bioavailable. Look for 'BCM-95' or mixed with black pepper. I took 3 daily (1200mg) until one year after being N.E.D, then 2 daily for 6 months and now 1x daily.

2. Quercetin

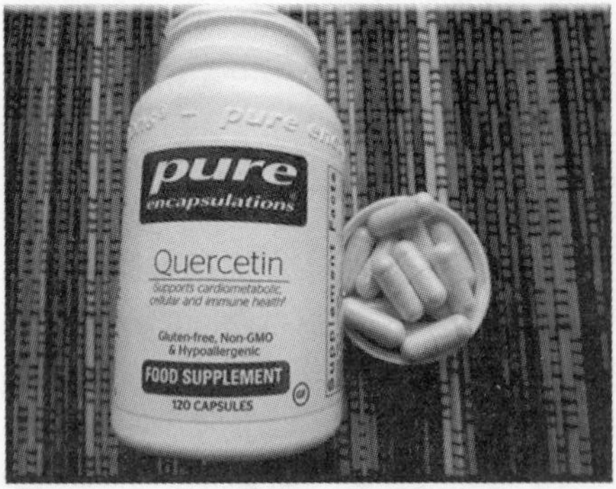

The anticancer effects of quercetin have been confirmed in many studies... Specifically, in vitro *and* in vivo *studies have suggested that quercetin possesses anticancer activity against different tumors; e.g. colon, lung, breast and prostate cancer. Quercetin can exert its anticancer effects through different mechanisms...*[266]

Quercetin is tested as standard and scored very high sensitivity against my cancer cells in the test tube in my RGCC blood test. I took 4 daily for one year past NED, a dose of 2000mg now down to 500mg. Available from: www.purebio.co.uk

3. CoQ10

According to the National Cancer Institute:

CoQ10 may be useful in treating cancer because it boosts the immune system. Also, studies suggest that CoQ10 analogs (drugs that are similar to CoQ10) may prevent the growth of cancer cells directly. As an antioxidant, CoQ10 may help prevent cancer from developing.

[266] https://www.ncbi.nlm.nih.gov/pmc/articles/PMC5561933/

The Gerson Therapy relies on nutrition primarily with a few supplements added in, Dr Nicholas Gonzales would use upward of 300 supplements a day including large doses of pancreatic enzymes with organic plant nutrition as the staple. It's not so easy to quantify the comparable success rates but it is easy to see that both approaches work tremendously well and they like many others use CoQ10.

This from The Cancer Tutor, one of our most trusted resources:

> *Coenzyme Q10 is an antioxidant that stimulates the heart muscles and the immune system in several different ways, mainly through higher antibody levels, and greater numbers and/or activities of the cancer fighting macrophages and T-cells. There may be other ways Co-Q10 aids in the fight against cancer that have not yet been isolated. Antioxidants help the body use oxygen more efficiently.*
>
> *CoEnzyme Q1O (ubiquinone) is a naturally occurring substance and a necessary part of the cell's energy metabolism. Without it, cells cannot produce the energy that is needed for the multitude of activities... and a cell that lacks CoEnzyme Q10 is comparable to an engine without spark plugs – even the most exclusive car on the market cannot run without its spark plugs!*
>
> *The word ubiquinone is derived from the Latin 'ubique' which means omnipresent or everywhere – hence the English word 'ubiquitous' – because it is present in every cell of the human body. As the human organism requires energy for all its functions, and as Q1O is a necessary part of the energy producing system in every single cell.*
>
> *Although the liver naturally provides much of the body's Q1O requirement, its ability to synthesize the relevant amino acids is greatly reduced by illness, and more significantly, the ageing process. This is why extra QIO in the form of a supplement can become a critical factor in some people's ability to make optimal use of Q1O's beneficial effects Q1O functions at a very fundamental level as a carrier in the 'electron transport' chain. This is the final stage of a very complex process in which energy is produced from food, leading to the production of Adenosine Tri-Phosphate, ATP. It is ATP which the cell uses as a 'fuel'.* [267]

I took 6x daily at initiation (360mg) and for one year past NED reducing to 2x daily (120mg) on maintenance.

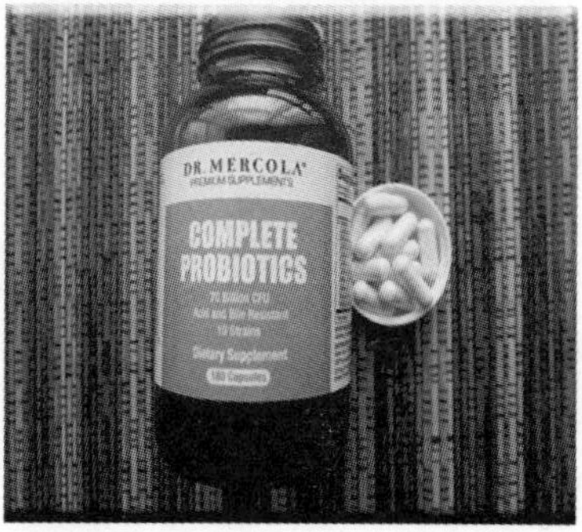

General:

Probiotics

267 https://www.cancertutor.com/q10/

Also called friendly bacteria or good bacteria, probiotics are live microorganisms that are similar to those found in the human gut. Useful for most of us particularly to restore balance after antibiotic use and when using enemas and colloidal silver, as one must. One capsule twice a day.

Potassium

One of our goals is to remove the burden of sodium (salt) at the cellular level and replace it with potassium, as it is meant to be.

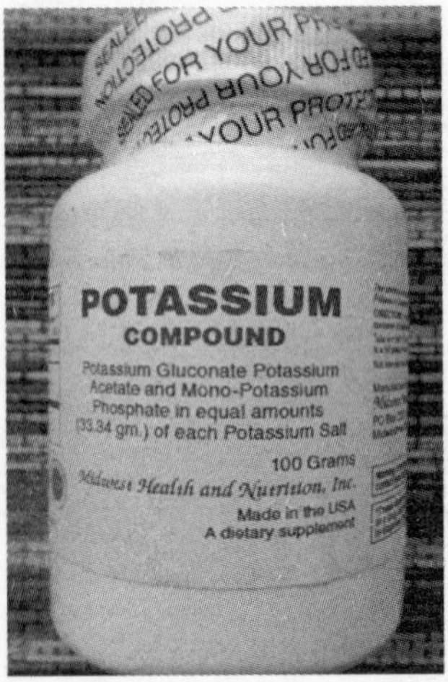

Dr Gerson found a clear correlation between potassium depletion in cells and chronic degenerative disease. This displaced element causes enzyme disruption and a loss of electrical potential. Where we once held a store of potassium delivered from our plant foods, the sodium we load up on in every meal is absorbed and the potassium is displaced. We are going beyond cutting back on adding it to meals – all the salt hidden and seen is removed. The juices and the potassium in the fresh food help us achieve this end but we also add a teaspoon of potassium to our juice. In a balanced diet there is no risk of a sodium deficiency as it occurs naturally in plant food and in only rare cases would salt be a vital supplement, and then in a more natural form, such a Himalayan pink salt.

According to Yushiro Watanabe M.D in 'You Can Eliminate Your Cancer. Healing Through the Gerson Therapy':

> *Modern eating habits result in the production of mutated cancer cells when intracellular DNA repair enzymes cannot function normally. At the same time, the cancer suppression gene cannot be activated in an intracellular environment of increased Na (sodium) and decreased K (potassium) levels. Thus, cancer cells evade apoptosis, divide, and proliferate. When the intracellular K/Na ratio returns to the original state by the rigorous Gerson Therapy, DNA repair enzymes and many other enzymes in the cancer control pathway for apoptosis are activated.*

We dissolve pure potassium power in distilled water and store in a dark glass bottle adding a teaspoon to the juices. I began adding two teaspoons to 10 juices a day for 2 years through Gerson to build up stores. I have since reduced to adding it to 2 juices as maintenance. The regular GP blood test monitors potassium/sodium levels and this is useful. Available here: [268]

---

268 https://www.healingnaturally.co.uk /potassium-compound-salts-100g?search=potassium

Vitamin K2

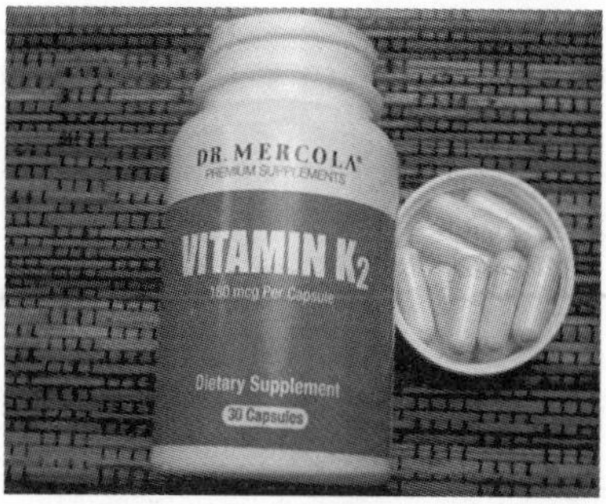

Vitamin K1 is in green leafy veg. K2 isn't and is typically found in meats, some cheese, and fermented foods. Vitamins D and K have a synergistic effect and have also been shown in research to help fight cancer. Chemotherapy depletes vitamins specifically B1, B2, K, B3 and folic acid so supplementation is a must. I took one capsule @ 180mcg daily. Available from Ancient Purity.

Barley Power

One ingredient. Our suppliers tell us: *The young barley leaf is a gluten free green cereal grass which contains the greatest and most perfectly balanced concentration of nutrients found in nature.*

Our preference is Green Supreme from the Dutch Amish in the heartland of the US. It's organic (this is not so easy to achieve in our supplement needs) and contains protein, beta carotene, vitamin C, thiamin, riboflavin, niacin, folic acid, biotin, B6, panththenic acid, iron, copper, zinc, calcium, potassium, magnesium, fibre, amino acids, enzymes, chlorophyll and loads of the micronutrients we don't get from many sources in the modern diet. This type of barley is also good for balancing pH.

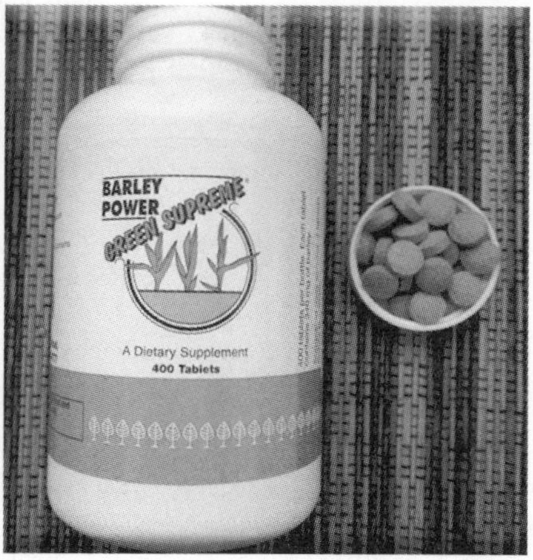

People often ask when I say I'm vegan, where do I get my protein. I ask where do you get your micronutrients. Not from takeaways or over-cooked vegetables and they ain't in those plastic pots of noodles.

I started out taking 20 and steadily increased to 30 a day while chasing my pH. I don't doubt that this bundle of nutrients has helped me create a balance now I have overcome the cancer but it didn't help slow the acid cascade at the height of cancer growth and that continued to deteriorate. Once we addressed the cause of that - by targeting the cancer microbes and the lactic acid cycle - my requirement for Barley Power has returned to 20 per day for my 12 months NED where I am sticking. [269]

---

[269] http://www.greensupreme.net/

Iodine

Iodine deficiency is a common problem equal to vitamin D and is little considered by most of us as we obsess with protein and calories. I was very low at diagnosis and I supplemented with Lugol's Solution at one drop a week. This is a low dose, all I needed, but individual requirements vary greatly. VEGA can help monitor levels so can a biolabs [270] urine test which costs around £30 and can be done via the post.

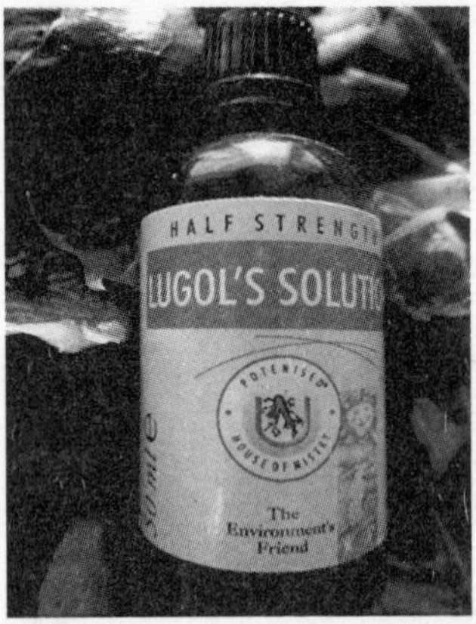

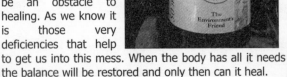

Multi Vitamins, Vitamin B2

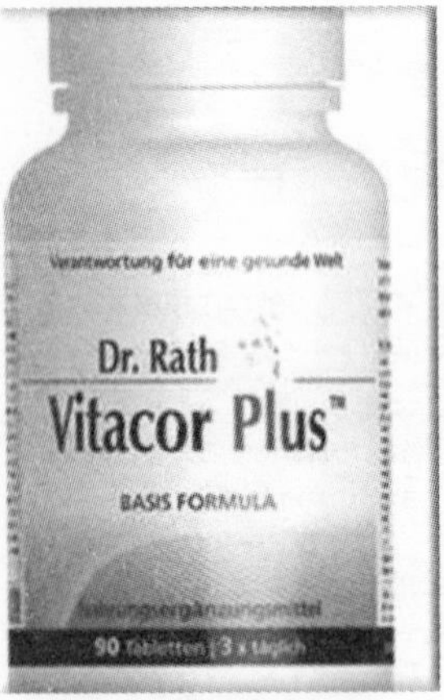

It's important to identify nutritional deficiencies that might be an obstacle to healing. As we know it is those very deficiencies that help to get us into this mess. When the body has all it needs the balance will be restored and only then can it heal.

I'm not instinctively a fan of vitamin supplements and was not drawn to including them in my protocol. There isn't an ideal brand but we wanted that little bit extra of everything so researched the best sources. I developed a B2 deficiency from chemo and our ever trusted VEGA linked that as the cause of an underlying tiredness. The instant I supplemented I bounced back. Viruses also deplete B vitamins and supplements were helpful for me in managing chronic infections brought on by the damaging effects of the chemo.

> *Cancer often causes malnutrition and specific vitamin and protein deficiencies. Chemotherapy also causes deficiencies by promoting anorexia, stomatitis, and alimentary tract disturbances. Antimetabolite drugs in particular inhibit synthesis of essential vitamins, purines, and pyrimidines. Because vitamin levels in the blood are often nondiagnostic, nutritional deficiency is identified almost exclusively on the basis of clinical signs and symptoms and the patient's response to therapy. Signs and symptoms of cachexia and hypoalbuminemia are common in patients with advanced cancer. Deficiencies of vitamins B1, B2, and K and of niacin, folic acid, and thymine also may result from chemotherapy. Nutritional deficiencies are chemically correctable; however, the tumor must be eradicated to relieve cachexia.* [271]

---

270 http://www.biolab.co.uk/

271 https://www.ncbi.nlm.nih.gov/pubmed/2296564

It's true in order to stop the patient dying of malnutrition the tumour must be eradicated but ideally not with chemo! Chemo causes all those deficiencies, any one of which can lead to more disease. We are seldom advised to address deficiencies only encouraged to load up on the calories that led to the mess we are in! Blood tests often miss deficiencies until the patient is further diseased and even then only the isolated deficiency is in view and not what caused it.

Bill Henderson recommends Dr David Williams Daily Advantage for customers in the US. For European and UK customers we found the Rath formulations fit for purpose. Both are loaded with essential micronutrients but Rath's is suitable for vegans and DA isn't. The Rath brand also has a synergistic effect with others in the complete product range. An excess of calcium is to be avoided in vitamin supplements and is found to contribute to cancer.

pH Restoration:

Sodium Bicarbonate/Magnesium Chloride

Returning body pH to 7.2 -7.4 is our aim and I did this with some determination so I drank 1 teaspoon of bicarb daily for one month and bathed in this combination for 45 minutes every 2nd day. Two years of eating green didn't balance my pH which was steadily acidic in the face of cancer growth. We concluded it might kick start my flagging pH level so I'd dissolve one teaspoon last thing at night. It could be worse, it could be castor oil. Last thing at night meant it wouldn't interfere with any other supplements or nutrients. After one month I reduced to once a week last thing at night and gradually to not needing it at all. Repeating the daily dose for one month once a year.

Dr Boris Veysman specialist in emergency medicine at the Robert Wood Johnson University Hospital in New Jersey described one emergency room experience of sodium bicarbonate:

> *The emergency department is always noisy, but today the triage nurse is yelling "not breathing," as she runs toward us pushing a wheelchair. A pale, thin woman is slumped over and looking grey. Without concrete proof of a "Do Not Resuscitate" order, there's no hesitation. Click, klang, and the patient has a tube down her throat within seconds. I do the chest compressions. On the monitor, she is flat-lining — no heartbeat. I synchronize my words with the compressions and call out for an external pacemaker. Pumping... thinking: Cardiac standstill... after walking in... with cancer... on chemo. This resuscitation isn't by the book. "Get two amps of bicarbonate," I say to the intern. The jugular line takes seconds, and I flush it with sodium bicarbonate. This probably will correct the blood's extreme acidity, which I suspect is driving up the potassium. The external pacemaker finally arrives. Potent*

electric shocks at 80 beats per minute begin to stimulate her heart. The vitals stabilize. [272]

I soon get bored in a bath but since we discovered the potential benefit of bathing in a warm vibrant combination of bicarb and magnesium I was obliged to take the plunge and more than willing.

Magnesium is one of the six essential macro-minerals that comprise 99% of the body's mineral content.

Magnesium chloride is highly absorbable through the skin and too little magnesium may be considered as carcinogenic as too many toxins; it's that significant! Magnesium is essential for survival and our cells, particularly if we have cancer, are literally dying for it! Magnesium protects cells from aluminium, mercury and other metals. Hundreds of enzymatic reactions rely on the presence of magnesium and without it cell walls become weakened and ATP energy production drops off. Magnesium helps build bones, enables nerves to function, and is essential for the production of energy from food. And it isn't just cancer, low magnesium levels have been associated with a wide variety of disease states.

Alcohol and dozens of pharma drugs including of course the chemo range interfere with magnesium absorption and retention.

Increasing evidence supports the anti cancer activity of magnesium, particularly at high saturation and I consider this absolutely crucial. According to our lead guide in this valuable element, Dr Mark Sircus, "It can take 3 or 4 months to drive up cellular magnesium levels to where they should be when treated transdemally but within days patients will commonly experience its life saving medical/healing effects."

But magnesium is not perfect and doesn't readily reach the mitochondria of the cell unless we add in sodium bicarbonate and that appears to do the trick! So we submerge our body in a warm chlorine-free, magnesium/bicarb bath (filled it up through the filtered shower or buy a bath tap filter) and soak it up. Transdermally we can load much more than taken orally. I made a point of bathing for 45 minutes every other day for 18 months using between 2 and 4 pounds of the magnesium and a handful of bicarb, reducing to twice a week.

Magnesium chloride and sodium bicarbonate is the ultimate mitochondrial/ATP/cell regeneration cocktail and all you have to do is lie in it! We do not use Epsom salt (which is magnesium *sulphate*) or any other substitute.

Helpfully for Mr Fidget here my healing was apparently significantly affected by these baths with abdominal cramps and nausea forcing me out of the bath early. Over time as the cancer receded I was able to stay in for my 45 minutes.

Dr Sircus informs us:

---

[272] https://drsircus.com/medical-news-comentaries/sodium-bicarbonate-full-medical-review/#_ednref2

Magnesium chloride administration possibilities are versatile: intravenous, oral, transdermal, in lotions and baths, via catheter; it can also be vaporized directly into the lungs and be used in enemas and douches. ***It is not a substitute for dietary corrections that leads one eventually into a healthy alkaline existence but it can be used quite effectively to change the terrain of tissues and cells quickly.*** *One of the greatest secrets in medicine is that bicarbonate and carbon dioxide are really two forms of the same thing and change into each other at the speed of light in the blood. One of the greatest tragedies of our time is brewing around the insanity of governments and their paid scientists and health officials, who are scaring the wits out of everyone with fear of carbon dioxide and the taxes they want to place on its production.*

Plants love carbon dioxide; we love carbon dioxide (it's what makes exercise so healthy) but others hate it because they can sell their souls and make money by deceiving everyone about it. The real danger coming out of the coal stacks of the world is not the carbon dioxide but the huge tonnage of mercury that is released into the air each day, which I calculate to be about 20 tons. [273]

By March 2017 I had no sign of cancer and my pH was for the first time in years a very healthy looking dark green 7.2/7.4. It's a curious observation to the uninitiated but by now for the first time in years I was also noticing my poo was formed and was leaving my body first thing in the morning in a very orderly fashion. This was a clear indicator that my gut was healed. So I'd now wake up to dark green pH readings, a formed poo and no sign of cancer instead of yellow pH readings, sloppy discharge and lumps all over me. How could I have anything but pure gratitude and a firm desire to continue doing right by my body?

It is critical to source a clean supply of magnesium. You can buy 25 kg Magnesium Chloride Hexahydrate Flake for around £30 from Bio Aquatek Ltd [274] or on eBay. Ancient Minerals also supply but it's more expensive: [275] Bicarbonate of soda is available from here in bulk [276]

Cayenne pepper is another readily accessible tool for helping to balance pH (which I didn't try).

---

[273] http://drsircus.com/sodium-bicarbonate-baking-soda/healing-power-baking-soda/

[274] http://www.bioaquatek.com/en/magnesium-chloride-hexahydrate-flake/248-magnesium-chloride-hexahydrate-flake-25kg.html

[275] http://www.ancient-minerals.com/products/

[276] https://www.buywholefoodsonline.co.uk/bicarbonate-of-soda-5kg.html

Darkfield Microscopy

Darkfield microscopy reveals that clustering in the red blood cells can be cleared with blood pulsing and ozone. Before and after observation show increased white cell activity, free moving red cells and increased oxygen levels.

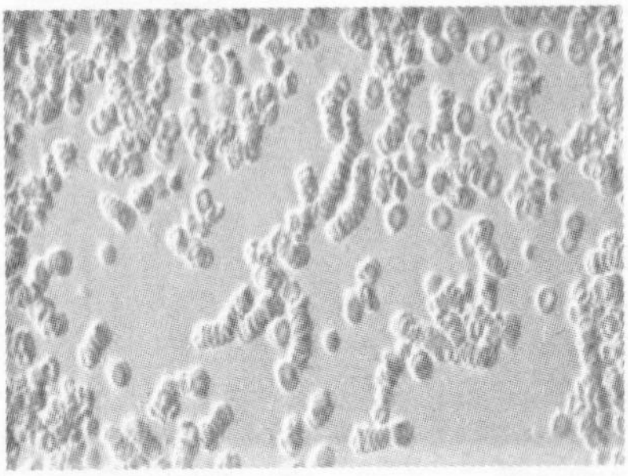
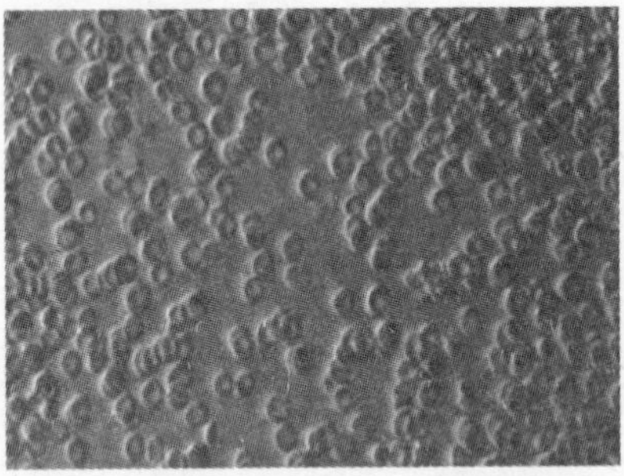

Images before and after. We don't have images from early diagnosis. Early shots at diagnosis would have been fascinating to compare to. We discovered that a diseased body transports the mess through the blood and in those that have gone through a detox and replenish, something remarkable has occurred. On the left you see red blood cells stacking due to a lack of oxygen and on the right a few weeks later, a pattern that continued.

Water, Wetiko, Wifi, Pots & Pans & Teeth

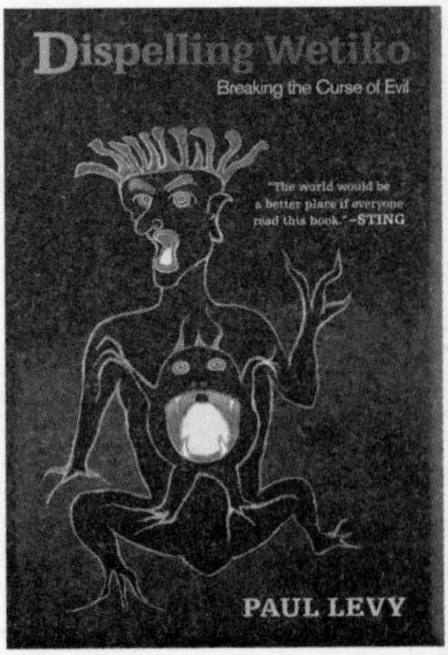

Detoxing emotional baggage is as important as fresh air and features in every successful protocol. I hadn't noticed just how much energy the vampires, trolls and hangers on were taking from me until I climbed out of their sludge bucket. The control freaks and parasites can be just as toxic as the pesticides and we are well advised to step away and allow them to fester on their own. I now separate myself as soon as instinct advises and prefer to be surrounded by the more positive, balanced human energies. Our thoughts create everything in our world and negative thoughts lead to negative outcomes, which is particularly unhelpful when healing. We need to be focussing on our issues not those of other people and any issue anyone else has with you is their issue. Leave them to it; you have an example to set.

There's a heap of chlorine and other contaminants in the regular water system supply that should be avoided. Chlorine alone is poisonous in the human body and displaces iodine. This in turn compromises the thyroid gland which is our internal thermostat. The shower filter removes the chlorine.

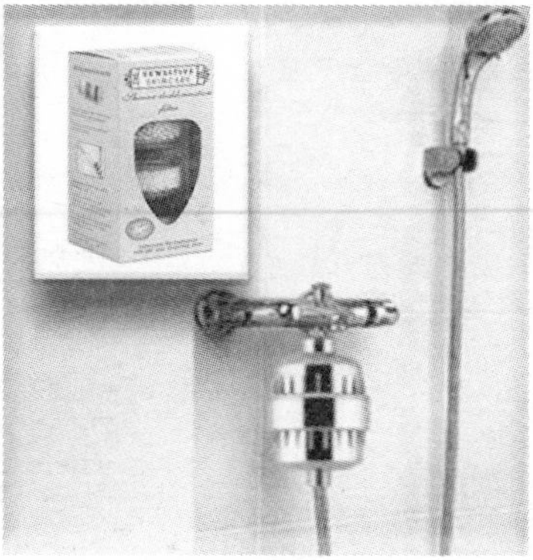

We use Reverse Osmosis a tank/filter system which is fitted under the sink and gives you a second tap and cleaner water. A second supply, this time distilled is even cleaner albeit lacking in mineral content. Both are safe for enemas and drinking.

We dumped our aluminium cooking pans and replaced them with glass and stainless steel. Aluminium is a poison and it leaches into food. Non-stick is a no no. Teflon makers Du Pont and their nasty little secret C8 PFOA - short for perfluorooctanoic acid - are in the firing line over the damage done by this poison to its factory workers and local residents. Those victims were subjected to concentrated doses and the effects are provable, but what of the end user? The toxic trickle feed. We are under such a bombardment of toxins there's no knowing what's causing what although our shared experience might give clues. C8 is used to create non-stick, in fact C8 was a critical ingredient in the manufacture of hundreds of products including Teflon. Non-stick not good. C8 is linked to a vast range of health impacts, including lymphoma, ovarian cancer, prostate cancer, reduced fertility, arthritis, hyperactivity and altered immune responses in children; and hypotonia, or "floppiness," in infants.

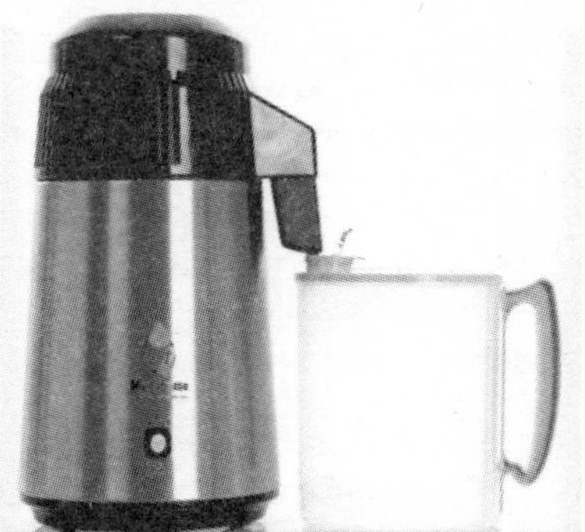

We should also become conscious that we are being literally trapped in a WiFi spider's web that is set to get more damaging the more they speed up the network. This dirty electrical interference is not vibrationally compatible and wreaks havoc on DNA. It is hard to avoid but we can become conscious of our daily uptake and limit it where possible especially when sleeping and trying to heal, and not get ill, and around young children, and the elderly, and so on and so forth. Turn off the router and tell them where to stick their smart meter. Utilities claim smart meters are safe, and compare them to cell phones. More like cell towers! But whatever, cell phones aren't safe, we don't sleep with cell phones and all wireless devices can affect health and the more we are bathed in this unnatural radiation the more we are suffering the effects. And since the WHO classifies wireless radiation as carcinogenic, based on studies linking cell phone radiation to brain tumours, and since brain tumours are the leading cause of cancer-related deaths in children we might want to think about this. [277] [278]

This more recent lab research on animals continues to suggest that we need to be alert when they shove this technology in our faces, or better come up with testing methods that don't involve animals and less lethal technology .

> *Under the conditions of these 2-year studies, there was equivocal evidence of carcinogenic activity of GSM-modulated cell phone RFR at 1,900 MHz in male... mice based on the combined incidences of fibrosarcoma, sarcoma, or malignant fibrous histiocytoma in the skin and the incidences of alveolar/bronchiolar adenoma or carcinoma (combined) in the lung. There was equivocal evidence of carcinogenic activity... in female... mice based on the incidences of malignant lymphoma (all organs). There was equivocal evidence of carcinogenic... based on the incidences of hepatoblastoma of the liver. There was equivocal evidence of carcinogenic... incidences of malignant lymphoma (all organs).* [279]

Other experiments on rats investigating chronic low-intensity microwave radiation exposure from mobile phone usage at frequencies as low as 900 MHz revealed neurogenotoxic and cognitive impairment described as "hazardous.... on the brain." [280]

Teeth come up a lot in natural cancer therapies. Mercury is a no brainer. Indeed it is bad for the brain. VEGA detected mercury toxicity in Alice's brain, we assume from fillings which have since been replaced and from vaccines in her childhood. Since chelating this heavy metal with homeopathy she has given off no mercury toxin signal but brain lesions and neurological symptoms remain at present. It's well-known as a poison at the extreme end yet by some extraordinary logic the one place mercury is claimed to be safe is inside the human body - in our teeth and in vaccines! This is idiotic. Lose the mercury. Lose the quacks. We found a holistic dentist with the equipment and the passion to remove the metal fillings safely. This has to be paid for as the NHS will never admit to the risks and it matters that they are replaced by a professional who understands the dangers of the traditional way of drilling into mercury based fillings to remove them. That process inevitably releases a cloud of poisonous vapour that is inhaled into your lungs. Root canals need consideration too. Seriously. I'm no dentist and no big fan but there is a growing body of evidence to show that a dead tooth in situ cannot be thoroughly filled and minute hollow capillaries are able to trap bacteria inaccessible to the immune system from which germs constantly leach in to the blood. This process could be an obstacle to healing or a cause of disease.

---

277 http://www.abta.org/about-us/news/brain-tumor-statistics/

278 http://emfsafetynetwork.org/smart-meters/smart-meter-health-complaints/, http://www.environmentalradiation.com/

279 https://ntp.niehs.nih.gov/ntp/about_ntp/trpanel/2018/march/tr596peerdraft.pdf

280 https://www.ncbi.nlm.nih.gov/pubmed/25749756

I had my one root canal filled tooth removed and the jaw cleaned out of the bacteria I had harboured for who knows how long. The tooth had been filled 30 years earlier and was diseased in 2015 when I had it removed, as I had learnt from the natural health community that it would be. They all are to some extent. I took the antibiotics the dentist advised and then loaded up on probiotics to restore my losses. I had 5 amalgam/mercury fillings removed and replaced. The x-ray equipment in modern holistic dentist surgeries are computer generated with minimal radiation.

They don't mention the mercury in the energy saving light bulbs we have all been persuaded to light our homes with. Anyone tell you of the danger to you and your family if you should break one and vacuum it up? The low-life 'environmentally friendly' bulbs aren't good for brain function either, emitting as they do dirty electricity. LED bulbs may be less hazardous to health and the environment and generate a much more natural light. We stocked up on the good old fashion bulbs before they were banned from sale.

The restoration of the teeth is an absolute requirement for the treatment, to prevent infection and toxic disturbances from defects of the teeth and inflamed gums.

Max Gerson

Toiletries & Perfumes

Our skin is a large porous organ through which toxins leave but may also enter our body. We therefore apply the same principle to that which we consume orally. If you wouldn't eat it don't rub it on your skin so there is no risk that it enters your blood and organs and adds to the toxic cellular burden that created disease in the first place.

Soaking armpits in deodorants laced with nano aluminium is obviously asking for trouble. Sodium Laurel/Laureth Sulphates are used to make the froth in shampoo, soap & toothpastes.

SLS/SLES go by many other names (including sodium dodecylsulfate & Gardenol) and have many other uses. The main industrial use is as an ingredient in floor de-waxers, engine degreasers, garage floor cleaners, and is a component of Agent Orange, the notorious weapon of mass destruction sprayed over the people and forests of Vietnam. Perhaps an even bigger red flag is the fact that its chief non-industrial use is as a controlled skin irritant in laboratory tests.

As is often the case there is no clear evidence of safety in the scientific literature just the usual confusion. According to the Journal of American College of Toxicology's

Final report of the amended safety assessment of sodium laureth sulfate and related salts of sulfated ethoxylated alcohols:

> ***The Expert Panel recognized that there are data gaps regarding use and concentration of these ingredients.*** [281]

Nevertheless their animal testing as reported in the 'Final Report on the Safety Assessment of Sodium Lauryl Sulfate and Ammonium Lauryl Sulfate' revels all manner of harm, including:

> *Acute animal skin irritation studies of 0.5%-10% Sodium Lauryl Sulfate caused* ***slight to moderate irritation.*** *Applications of 10%-30% detergent caused* ***skin corrosion and severe irritation****. Solutions of 2%, 10%, and 20% Ammonium Lauryl Sulfate were* ***highly irritating and dangerous****. One percent and 5% Sodium Lauryl Sulfate produced* ***a significant number of comedones*** *when applied to the pinna of albino rabbits.*
>
> *Both Sodium and Ammonium Lauryl Sulfate* ***appear to be safe in*** *formulations designed for discontinuous,* ***brief use*** *followed by* ***thorough rinsing*** *from the surface of the skin. In products intended for prolonged contact with skin, concentrations should not exceed 1%. Sodium Lauryl Sulfate had a degenerative effect on the cell membranes because of its protein denaturing properties. Low levels of skin penetration may occur at high use concentration.* [282]

Of course most of the wide variety of cosmetic products that contain SLS have far more than 1%! More disturbing when you consider cosmetic products can have concentrations as high as 50%! And what of the hot water we use with these products when showering or bathing, what impact does that have on absorption into the skin and eyes? No mention of that in the settled science.

Other research suggests that SLS and SLES may cause potentially carcinogenic nitrates and dioxins to form in shampoos and cleansers by reacting with other commonly used ingredients which are easily absorbed by the body and may enter the bloodstream from even a single wash. They may also mimic oestrogen. Hormone imbalances may develop into cancer and they are not good for healing either! There are many other ingredients in these products which do not aid healing.

Too many iffs buts and maybe not worth the risk, you may think.

There are many natural products to choose from, such as the Faith in Nature range but best of all, I think: soap nuts are a simple soap that grows on trees, and have been used for centuries as a 100% natural laundry detergent. They are non-polluting and compostable and can be scented to personal choice with essential oils. Look them up.

281 https://www.ncbi.nlm.nih.gov/pubmed/20634505

282 http://journals.sagepub.com/doi/abs/10.3109/10915818309142005

In reality, it is not the bacteria themselves that produce the disease, but the chemical constituents of these micro-organisms enacting on the unbalanced cell metabolism of the human body that in actuality produce the disease. We also believe if the metabolism of the human body is perfectly balanced or poised it is susceptible to no disease.

Royal Raymond Rife 1953 (1888 -1971)

Taking Time to Heal

Cancer, above all other diseases, has countless secondary causes. But, even for cancer, there is only one prime cause. Summarized in a few words, the prime cause of cancer is the replacement of the respiration of oxygen in normal body cells by a fermentation of sugar.

Otto Warburg (1883 -1970)

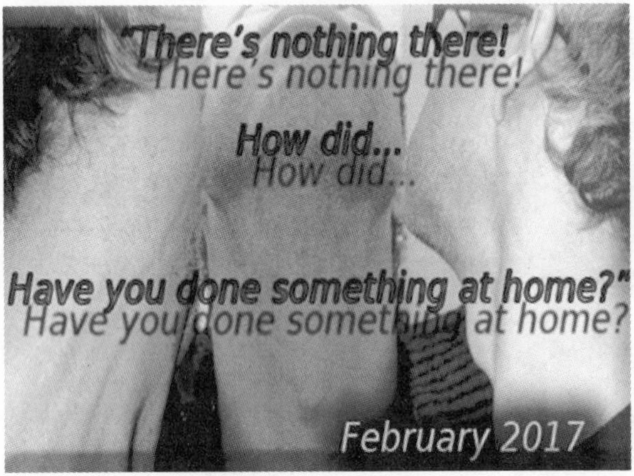

Here is my approximate daily treatment timeline from October 2016, this kickstarted the complete reversal of an orthodox deemed "incurable" disease through to the following summer. I have since, one year in, adapted it accordingly, partially reducing some supplements. I must stress I am in no rush to detach myself from this life-saver and I believe the reason I am in a position to pull back at all is because of the foundation we established in building up to our creation. I am my own creation! It is one of the absolute essentials of all cancer therapies that we do not pull back from immune restoration too soon. I will link the relevant research for key elements at www.iamkeithmann.com.

The time gaps allow for the specifics to do their thing. Cramming is unfortunate. The MSM sulphur requires a 15 minute gap to get the cancer cells to open. We don't mix the ozone - an oxidant - with anything else and leave a time gap both sides of the ozone so it has a window to focus on toxins on the inside and not food and juice and supplements coming from the outside. Homeopathy works better with a time gap and so do some supplements. I wear the blood cleaner while getting on with my day. All I have to remember to do is keep some batteries charged and keep the wrist bands wet. And to take it off before I get into the shower. Idiot.

I use the magnetic pulser while sat down eating, during enemas, typing this and/or I make time.

I do a minimum of two hours a day. Likewise with the blood cleaner.

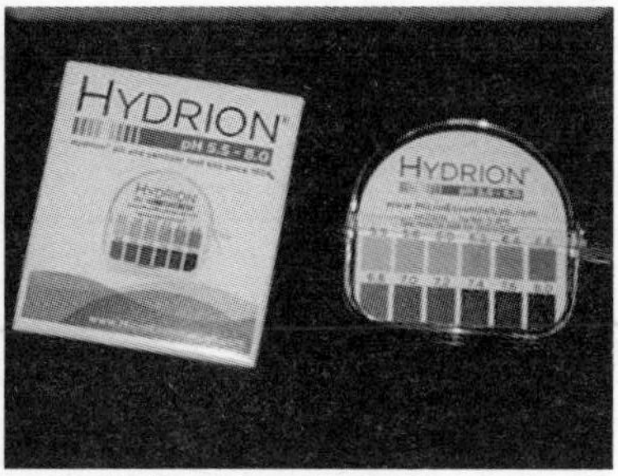

1st thing in the morning once a week I check saliva pH. Aiming to get it nice and green 7.2 - 7.4 and keep it there. A change in diet, too much vinegar for example can affect pH.

Rebounding. For lymph circulation (10-15 minutes 2xday).

Cold ozone water 1 or 2 pints. A refreshing start to a healing detox day.

30 minutes later **beta glucans,** then 30 minute gap before any other supplements or food. Dose by body weight.

Homeopathy/other herbs/no food supplements e.g. quercetin.

7.00am **enema + magnetic pulse**. Shower: **body scrubbing** is a good habit after shower to help open the skin pores. Long handled brush to clear the skin. Big detox organ.

8.00am a tablespoon of **MSM organic sulphur** dissolved in water. MSM takes 15 minutes to open access into cancer cells and likely after 30 minutes the opportunity to transport a substance in has passed. MSM also corrects the lactic acid cycle/ph balance. Build up to 3 x daily. The MSM dose is active for only 12 hours in the body.
8.15am 200ml home-made **colloidal silver** to follow the sulphur.

9.00am **16oz green/carrot juice, Barley Power**
9.15am **Breakfast + vitamin D + K2, NK Cell Activator, multi-vit, probiotics, Agaricus Blazei mushroom, kidney support, CoQ10 & Rath supplements.**

10.00am **16oz green/carrot juice + tsp potassium.**
11.00am **carrot juice/tsp potassium + liver support.**

12.30pm **Lunch + CoQ10, mushroom, B2, kidney support, Rath, NK, vitamin D, curcumin, probiotics.**

Enema.
2.30pm **ozone water.**

3.30pm **MSM sulphur in water (1 tbsp)...**
3.45pm **200ml colloidal silver.**
4.00pm **16oz green/carrot juice + tsp potassium, liposomal vitamin C. Alternate daily between magnesium chloride/bicarb bath or blanket sauna.**
6.00pm **16oz green juice + Barley Power + liver support.**
6.15pm **Enema and pulsing.**
7.00pm **dinner + vitamin D, Agaricus Blazei mushroom, Rath supplements, CoQ10, probiotics, kidney support, NK cell activator, multi-vitamin.**

Homeopathy/herbs. Allow 15 minutes either side.
Enema and pulsing.

Half an hour before bed:
9.30pm **MSM sulphur...**
9.45pm **200ml colloidal silver with 15ml DMSO** opens cancer cells and carries agents in. Very powerful combination. We use MSM, colloidal silver, bicarbonate of soda and vitamin C.

10.00pm **Enema.** I took **bicarb** last thing to chase down that MSM/DMSO. Kills cancer but can affect other supplements and stomach acids briefly. It is useful in bringing up pH but it is also an agent that can be used in a Trojan horse as the substance we are trying to get inside the cancer cell.

I maintained the MannIcure at the full protocol for one year past the point of No Evidence of Disease (N.E.D). That process in me, the elimination of dozens and dozens of these cancerous tumours, took around 5-6 months to achieve from full initiation in the fall of 2016. One of the biggest palpable lumps in my neck that we chose to monitor, of approximately 6cm x 4cm, took 5 months to dissolve completely. In that time I went through three 25 kilo sacks of magnesium. There was also an obvious correlation through this process between the amount of tumour I had and how toxic I felt. Early on with a large burden breaking down I would need, and would do, 4 enemas through the day and maybe another in the night, but as time went on I could easily half this number and still feel well. With no sign of tumours I could do just one enema to start the day and function as I used to before I got ill, for 18 hours non-stop (but nevertheless I choose to do two a day).

After one year of being N.E.D we reduced gradually all elements to a maintenance level – 1x beta glucan daily, 1x NK, 1x quercetin, 2x mushroom, 1x curcumin, 4 x 16oz green/carrot juices, 2 enemas, 2 saunas per week, 1x magnesium + bicarb bath, 1 spoon Rath LyCin daily (other Rath collagen product dropped) 1x liposomal vit C daily, 9x vit D daily (monitored and adjusted accordingly by VEGA and blood tests), 2x60mg CoQ10 daily, 20x Barley Power, 2x kidney, 2x liver support, 1x K2 per day, 1 probiotic a day, half the dose of multivitamins, 1 tbsp MSM twice a day (approximately 12 hours apart) including 3x a week within the Trojan horse (colloidal silver + DMSO). I continue to use the blood pulser and magnetic pulser for at least 2 hours daily and drink as many ozone waters as I can fit in. My healing has been in no way affected. Annually I intend to up all supplements for a one month period back to the full protocol (specifically immune support, Trojan horse and detox but excluding high dose liposomal vitamin C). We may call this a spring clean or MOT. I have no science to back this up and no one to compare to. I am an experiment but I have no sign of cancer and just as the protocol does, this makes perfect sense.

More potassium may be necessary for others than I took on the MannIcure as I had created a foundation with 2 years of supplementing on Gerson.

Sleep, sleep, try and sleep. Sleep time is healing time. *You don't need any more apples. You don't need any more apples... the dog doesn't want to go out at 2.00am... the book can bloody wait...*

I get there's an instinctive response that say this is a lot of work or put it off for costing too much. Such is life? We might do well to remember what we are trying to achieve here. We spend decades mistreating our body to please the mind and now we need to take control of the chatter and focus our mind on our body. If it matters enough, and makes sense, it will happen. People get medals and awards for what we did with cancer, and isn't that the goal of our huge medical research institution? I don't want a medal by the way I'm happy with what I got for my efforts.

SV40's knocking at the door
The polio vaccine's gravest flaw
There's cancer in the needle
No informed consent
We said there was a plot
This is what we meant
Babies are dying
Doctors are lying
Speak out
Stand up
Look up and see

The writing on the wall
For the drug industry

Keith Mann

A Glimpse at the other (us)

Truth is born into this world only with pangs and tribulations, and every fresh truth is received unwillingly. To expect the world to receive a new truth or even an old truth, without challenging it, is to look for one of those miracles which do not occur.
Alfred Russel Wallace (1823 - 1913)

You have to love the irony. For all the superiority and guile, the research grants and the prestige, here we are with none of the above yet we have revealed a cause of cancer and discovered the Holy Grail of medical research long before the vast hoards of employees of orthodox medicine have even gotten out of bed, let alone smelled the coffee, which we've had swilling through our colon and sucking out toxins since the crack of dawn.

It is beyond the scope of this story to go into any more detail on the wide array of natural therapies available to us, but hidden in the healing underground lies the answer to your cancer. I suggest you work with what I have laid out in this book, but whatever you do remember you have a choice. So what if someone else doesn't approve? It's your body. You decide on the information you have gathered. Once upon a time the same controlling mentality that denies this choice burnt witches. Witches weren't evil, witches were usually women who had insight and vision and a deep connection to the natural and spiritual worlds, who could heal and who were conscious. Nurturing and cooking threatens the weapon-wielding macho obsession with hacking, burning and poisoning everything. In modern times the same angry ego is harassing and killing natural healers, revealing for the world the strength of their argument the only way they can.

It's easy to figure out who 'they' are by observing with an open mind what they say and comparing to their product. We hear them most often when they seek to deny or go on an offensive. They typically prioritise attacking the other over proving their own worth. Natural therapies are targeted like this not because they lack worth but because they are worthy! Under these circumstances with no defences the only resort is to attack. It is the modus operandi of that which lacks credibility.

Death is not caused by immune restoration yet they make natural therapies sound like weapons of mass destruction. Ours is innovation and inquiry replacing dogma, textbook training and compliance with the rules of drug medicine replaced by humility and a search for the truth. They can't handle it!

There are clinics in Europe and Mexico providing various cancer therapies. If you have the money and the energy enjoy the ride. But if not, if you have the belief and the desire to make it work you can do this from home and trust me you will need all your resources for that anyway. Whoever you are and whatever you own you can't stay in these clinics for the extended time it takes to heal and will still need to heal at home if you want to succeed. Seeking help out there and blaming others is a critical flaw of humanity as the answers lie within.

Italian oncologist Tullio Simoncini gained a reputation for treating cancer with sodium bicarbonate, direct into the tumour, on the assumption he is treating a fungus. He is of course ridiculed and persecuted for his efforts.

> *Sodium bicarbonate, unlike other anti-fungal remedies to which the fungus can become immune, is extremely diffusible and retains its ability to penetrate the tumor due to the speed at which the sodium bicarbonate disintegrates the tumor. This speed makes fungi's adaptability impossible, rendering it defenceless. For each treatment, take into consideration that tumour colonies regress between the third and fouth day and collapse between the fourth and fifth, so that a six day administration is sufficient. A complete, effective cycle is made up of six treatment days on, and six days off, repeated four times.* [283]

Gaston Naessens is now an elderly man who has hurt no one yet is fearful of the authorities if he mentions curing cancer. He is derided and has been hounded by the medical mafia, arrested and fined for illegally practicing medicine, arrested again prosecuted and tried, yet is innocent! Innovator, life-saver, threat. He developed 714-X made from camphor to be injected at home into the groin for lymph node uptake. This is a safe and unique tool for immune support.

> *In liquefying the lymph, 714X promotes cleansing for a better disposal of metabolic waste circulating in the blood (toxins)... it brings to the blood circulation particular elements (structured and organized molecules including nitrogen fixed to camphor) to directly address white blood cells (leucocytes) to resume their respective defense functions.* [284]

Essiac tea was used successfully to treat thousands of patients between the big wars by Canadian nurse Rene Caisse, following a native Indian herbal formula she was handed by a cured cancer patient she treated. The specific blend of burdock root, sheep sorrel (whole herb), slippery elm (bark) and turkey rhubarb root was popularised by this kind lady as Essiac tea and used to cure thousands of cancer patients. She was hounded mercilessly by Canadian authorities and had her clinic closed by the state, for harming or misleading people? Nah. The people were queuing up to get in! You can see this story told at iamkeithmann.com

Scenes in this film of cancer patients once sent home to die by a fraudulent medical system show them knocking hopelessly on the padlocked doors of the herbal clinic that offered their only hope. Few realising they had been condemned by the mafia for the second time or that they represent the next one hundred years of medical fascism. There was not a doctor among them who stood up and said 'No, these patients must be allowed to drink herbs!' Death by omission, this too is common among quacks. When Hippocrates entrusted the doctor must first do no harm he was not referring to ones' career.

---

[283] http://www.curenaturalicancro.com/en/simoncini-therapy/

[284] https://www.cerbe.com/714X

Royal Raymond Rife was an American scientist and much more. Born in 1888 he was an inventor of the Universal Microscope, the world's most powerful optical device which outstripped standard research microscopes by light years - and to this day - and meant Rife was able to magnify live specimens 60,000x in colour and became the first person in modern human history to see a living virus and the first to identify the cancer virus which he named *Cryptocides primordiales.* And then because he could see them he figured out how to kill them. **By the end of 1932, Rife could destroy the typhus bacteria, the polio virus, herpes and cancer viruses.**

For perspective, he achieved this nearly 100 years ago yet today's standard Mickey mouse medical microscopes can still only manage around 2000x clear magnification, with exceptions but of dead material only. Rife was a genius and an inventor, engineer, biologist and microscopist, who understood pleomorphism. Crucially he had the expert ability to weave all these skills into fantastic inventions. Rife was humble and unassuming and has left a legacy that will one day be properly recognised.

The Rife Universal Microscope

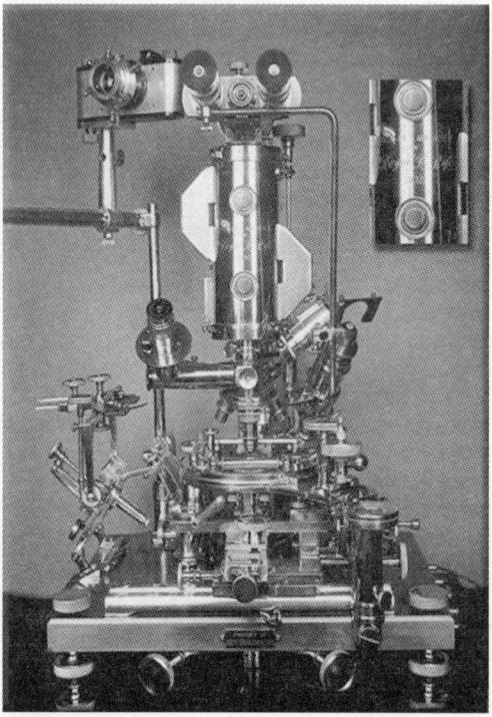

In time Rife won more than a dozen government awards for scientific discoveries, he was granted an honorary medical degree from the University of Heidelberg for his work in bacteriology and crucially, we might think, Rife discovered that those microbes at the centre of his optics and of our discussion would die when exposed to specific ultrasound frequencies, for which he invented a method of delivery. Rife's super multi-task microscope invention was elaborate, made of 5,682 parts and cost $¼ million. The invention was based on a novel method of illumination using a very long optical path with specially ground counter rotating quartz prisms enabling him to bend light and tune his light frequency into the electromagnetic frequency of the target organism thus creating a feedback loop and as a reward the target was brought into view.

Alive!

The principle sounds logical to me but the medical experts of the 1930's were dumfounded, blinded by science we might say. This we might be able to excuse with the benefit of 100 years of human advancement especially in the realm of medicine, right? Except that the medical experts of today are no closer to tuning into the genius of Rife. Perversely the standard electron microscopes still in use today not only fail to achieve anything like the magnification Rife achieved, but in order to pinpoint their specimen the researchers kill everything with electrons leaving only dead stuff to study! Living organisms at the microscopic level are as alien to the experts who have painted themselves into a corner with theoretical limitations on another settled science as cures are. What can we expect from experts who haven't yet progressed beyond merely performing autopsies on once complex life forces?

> ***As far back as 1920 I conceived the idea and the possibility of when the causative agent of malignancy, so called cancer, would be discovered and found and proven that it would be caused by a microorganism. Of course, reception that I received that far back from the medical profession and scientists was nil but I kept at the work and I succeeded in eventually isolating a virus.*** [285]

Rife discovered our target microbes were smaller than the dye particles traditionally used to stain life to death for orthodox research purposes. Once a virus was identified Rife experimented for years in his own laboratory until he found the exact resonance needed to destabilise them. In early experiments Rife was able to isolate fungus from the blood of a cancer patient and from that he grew a virus. By simply adjusting the medium in which he fermented these various forms he was then able to revert the cancer virus back to a cancer fungus.

Each entity also has its own colour code making sense of using light to heal as some do. Rife was able to tune his microscope to reflect back their colour signal. The carcinoma virus he first identified as 'BX' was purple-red in colour, the typhoid bacillus turquoise-blue. Then he worked tirelessly to build a device to deliver the exact resonance or vibration for each organism, which he called the Mortal Oscillatory Rate, causing the microbes to tear apart due to structural failure within his directed energy field. We saw this principle magnified greatly on 9/11. Rife's personal dream was realised thanks to the belief and benevolence of a wealthy benefactor who sponsored his independent research meaning he was eventually able to see live for the first time ever a cancer microbe and watch it die.

> *These results are observed under the high power of the universal microscope and when the mortal oscillatory rate is reached, the BX forms appear to "blow up" or disintegrate in the field.* [286]

This is amazing. In humans it took no more than **one half hour of treatment**, in three minute sessions for Rife to achieve N.E.D - no evidence of disease. Remember this when someone says they have a Rife machine, which is not to say they don't. In

---

[285] http://www.rifevideos.com/dr_rife_talks_about_his_work_on_the_cancer_viruses_of_bx_and_by.html

[286] http://users.navi.net/~rsc/cancer/rifebook.txt

1953 Rife documented in his findings, that by staggering the microbe killing treatment this gave the lymphatic system "an opportunity to absorb and cast off the toxic conditions which is produced by the devitalized dead particles of the 'BX' virus". This achieved better results than daily treatment. I agree detox takes time and requires management.

> *No special diets were used in this clinical work but we sincerely believe a proper diet compiled for the individual would be of benefit.*

I'm getting good at this. I agree again! As incredible as all this is, long-term follow up of Rife's 'cured' is poorly documented and of course cancer will return if no consideration is given to leaving behind the cancer lifestyle, a concept Rife understood.

During research Rife would adapt the environment of the microbes under his microscope and observe them evolve or devolve accordingly. Pig meat and mushrooms were found to be mediums on which the cancer virus liked to grow and with the use of radiation he was able speed up their growth and therefore his work. He described tissue killed by X-ray as a "natural parasitic feast".

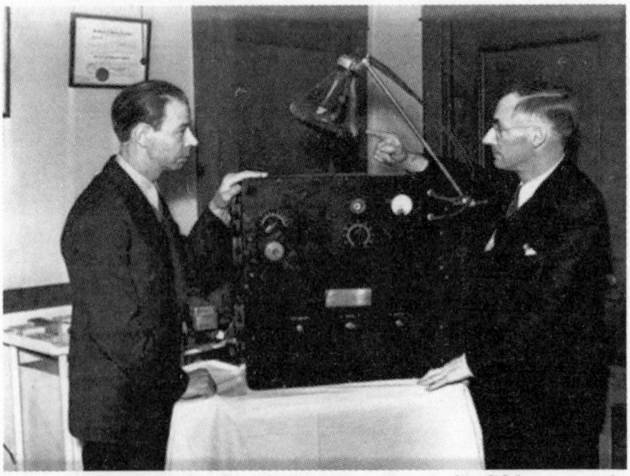

Rife and Phillip Hoyland with the Beam Ray 5 the fifth generation of his microbe killing technology.
Photo: http://www.royal-rife-machine.com/

The media of the day warmed to Rife and he was headline news, for a while. He told the San Diego Evening Tribune in 1938:

> *We do not wish at this time to claim that we have 'cured' cancer or any other disease, for that matter. But we can say that these waves, or this ray, as the frequencies might be called, have been shown to possess the power of devitalising disease organisms, of 'killing' them, when tuned to an exact wave length, or frequency, for each different organism.*

He may well have sold himself short here since 4 years earlier in the first clinical trial of Rife's device a 100% 'cure' rate was achieved when treating 16 terminal cancer and TB patients using the device on them for just 3 minutes every third day over 70 days (for two of the patients it took a few weeks longer to show no disease). Later trials would achieve around 90% cure rates of multiple diseases.

Rife was born in 1888 the same year as Gerson. Rife died in 1971 the year US President Richard Nixon announced the launch of their ongoing war on cancer. Dr Livingston-Wheeler summarises the early days of the long war in 'Cancer: A New Breakthrough':

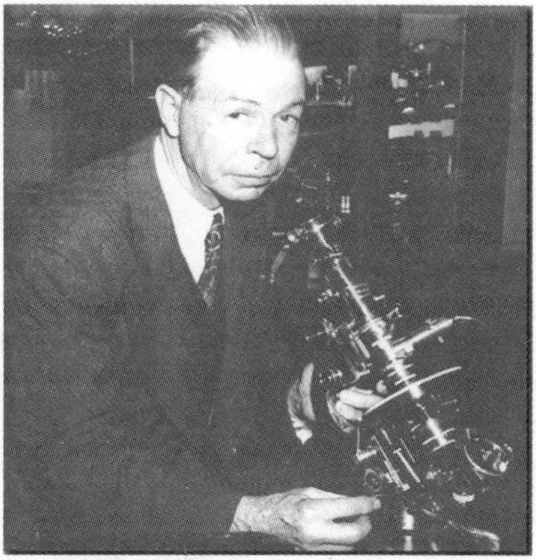

> *In thirteen years the NCI has spent five hundred million dollars and has tested 170,000 poisonous drugs for possible use in the fight against cancer. The results have been zero except for a few rare types of cancer. Over 100,000 cancer patients have been used as guinea pigs without their full knowledge and informed consent.*

The numbers got bigger and the stench of death permeates.

At the peak of his invention and with due admiration Rife's genius shone from the front pages, seen here in the San Diego Evening Tribune in 1938. But by the end of the 1930's Rife's threat to production line consumables was causing concern and he was being edged out of the limelight. He'd only saved lives and threatened to revolutionise healthcare, so the funding was stopped and the sabotage started. Over the coming years as the war against fascism raged in Europe fascism was on the rise in the US. Photographs, film and mountains of other data were stolen from offices linked to Rife as the mafia sought to crush all opposition to Big Pharma's plans for humanity.

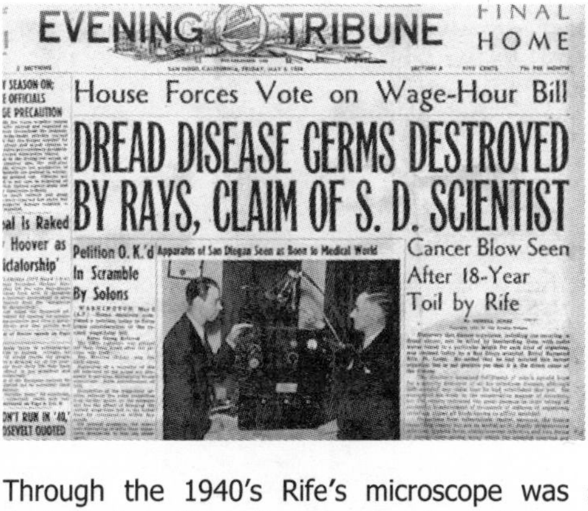
EVENING TRIBUNE FINAL HOME

House Forces Vote on Wage-Hour Bill

DREAD DISEASE GERMS DESTROYED BY RAYS, CLAIM OF S. D. SCIENTIST

Petition O. K.'d In Scramble By Solons

Apparatus of San Diegan Seen as Boon to Medical World

Cancer Blow Seen After 18-Year Toil by Rife

Through the 1940's Rife's microscope was sabotaged, parts stolen and arson destroyed a New Jersey laboratory just as scientists were set to announce confirmation of his achievements. The police later took much of Rife's research in an illegal raid. By the end of the 1950's with a story being told of fascism crushed by the 'free world', any doctor in the free world model of the USA who crossed into Pharma territory was being reined in, harassed or eliminated. Dr Royal Raymond Rife aged 72 was a gentle man who only achieved great things, but with raids on doctors, confiscations of equipment and criminal prosecutions, the good ole USofA was no place for crazy talk about healing. Rife had gone to ground and was keeping his head down in Mexico.

Milbank Johnson, MD., a multi millionaire medical politician & Medical Director of the Pacific Mutual Life Insurance Co. hosted a dinner to honour the accomplishments of Royal R. Rife. The dinner party to celebrate the 'end to all disease' was attended by America's medical elite. November 20 1931.

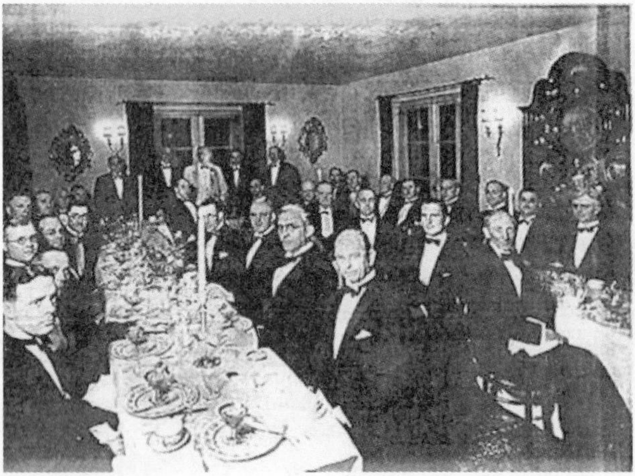

In time, as was the game plan, Rife and his inventions had drifted into obscurity. The truth buried! Rife's dead now too, like the countless millions treated to an early grave by the chemo quacks.

But you can't kill an idea. Rife's genius is reincarnating in the Bob Beck/Sota devices and Rife's vision of a brave new world is re-emerging.

Another tool for which the evidence is clear is that the simple herb made into cannabis oil. That has an incredible role in healing and not just for cancer. CBD oil is not the same, and while that product is becoming less restricted by authorities and it is being manufactured by pharmaceutical interests it has less medical value. The effect of cannabis oil, with THC & CBD elements intact, and its immediate control of Parkinson's disease is really neat to watch. I'll post all this video material on the website so you can see for yourself. It's beyond sick that this plant food is criminalised as a dangerous gateway to harder drugs, and denied to desperate people, in some parts of the world at least, where the really hard chemical drugs flooding society are a gateway to the mortuary. Canadian Rick Simpson has given legs to this amazingly simple albeit generally illegal nutritional solution to some serious health issues, through his film Run from the Cure.

When one claims a necessary evil but cannot sustain necessity all one is left with is evil.
Keith Mann

A Glimpse at the other (them)

They don't really care about us.
Michael Jackson

It's perhaps fitting in our confused human state that while none of these natural cancer treatments are toxic or do harm they are wreaking havoc on those practicing them! None of the practitioners in the next story were promising a cancer cure, because that's illegal in modern medicine and will guarantee a practitioner be harassed, raided and shut down, yet actually delivering a cure may constitute a capital offence. We have seen how the clinical trials are loaded with drugs, the placebo killed off, how the drugs are as deadly as the disease and how the vaccines cause disease, yet there are more layers to this archaeological dig through the dirt. This here shows how desperate they are to keep us from seeing the truth in their long lost battle for hearts and minds and our physical self.

In the US in 2017 a 56 year old Amish farmer who made and sold herbal skin salves successfully for 20 years and harmed no one, was sent to prison for 6 years. Herbs. No dead, only healed.

Oh no sorry there have been deaths. Loads of them! And I am sorry. In the US in the space of just 14 months between June 2015 and August 2016 over 60 well known doctors and researchers in the natural health field were murdered, disappeared or suicided. Some were high profile figures in the natural health community who we had been following during our journey. As of June 2018 the number has risen beyond 90. Being suspicious makes me suspect this is no coincidence. According to the investigation timeline recorded by Erin Elizabeth of healthnutnews.com, on three separate occasions two doctors died on the same day. That's six doctors dying in pairs on three different days. The renowned Dr Nicholas Gonzales died on the same day as a holistic dentist, both of "natural causes". Others have been gunned down at home, stabbed, driven off cliffs, into rivers, jumped from high-rise buildings, and a few had fatal heart attacks.

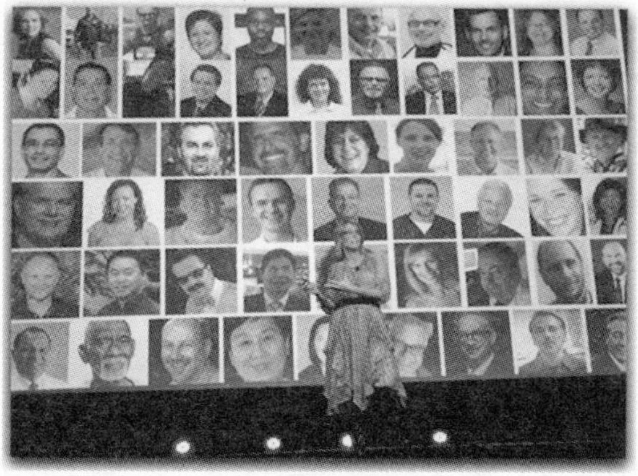

Just a coincidence [287]

[287] https://www.healthnutnews.com/recap-on-my-unintended-series-the-holistic-doctor-deaths/

It's seldom mentioned and he doesn't appear in this catalogue of suspicious deaths but for the record I think they killed Max Gerson too. I also think it's clear we're onto something with this natural leaning toward healing, but other than attacking free thinkers what else are they up to in their war on cancer?

As I finished my first draft I saw Cancer Research UK loading the TV with adverts, as they do every year, showing happy patients fresh out of treatment and as cancer free as they will likely ever be. The deception they deliver is 'living happily ever after', in this moment in time on the word of an oncologist. At the same time CRUK is promoting toxic sun cream with cancer causing ingredients! This liquid chemical concoction is to be spread over that large, porous organ protecting our innards and its purpose is to block out the sun. The life-giving sun is a greater threat to our health than this?

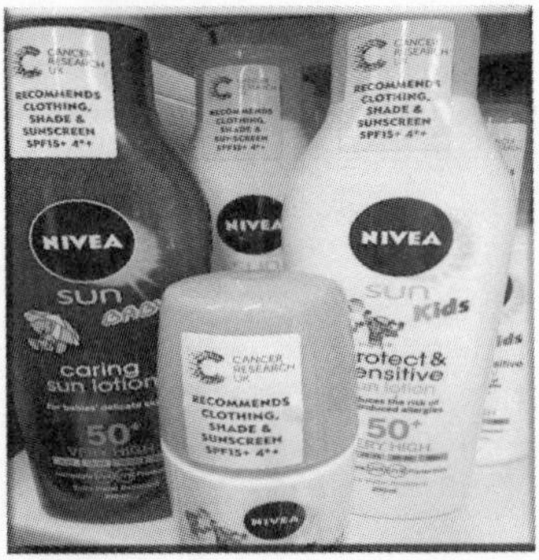

Aqua, Homosalate, Octocrylene, Glycerin, C12-15 Alkyl Benzoate, Ethylhexyl Salicylate, Alcohol Denat., Butyl Methoxydibenzoylmethane, Glyceryl Stearate Citrate, Panthenol, Hydrogenated Coco-Glycerides, Myristyl Myristate, Tocopheryl Acetate, VP/Hexadecene Copolymer, Xanthan Gum, Sodium Acrylates/ C10-30 Alkyl Acrylate Crosspolymer, Cetyl Alcohol, Stearyl Alcohol, Sodium Citrate, Silica Dimethyl Silylate, Citric Acid, Trisodium EDTA, Ethylhexylglycerin, Phenoxyethanol, Methylparaben, Ethylparaben, Linalool, Limonene, Butylphenyl Methylpropional, Benzyl Alcohol, Alpha-Isomethyl Ionone, Citronellol, Eugenol, Coumarin, Parfum.

Are we insane? This is a charity supposedly seeking a cure for cancer. These compounds block the production of vitamin D, which we need for survival and cancer prevention; they are heated by the sun, pass through the skin and circulate through the blood and the organs. Are we experiencing a 1-in-2 cancer incidence because of this kind of stupidity? We could compare this to the introduction of chemotheraputic toxins into the body instantly killing cells, and causing cancer. We tend to drip feed the death of our cells through our mouths and our skin taking longer to reveal the damage but the outcome is similar.

The main ingredient after water is Homosalate. Described on pesticideinfo.org as an insecticide, fungicide, microbiocide. This UV-absorbing ingredient helps the other sunscreen ingredients to penetrate the skin. Once absorbed, Homosalate's toxicity accumulates and generates free radicals, which lead to cell damage. Which is what leads to cancer, right? And it's an antiandrogen, a sex hormone antagonists. Homosalate disrupts hormones. Remember that. Disruption is not something we are looking for in health restoration, but if we can stay in the sun for longer and not have the worry about skin cancer then maybe that's a good thing? We are invited to another trade off. We are invited by these morons to buy a perceived protection from one disease while risking others.

I looked for the safety data on Homosalate (salicylic acid). The safety data is slim for Homosalate used on its own, and in combination with the other dodgy ingredients forget it. This is common where toxic chemicals and toxic drugs are concerned and the less said the better, but what is for sure is that we are guinea pigs too, if we want. There is minimal data but there are big clues to the damage this stuff can do. On the European Chemical Agency website I asked about Homosalate and carcinogenicity. This is what they rely on, from 1963:

> *Webb and Hansen (1963) administered* ***methyl salicylate*** *in the diet to groups of 24-25 male and 25-26 female Osborne-Mendel rats at dietary concentrations of 0, 0.1%, 0.5%, 1.0% or 2.0%, providing doses of approximately 0, 50, 250, 500, and 1000 mg/kg body weight/day for two years. All rats in the 1000 mg/kg group died by the 49th week. Body weight of both sexes were significantly decreased in both the 500 and 1000 mg/kg group body weight/day groups.*
>
> *Gross pituitary gland lesions were found in* ***10 rats at 250 mg/kg bw/day compared to 4 rats in the control groups****. Incidence in the 500 mg/kg/day group was similar to controls, while all animals of the 1000 mg/kg/day group died before the usual age at which many spontaneous lesions develop.*
>
> *Similar kinds and numbers of tumors occurred in rats of all diets except the 1000 mg/kg/day group (premature decedents), with mammary tumors of the females being the most common. Benign pituitary tumors occurred in similar numbers of surviving rats on all diets, with occurrence predominantly in females. Malignant pituitary tumors occurred in one male and two females receiving 250 mg/kg/day. Since no such tumors were reported in either the lower or higher dose groups (50 and 500 mg/kg/day), this low incidence does not clearly indicate any relation with methyl salicylate treatment.* [288]

That's it! From this oral poisoning of rats, from which large numbers developed tumours or died, our safety experts conclude that Homosalate into the bloodstream is good to go. Is that what we learnt? It's hard to see what's being learnt.

All safety tested on animals, they say. But further experiments show:

> *... developmental toxicity in offspring with high fetal mortality high frequency of complex anomalies and dose-related foetal growth retardation. At the dose of 0.2%, the body weight and length and the tail length were statistically significantly decreased. At the dose of 0.4% litter size and body weight and length as well as tail length were statistically significantly decreased. The general conclusion of the authors was: "It is clear from the results obtained in the present and previous experiments that salicylic acid through oral route has a teratogenic effect on rat". The teratogenic effects of salicylic acid may be attributable to a direct action of the compound on fetal tissues.* [288]

---

[288] https://echa.europa.eu/registration-dossier/-/registered-dossier/13246/7/8 s

Teratogenic means it makes a mess of an embryo or foetus, causing deformities.

Best not absorb too much then, eh? Ask the National Center for Biotechnology Information about Homosalate and they flash up these warnings:

> *Warning: Skin corrosion/irritation - Category 2*
> *Warning: Serious eye damage/eye irritation - Category 2A*
> *Warning: Specific target organ toxicity, single exposure;*
> *Respiratory tract irritation - Category 3*
> *May cause long lasting harmful effects to aquatic life. Hazardous to the aquatic environment, long-term hazard - Category 4* [289]

No matter where you look, it doesn't sound like something you would want to absorb into the skin, but don't worry it might not be so bad after all because scientists have found a way around this problem of animal toxicity. They ignore it. We can find their loophole or get-out clause within the very same horrific experimental reports here with the observation that **"the rat is not a relevant species to extrapolate developmental effects to humans".** It's also reported that "bone effects" were seen in rats exposed to salicylic acid. That doesn't sound good either! In the world of the crazy this actually means it's doubly safe because they claim it's actually rabbits that are "more like humans with high protein binding capacity" and when pregnant rabbits were poisoned with "high maternally toxic doses", their babies came out unscathed. Safety tested on animals! Gobble it up peeps! [290]

Octocrylene is the second most prolific chemical in this product that CRUK invite us to rub into our skin to protect us from cancer. This one is described by the European Chemicals Agency as a substance: "of very high concern" due to its endocrine disrupting properties, and we should be concerned because it's lethal!

> *UV filters act as endocrine disruptors and exert developmental and genotoxic effects, thus posing a potential risk to ecosystem and human health... several reports have focused on the impact of these compounds on human or mouse cancer cells, germ cells, or embryonic stem cells.* [291]

Off to a shaky start with more disrupting and not a single long-term study has been carried out on the accumulative effect in humans. But we do know what endocrine disruption does to animals. In the short-term human testing that has been done we find

> *In a monitoring study on human breast milk we found 6 out of 8 analyzed UV filters in mother/child cohorts from 3 different years. Use of sunscreens or*

---

289 https://pubchem.ncbi.nlm.nih.gov/compound/8362#section=GHS-Classification

290 https://echa.europa.eu/documents/10162/13626/clh_additional_report_salicylic_acid_en.pdf/a87638d8-c478-470e-8bc6-b877a7899964

291 dpi-proceedings.com/index.php/dteees/article/download/15561/15072

other cosmetic products containing these UV filters was significantly correlated with their presence in human milk. [292]

So the babies get it through our skin, of course!

The risks are clear so what do we have to prove the benefit of these sunscreens?

The only randomized trial examining the risk of M[alignant] M[elanoma] after regular sunscreen use, found borderline statistical significance for a reduced incidence of new primary melanoma. [293]

What? What did we learn from this trial about the safety or risk of chemical sunscreen? Same old nothing! Whatever it means it is not much of a trade off.

In 'Cancer - The Wayward Cell - It's Origins, Nature & Treatment', Victor Richards M.D explains Experimental Endocrine Carcinogenesis:

Direct Action of Hormones. Some pituitary tumours can be induced in mice by obliteration of the thyroid after irradiation, thyroidectomy, or prolonged administration of a drug stopping the production of thyroxine hormone. Pituitary tumours in mice can appear following gonadectomy at an early age. ***A whole host of experiments involving endocrine manipulation indicate that the reduced function of a target organ alerts its reciprocal relationship to the pituitary causing ultimately neoplasia, or cancer, of the target organ.*** *The sequence of events seems to be as follows:* ***the endocrine imbalance produces hypersection of the pituitary, which in turn provokes overstimulation of the target organ, and ultimately neoplasia. Cancer of the breast is not purely an autonomous growth but depends on the hormonal environment of the body.***

Thinking like we do Richards concludes:

Hopefully the neoplastic transformation could be prevented if a normally functioning hormonal state were to be restored.

See how we started with a Cancer Research UK sponsored chemical sun block and ended up with cancer?

I am not going through the entire list of ingredients you'll be pleased to hear but I must mention perfum, the last but not the least significant by any stretch of the imagination. And it takes some imagination to bring to mind the bewildering swamp of poison they fit into that small word. Literally thousands of undisclosed scent chemicals and other ingredients are concealed under a few simple words such as

---

[292] https://www.ncbi.nlm.nih.gov/pmc/articles/PMC3084961/

[293] https://www.researchgate.net/publication/225051747_Sunscreens_Are_they_beneficial_for_health_An_overview_of_endocrine_disrupting_properties_of_UV-filters

fragrances, parfums, perfumes, polycyclic musks, many of which are carcinogenic. Most have not been tested for safety, neither in isolation nor in combination. What we do know from the human experience/experiments is that they trigger asthmatic reactions, migraines, skin irritation, respiratory distress, central nervous system disruption and other life changing events. We also know that diethyl phthalates (DEP) are hormone-disrupting and potential carcinogens and are widely used in these concoctions to leave that thick lingering stench of artificial chemicals in the air long after the wearer has wandered by.

And they do make money for CRUK to search for that ever elusive cancer cure. The European Commission on Endocrine Disruption has listed DEP as a Category 1 priority substance, based on the fact that it interferes with hormone function.

The irony is of course that while we risk hormone disruption and cancer, and who knows what else, there is no good evidence that the sun causes cancer when enjoyed in moderation and if we keep our defences in optimum function cancer will struggle to establish a home. We need the sun for life. Tanned skin, if you are lucky enough to have a choice, serves as a protection against sunburn, if used sensibly.

And of course it doesn't have to be chemical, brown or burn, there are always other options. For CRUK maybe a commercial product of dubious necessity that causes developmental malformations when tested on traumatised animals is a good choice, but they also choose to ignore the other cancer treatment options that are healing people and that might suggest they got this wrong too.

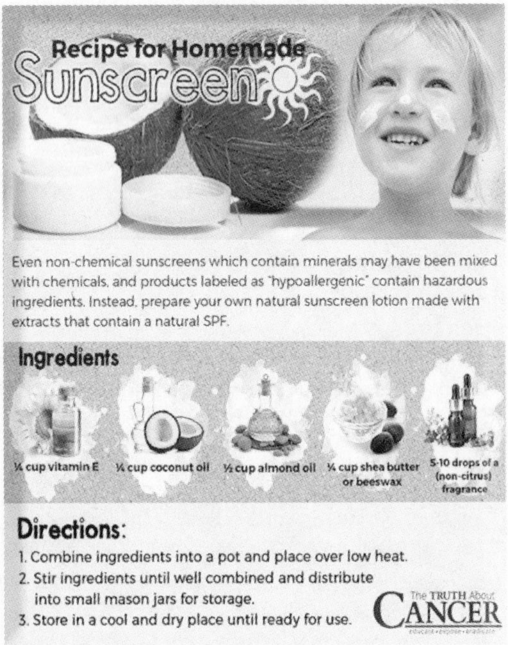
Recipe for Homemade
Sunscreen
Even non-chemical sunscreens which contain minerals may have been mixed with chemicals, and products labeled as "hypoallergenic" contain hazardous ingredients. Instead, prepare your own natural sunscreen lotion made with extracts that contain a natural SPF.
Ingredients
¼ cup vitamin E
¼ cup coconut oil
½ cup almond oil
¼ cup shea butter or beeswax
5-10 drops of a (non-citrus) fragrance
Directions:
1. Combine ingredients into a pot and place over low heat.
2. Stir ingredients until well combined and distribute into small mason jars for storage.
3. Store in a cool and dry place until ready for use.
The TRUTH About CANCER

So what did these high profile high income charities do with all the money they already collected over decades from their products and projects? We know about all the clinical trials comparing junk drugs, and all the very expensive junk drugs and the gimmicks, the diagnostic testing machinery and advertising and shop rent and staff salaries and bonuses. In the many varied cancer TV adverts we see patients and actors begging for more, with no mention of a cure. More like: 'here are some people we just treated but can't cure, gives us more money'. CRUK have recently handed comrades on the cancer gravy train £100 million to spend looking at "seven unresolved challenges in cancer research". At Cambridge University £20 million of this bumper harvest of public contributions is being gobbled up to play with 3D models of breast tumours.

> ***This new way of studying breast cancer could change how the disease is diagnosed, treated and managed. We want to create an interactive, faithful, 3D map of tumours that can be studied in virtual reality that scientists can 'walk into' and look at it in great detail. By doing this, we could learn more about tumours and begin to answer questions that have eluded cancer scientists for many years.*** [294]

Seriously!

These vast resources are being spent to look at a 3D model of one symptom of one branch of one disease with a view to treating or managing that one symptom! Maybe!

I say keep an eye on this going nowhere slowly and then leading to the need for further public money for more research grants (salaries) to study 'artificial intelligent micro-scientist delivery systems' for the next generation of wonder drugs. I made that up but that's all they're doing.

CRUK responded briefly to me, when I begun pestering them, with the party line and then, clearly irritated, directed me to the website of the National Cancer Institute, which sounds professional and impressive and this was a useful lead in my investigation but not so helpful for CRUK. Debunking is an ugly word and those who engage such as the NCI don't inspire confidence in their ability to provide solutions. We hear it said that the best form of defence is attack, but then we do say some stupid things. That's that macho thing going on again. The best form of defence is defence. They've been attacking us for years with chemo and radiation and all kinds of shit, they attack anyone using safe and effective methods to treat disease, anyone who protests or who comes up with a new idea or an old idea and to what end? Attack-attack-attack! Chill out! Is it really about science or is it about ego, status and status quo?

I know, I know, but I have to ask.

---

[294] https://www.cam.ac.uk/research/news/virtual-reality-journey-through-a-tumour-cambridge-scientists-receive-ps40-million-funding-boost

The NCI have an extensive list of natural therapies and products they try to rubbish. On the NCI's Gerson Therapy exposé page that I was invited to browse they helpfully inform inquiring cancer patients, such as I, that of this the oldest and best recorded human cancer cure:

No results of laboratory or animal studies have been published in scientific journals.

That's it! Blame everyone else for something that cannot be done in order to prevent you from having to move forward. A hat-trick of negatives! From that self-confessed lack of intellectual scrutiny, what Gerson actually is capable of gets dismissed by generations of ignorant medical experts as quackery. Go scientists!

Regarding coffee enemas, they warn:

> ***Reports of three deaths that may be related to coffee enemas have been published****. Taking too many enemas of any kind can cause changes in normal blood chemistry, chemicals that occur naturally in the body and keep the muscles, heart, and other organs working properly.*

Or the opposite might happen. See how published becomes proof! How silly. Let's face it too much of anything is usually harmful, such as chemo, on which bucket loads have been published and which they also fail to mention **is directly related** to millions of deaths. And there **may be** something to the Gerson Therapy but they keep that quiet, until it's time for debunking.

Here they refer to four studies, of sorts, which are all they can find and are meant, I think, to convince us the science is settled on the Gerson Therapy. The first study they tell us was regarding 38 patients in some retrospective interviews but since the interviews contained no accompanying medical records there was no value in this information, so we don't get to see it. No idea who did or didn't do it or what it found. This leaves 3 studies left to rattle the foundations of the Gerson Therapy.

Number 3:

A study of a ***diet*** *regimen* ***similar*** *to the Gerson therapy was done in Austria.* That's it. A diet? Similar? Is that a bit like science? This isn't a joke, this is as serious as cancer and people are dying. The Gerson Therapy is not a diet, it's a way of living and much like that airplane engine parts, you don't use similar lifestyle choices because you can't be bothered or you think you know better. Funniest bit of all, the patients on this Gerson-like 'diet' also received the orthodox treatment and yet still the authors of the study reported that "the diet appeared to help patients live longer than usual and have fewer side effects" and concluded it needed further study. Screaming out for it if you ask me!

Number 2:

In keeping with the trail of tragic comedy, this one laughingly refers to the rather impressive retrospective Gerson melanoma study I covered earlier of Gerson patients who at all stages of disease lived much longer than patients treated to orthodox protocols. See the pattern they insist on ignoring? That isn't science, science is about pattern recognition.

Unashamed in their disinterest, they brush past this clue to the cause and cure of cancer with another one of their negatives

> *There have been no clinical trials that support the findings of this retrospective study.*

Happy to leave scientific inquiry and any hint of a cure for another time, we move on to what must be something really special.

Number 1:

> *Case review of* ***6 patients with metastatic cancer who used the Gerson therapy reported that the regimen helped patients in some ways, both physically and psychologically. Based on these results, the reviewers recommended that clinical trials of the Gerson therapy be conducted.*** [295]

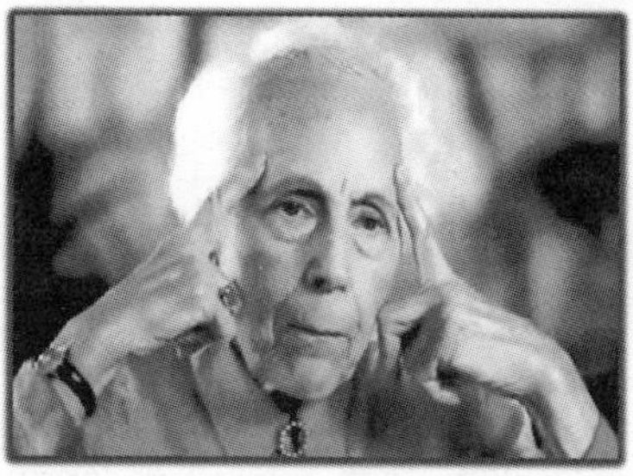

I recognise a pattern when I see one! And again in trying their hardest with all the science written in their books, all they can come up with in debunking Gerson is confirmation it works.

My browsing of this orthodox cure-debunking website taught me more about the potential in healthy eating than it provided proof our way doesn't work, yet they have all been telling me something different! There will of course be no clinical trials anytime soon, but who do I ask in the meantime if I want to try living longer like all the Gerson-like people do? Unpersuaded I was eventually redirected by the NCI people to their CRUK and Macmillan comrades-in-arms in the UK! Call me incredulous - I was back on the bullshit roundabout!

And then to my exaggerated incredulity, I get an envelope through the door from Macmillan with a crappy flat plastic pen and a begging letter. Having dodged their trap door they were now after my money!

I'm not criticising the foot soldiers, the volunteers and fundraisers by the way, but the organisation at the heart of the machinery is as much a part of the obstacle to change as the likes of CRUK and the controlled opposition and the Pharma. I find their gentle guidance into the bowels of this monster quite nauseating. This process brings to my mind those inmates we hear of, repeated throughout history, who work

---

[295] https://www.cancer.gov/about-cancer/treatment/cam/patient/gerson-pdq

for their captors for privilege and help enslave their fellow prisoners. I met some of them.

Macmillan are on the TV a lot too. I crept up on them using a pseudonym having failed to get answers to my earlier queries as me. I talked about donating and asked of the discrepancy in time spent promoting the failed orthodoxy compared to that expended on natural protocols that work. In my pestering of the 'all knowing' I recognise a pattern in me: I get to the point, say what I see. I got their pattern response: the party line fob off.

> *Macmillan cannot highlight or advocate alternative treatments or diets that have not yet been proven to have any benefits. Alternative therapies can be very expensive and unscrupulous people do make a profit from vulnerable people wanting to believe they can cure them of diseases like cancer.*

Unscrupulous people! The nerve of it! They can't highlight but they can undermine? But that shows a bias. A lethal bias.

> *There are those who tell us that Macmillan does too much on Complementary therapies. Finding the balance in the context of supporting people affected by cancer is an ongoing challenge for the charity. We aim to do the best we can for as many people as we can.*

Really? The best? I'm irritatingly interested in complementary and alternative therapies but I'm still struggling to find much getting in the way of the regular must-do cancer treatments Macmillan invest heavily in. I was handed a 108 page booklet by my Macmillan nurse at diagnosis in which what they describe as "complementary therapies" are referred to just once near the end. They do encourage that hypnotherapy, massage, visualisation, reflexology, aromatherapy and relaxation classes "may help you feel better, reduce stress and anxiety, and improve some treatment side effects", but that is all the guidance on healing we are getting from the popular cancer charity shoved in our faces from the moment of diagnosis. They don't so much push the boundaries of cancer survival as erect a bigger fence. The rest of this document may as well be a sales brochure for chemotherapy.

I compared with my Macmillan contact the $billions in fines imposed on drug companies for their life destroying serial crimes including experimenting on humans, and asked how it is the unscrupulous healers they allude to actually benefit from encouraging cancer patients to do their own research and to go home and heal themselves. With the internet we can easily discover what treatments heal and what treatments don't. The reason authorities want to control the internet is because it allows us to see through the smog.

No one they bounced me around to at Macmillan could address my concerns and because I was being irritating they sent me away to Macmillan's website to see about all this money they want. And money is flowing. As a cancer patient I got a few hours free parking from Macmillan and was thoroughly misinformed about some very important things. So what are they spending all this generosity on? Not much on alternatives.

> *Alternative treatments*
> *... are unconventional and unproven therapies that aim to treat cancer. There is often no scientific evidence for their use and some alternative medicines can interact and interfere with conventional treatment. It is important that you speak to your doctor if you want to explore alternative therapies.*

You may as well speak to your plumber as your doctor. What's the doctor likely to say? He is in the same mind prison as Macmillan and CRUK and is not permitted to promote anything not on the list of patented products and everyone knows it. This is a despicable thing to advise a desperate cancer patient to do, knowing they will be turned away from any hope of a cure. Instead...

> *The University College Hospital Macmillan Cancer Centre is a* ***£100million*** *state-of-the-art facility equipped with the latest technology to diagnose and treat cancer. If cancer is diagnosed, a named key worker will be allocated to the patient to support them through their treatment and follow-up care.*

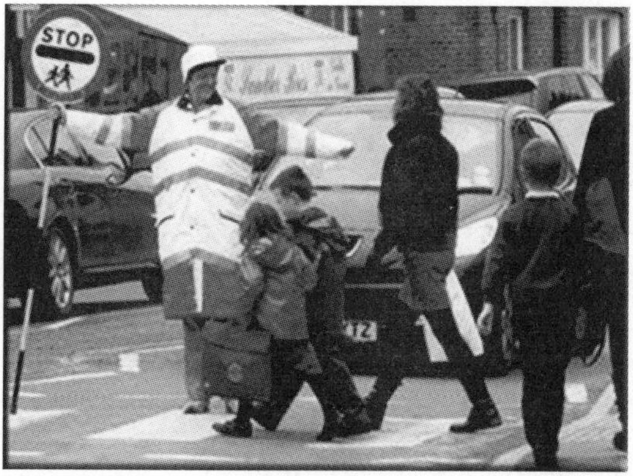

Not short of a little spare cash to invest then! Consistency of care is an important factor, but what this 'key worker' will do is guide you in the right direction and ensure you remain a loyal customer for as long as your body can handle it.

University College (UCLH) boast they were "the first hospital in the UK to develop a teenage cancer unit in 1990". Good to be ahead of the game I guess, but I don't think this is anything to be especially proud of. Teenagers with cancer? Why is that? Maybe we need a vaccine? Or greater emphasis on cancer prevention? There's a thought. No mention of that here though but there's an awful lot of that toxic treatment being churned out undercover of waffle:

> *The future of treatment for patients is* ***precision cancer medicine*** *– a* ***treatment package*** *that is specific to the individual and which applies our* ***whole suite of tools to the understanding*** *and treatment of a patient's* ***own unique cancer****. It is our vision that,* ***within five years****, every patient will have their own* ***personalised cancer pathway, from early diagnosis and screening, to imaging or biopsy, to genomic analysis of their cancer, through to state-of-the-art clinical trials.***

> *This second Institute will build on the* ***underlying cancer science*** *at UCL, and* ***will provide a physical focal point for cancer-relevant expertise across the medical, life and engineering sciences****. Patients will be* ***brought alongside the research process and real-time analysis*** *of patients will help* ***to continually refine and improve emerging treatments****. These plans underline UCLH's commitment to providing the best comprehensive cancer research and treatment in Europe. The aim of the new Institute is to* ***detect cancer earlier and more precisely,*** *to understand* ***the molecular biology of patients' cancers more precisely, and to develop and deliver clinical trials more precisely****. This is the future of cancer care – relevant to the individual.* [296]

Actions speak louder than words.

Drifting seamlessly away from and back round to that long lost pledge of a cure in 5 years time, these world leaders in the booming cancer sector are offering the same useless treatments they always offered with equal absence of ambition to even look for a cure. Now remarketed as "a whole suite of tools". This sounds enticing but that's chemo, radiation, surgery and those comparable death delivering mAbs. A personalised pathway to the cemetery! Sounds like a breakthrough just around the corner. One that will be targeting those tumours much more precisely than before while researchers investigate ways to "make chemotherapy kinder and radiation less destructive". It has taken 100 years of death delivering cancer treatment and thousands upon thousands of clinical trials to get them to the point of acknowledging they need to change something. And the best they can come up with? Business as usual! Always the outcome.

Personalised treatment protocols are the gold standard in genuine healthcare where the patient is treated according to the needs of the patient, whatever they might be, and not according to the failed orthodox disease-maintenance rules which command the recycling of junk drugs, cancer patients and cancer.

We see reference throughout the newly worded symptom treatment narrative of the need to progress from one size kills all to something more personal, but how? More personalised chemo? To what end? To save lives? They don't mention a cure or healing anywhere! And as has been demonstrated graphically a hundred million times over more chemo means more death. Less chemo, now that's seriously worth looking at, much, much less and never as a stand-alone treatment.

So what we have is business as usual and business is booming.

UCLH et al are currently expanding operations through a merger with the Royal Free haem-oncology unit. This was a "massive undertaking" says Dr Kirsty Thomson, Consultant Haematologist, and the good news is that this now makes them "the largest haemato-oncology unit in Europe and gives **an unrivalled opportunity to create teams of highly sub-specialised clinicians** providing specialist care for

---

296 https://www.uclh.nhs.uk/OurServices/ServiceAZ/Cancer/Documents/UCLH%20Cancer%20Strategy%202015-2020.pdf

their patients 24/7." The devil is in the detail and nowhere do we see kindly volunteer nurses juicing and prepping nutritious food and cleansing enemas, working to correct imbalance and pull people back from the brink of death and restore full health. Not even close. Rather, these cancer people have seen an opportunity.

And of course the breakthrough has hit the news where these baseless claims are repeated ad nausium to keep us dangling along, hoping. From the inappropriately named Independent newspaper in 2017 we find the glimmer of hope has returned (briefly).

> ***An effective cure for all types of cancer could be just five to 10 years away,*** *according to one of the world's leading experts on the disease. Advances in genetics mean doctors will be able to prescribe drugs to treat each individual's unique form of cancer,* ***turning the often deadly disease into a chronic, but treatable condition.*** [297]

Some professor said

> *"Understanding the molecular cogs that make cancer cells different to normal cells and therefore developing drugs personalised to the cancer would allow personalised, precision medicine... it would... suppress the cancer and convert cancer into a long-term chronic disease. Most patients with cancer tend to be in their 50s or 60s. If they live another 20 or 30 years, they would effectively live a normal lifespan".* He suggested this medical revolution would happen *"in the next five to 10 years. There will be, not a cure-all, but a much better predictive way of knowing which drugs to give to which patients".* [297]

There will not be a cure at all!

Dividing up the human being into smaller and smaller sections and creating specialities in each part is not what it means to personalise treatment! We are seeking to perfect protocols designed for the individual to heal, adding in what the individual needs. But as discovers the dealer who cuts his bag of pure cocaine endlessly, each cut further separating it from purity, there are benefits in the short-term in thinking of self. Our cancer treatment guides boast of bagging another £25 million investment in the second Macmillan/NHS/CRUK venture on a valuable piece of central London real estate next door to their existing cancer treatment centre. And:

> *During the last year the* ***CRUK-UCL CTC has generated new grant income of £4.1m, has 25 new trials open or in setup and published 31 papers related to clinical trials.*** [298]

And that's it in a nutshell. Clinical trials, status and cash! In amongst the waffle.

---

[297] https://www.independent.co.uk/life-style/health-and-families/health-news/world-cancer-day-2017-effective-cure-will-happen-five-to-10-years-expert-karol-sikora-a7558846.html

[298] https://www.uclh.nhs.uk/OurServices/ServiceA-Z/Cancer/Documents/UCLH%20Cancer%20Strategy%202015-2020.pdf

To base opposition to vivisection mainly on ethical grounds, as some societies and speakers are accustomed to do, is on the one hand to neglect the strongest and most vital argument at our command – on the other to postpone all prospects of success for at least 500 years to come.

London & Provincial Anti Vivisection Society 1919

The beginning of the story

The coming years will make it more and more imperative that organically grown fruit and vegetables will be, and must be, used for protection against degenerative diseases, the prevenetion of cancer, and more so in the treatment of cancer. According to present government statistics, one out of every six persons in our population will die of cancer. It will not be long before the entire population will have to decide whether we will all die of cancer or whether we will have enough wisdom, courage, and the will power to change fundamentally all our living and nutritional conditions. We will again need... homemakers who will devote their lives to the task of developing and maintaining a healthy family. Babies would no longer be fed by formula but would have the natural mother's milk; they would grow up without being afflicted with a fatal disease such as leukaemia, and without being mentally retarded, both conditions which are increasing rapidly at present.

Dr Max Gerson 1958

So what have we learnt?

- Quacks quack.
- The cancer industry serves self.
- There's nowt funnier than folk.
- Cancer is curable now.
- Is it fungal, is it bacterial or is it viral? It's systemic - focus on the system.
- Magnetic pulsing disrupts cancer tumours.
- Chemo helps around 2% to make 5 years.
- In real-life experience people labelled "conspiracy theorist" have shown a significantly greater chance of curing cancer than any other group, especially the group who use that killer phrase most often.
- Vaccines are dangerous, untested, unproven, pseudoscientific and speculative.
- Vaccines cause cancer and autism.
- Pesticides used in food cause cancer.
- Placebo is so 1980's.
- SV40 is an oncogenic monkey virus unleashed on hundreds of millions of humans by animal researchers from the 1950's to the present.
- Doctors and vets do do harm and don't train in nutrition or healing.
- Actions speak louder than words.
- It is not the patient's fault.
- In the search for a chemical cure left is right, right is left, sooner is later, maybe.
- Cancer is not just a tumour.
- Black salve eats tumours.
- We can't always trust what a scientist says.
- Cancer has always been curable.
- One size does not fit all.
- Other people's opinions are not your rules.

- Animal experiments teach us about how deeply traumatised animals react when traumatised and have led to devastating consequences for humans.
- Experts can be as stupid as the rest of us but they have a greater responsibility to the rest of us.
- The cancer environment is key.
- It's OK to say shapeshifter.

There is a great stigma attached to the concept of a cure and the idea that some uneducated smart arse thinks he can do what the world of medicine has failed to do does raise the hackles. Good. It's a done deal. Get over it. What's more important?

We can see that if we don't think for ourselves then someone else is going to think about themselves on our behalf. The medical profession has already left a trail of carnage bigger than all the dictators and democratically elected crackpots put together. If we are to get self-righteous and aggressive over chemical weapons killing people in far away places we might want to start with the vaccines and drug treatments in our own backyard. Not only does the death toll outstrip any perceived killing in foreign lands using chemical weapons but the toll of the maimed and the suffering is way off the scale.

We are told there's no work and society is broke and obese and 1 in 2 will get cancer. Now we have reminded ourselves how important clean food is, maybe we could think about turning the clock back to a time when poison free plant food didn't have a special name, where working the fields to grow our needs, not animal feeds, made sense. With this hippy ideal we would find work for idle hands, and heal, and protect and diversify our environment. Or we can allow Monsanto, Merck and McDonald's to drive us further into a toxic wasteland.

Have I captured the imagination of the big anti-vivisection, animal rights groups with this project? At the grassroots the backup has been genuine and gratifying, almost embarrassing, but I expected that. Our world is bursting with good people. Let's face it I set out to cure cancer, as a carer, with no income, with what was on the face of it a crazy idea and a heap of unknowns. Yet even when we had to start again with an even more ridiculous idea, we were guided through this experimental journey seamlessly by people motivated by love. Financially it has been a struggle but we have nevertheless achieved something quite remarkable because we had the belief and the desire.

Early on in the journey we contacted the alphabet soup of well-know vegetarian and vegan groups, the anti-vivisection groups, the non-animal medical research groups, even the 'cruelty free' high street firms and AR groups deemed more radical. We invited support, input, anything. You'd think wouldn't you that for a community trying to bring radical change through food and non-animal testing methods that its 'big guns' would be hungry for that something that makes a difference, like a natural cancer cure using organic non-animal nutrition and no vivisection. But it would appear this is not it.

Nearly two dozen of these organisations responded with not so much as a friendly word of support or encouragement. In my hippy ideal I see loving people standing together loud and proud with their innovators, their dreamers and home-made cancer survivors, fingers up to the medical mafia and their vivisectors and those who defend the status quo.

The New Zealand Anti Vivisection Society, the Animal Liberation Front Supporters Group and Animal Aid are the only three animal rights organisations worthy of praise for having the courage to step off the fence. I think that little list says quite a lot.

Together Against Cancer[299], Cancer Crackdown[300], Yes To Life[301], The Carrot Fund [302] and the Gerson Institute[303] and many affiliated supporters have been loyal to our cause from the beginning and our Riverford delivery driver saw what we were trying to achieve and went out of his way to ensure we never ran out of supplies during the Christmas meltdown. These people, curiously, appear to have more to offer the anti-vivisection/human health cause than many of the anti-vivisection/pro animal campaigning organisations and my advice to anyone serious about this cancer issue and the vivisection issue would be to work with these organisations instead of those currently juggling old ideas.

What is it we are warned? That which you fight you become? In the community I represent it's clear that almost all of the more established organisations have themselves become mere business operations using the animals to generate income and maintain status. One feature long looming large among these entities gathers our resources on the pledge of discovering alternative testing methods for the orthodox to integrate into their system to replace the animals in their endless search for answers to the mystery of disease. Key animal friendly organisations have normalised fundraising operations for the sole purpose of making financial awards to scientists to *search* for the alternatives, which can then be used in the never ending *search* for the drug cures, which the animals have failed to deliver. The advertising comes through emotive campaigns exposing more of the ubiquitous laboratory cruelty and disregard, with dogs on hotplates, cats being shot by the military, monkey self-mutilation, narcotic experiments, and the timeless distraction of cosmetic testing. Cosmetic testing is still a marketing tool used by the controlled opposition four decades after such horrors were forged on the public consciousness by the animal liberators covert creativity.

In what couldn't be a better example of this absurd state of affairs, this organisation promoting themselves as a Physicians Committee for Responsible Medicine claim to be:

---

299 https://togetheragainstcancer.org.uk/

300 http://cancercrackdown.org/

301 http://yestolife.org.uk/

302 https://www.facebook.com/carrotfund/

303 https://gerson.org/gerpress/

"leading a revolution in medicine" They advertise how they "promote" preventive medicine, conduct clinical research, and encourage "higher standards for ethics and effectiveness in research and medical training".

With an income of $22 million they boast of combining

> *... the clout and expertise of more than 12,000 physicians with the dedicated actions of more than 175,000 members across the United States and around the world... regularly works with federal agencies and other stakeholders toward the common goal of replacing animal tests.* [304]

Common goal? Working *toward* alternative tests for chemo, vaccines and mAbs, with government? What about the alternatives already in use, most recently by me, but for 100 years and more? Do revolutionaries work side by side with the likes of the Department of Defense: delivering health by stealth bomber; the Department of Health and the FDA: the monkey virus vaccinators crushing natural therapies for decades and the NCI: the debunkers? How do we imagine things are progressing on this particular road to animal liberation and human health? PCRM were one of the groups invited to give my idea of a suitable alternative a go, or to just say hello; help me, help the animals? Not their thing. Of course they know best, they are doctors after all, who only want to heal people and there appear to be a lot of them and they all like animals too. They're the best! And maybe, just maybe there is some hope just around the corner because in 2017 the PCRM announced their scientists had now, 30 years of campaigning later:

> ***Provided input that helped shape NIH's new Roadmap, which recommends*** *replacing animal tests with human-relevant methods to better protect human health.* [305]

I see through that bullshit straight away but if that doesn't raise suspicions for you regarding their true intent, they do make it very clear:

> *The Roadmap was developed to* ***guide the application of new technologies, such as high-throughput screening, tissue chips, and computational models,*** *to toxicity testing of chemicals and medical products. It* ***creates a framework*** *where the agencies* ***can work together to fund and develop new nonanimal methods, modify regulations to replace*** *current animal testing requirements,* ***and engage with the scientific community to facilitate the use of new methods*** *to assess the toxicity of drugs, chemicals, and other products.*
>
> ***We encourage them to commit funding and other resources to implementing the plan without delay, to ensure improved safety for all consumers.*** [305]

---

[304] https://www.pcrm.org/research/good-science/physicians-committee-provides-advice-to-government-on-strategy-to-replace

[305] https://www.pcrm.org/media/news/physicians-committee-applauds-nih-roadmap-to-replace-animal-testing

Sounds like things will be staying just as they are for that little bit longer if this all goes to plan. Compare again with the opposing team at the Macmillan Cancer Centre as they intellectualise the inevitable score draw:

> *The future of treatment for patients is* ***precision cancer medicine – a treatment package*** *that is specific to the individual and which applies our* ***whole suite of tools to the understanding*** *and treatment of a patient's own unique cancer. It is our vision that, within five years, every patient will have their own* ***personalised cancer pathway****, from early diagnosis and screening, to imaging or biopsy, to* ***genomic analysis*** *of their cancer, through* ***to state-of-the-art clinical trials****...* ***will build on the underlying cancer science****... and will provide a* ***physical focal point*** *for* ***cancer-relevant expertise across the medical, life and engineering sciences****. Patients will be* ***brought alongside the research process and real-time analysis*** *of patients will help* ***to continually refine and improve emerging treatments****.*

Pathways and roadmaps leading to a dead end.

Animal testing is a hopelessly failed hypothesis but equally lost causes are the makers of the drugs and the drugs themselves. One size does not fit all no matter how their chemical products are tested. It isn't a tweaking of the existing system we need but a new way of thinking.

We would be well served to view the problem of animal testing in a more holistic way. They test on animals because there is no other way to save humanity, right? It's a simplistic claim and a primitive approach but that's where we are at. So it's time to be somewhere else. We need to find the courage to look at the bigger picture and to question our service to the status quo which is wrapped around mind control, addiction and depopulation.

Another prominent feature of today's popular animal publicity campaigns, of which the PCRM also happens to promote vigorously, is the consumption of non-organic processed food products as healthy alternatives to the processed meat and veg staple. Alternatives they are, healthy they are not. We petition the fake food product makers asking they remove an animal ingredient so we can all tuck in to their trash and appear normal. Now I'm not saying we shouldn't, better junk food than corpses if you ask me but those aren't the only choices. If you want to recover or maintain good health then of course you have no choice! And when that bit of egg is removed from the recipe, we should still think about what they have left in the product. An army marches on its stomach, but those not so war-like feed the body and the brain. Vegan food-like products are the same junk science as the non-vegan products masquerading as food and delivering a steady supply of depleted consumers for the drug companies to treat with their same science vaccines and pharmaceuticals.

In the wide search for human health and animal liberation we can see how the pie can be shared out and the wheels keep turning. With the front line of 'activists' pushing back against all initiative and working with the enemy the status quo is safe. But why such resistance to even mention the route to health already long established and here now proven by me? No money in it? Requires we question what we shovel down our faces and other big issues? Makes us look like conspiracy theorists?

It's a choice.

In July 2017 I did a full VEGA follow up and with this a percentage comparison to my August 2016 reading. This shows where there are improvements or otherwise. My acid alkaline balance was restored, acquired toxicity was at 50% improved, lymphatic stress 90% resolved, immune deficiency 50% improved, lymph nodes 40%, liver 60%, kidneys 90%, blood 80% resolved, lymph 80% resolved. These are all huge leaps in no time at all.

By November following the MannIcure my health monitoring recorded the following pattern of improvement. Acquired toxicity a further 12% improved, lymphatic stress 6%, immune deficiency 25%, lymph nodes better by 15%, liver 20% improved, and kidneys 2%.

In these consultations with the magic box my biological age improves each time too. I'm getting younger!

It took a full eight years for Alice to finally get an accurate diagnosis for her structural mobility issues and the long process of resolving it has begun. We have had little else to do with our lives since she took ill and the drift into darkness began except to get by and hope to find solutions to her ills, then mine came, and ditto, but what an amazing experience! It turns out she was born with this duel complex pelvic/hip/femur misalignment that was missed for years by a lack of imagination, or something. Her saviour was an osteopath, Ben Cull near Brighton. He has untangled me over the years and has kept Alice at some level of comfortable and was spot on in figuring out where she needed to direct the ortho-docs, who had never thought to scan the right areas. Having an equally diligent and empathetic doctor who was happy to seek a referral to an excellent surgical team of Alice's choosing was all we needed to get the wheels in motion to get Alice in motion.

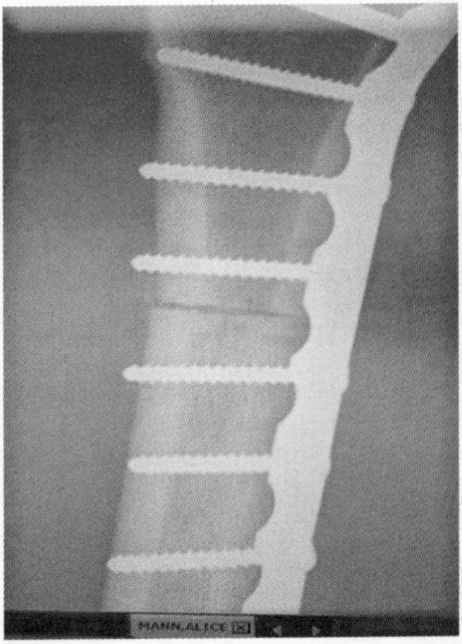

We've been lucky but we have worked at it and deserved a break! No one can deny her now and we have a good medical team whose work involves multiple invasive adjustments to reconstruct angles and realign joints. Sawn bones, metal plates, nuts and bolts and screws and crutches. She's actually excited as hell about her future and the fact I'm in it.

Alice for all she has been through and still has to endure has learnt enough to know that natural healing is her calling. Her life spiralled into something of a nightmare and because of that she fully intends to make a successful career of nutri-functional medicine, the science of nutrition and holistic healing. She is cut from the right cloth has some unique and invaluable experience on the front line of the new paradigm in health care, and she cares. Together we pulled her from the brink and she has neatly and professionally guided her aunt Evelyn and the man she fell in love with to that sacred place where, from my perspective, the fear of cancer returning has been replaced with pure gratitude. Evelyn kept her spleen thanks to Alice who proved the experts wrong. She was diagnosed in 2012, it's now six years later and she has recovered her health and has required no more destructive orthodox cancer treatment. The doctor who laughed in her face for choosing enemas over death by drugs has since apologised and has set a shining example for his peers to consider.

I have no sign of cancer however we look at it but I'm staying focussed on that extra mile to become as restored as it's possible to be. I'll continue to monitor and adjust accordingly. I'll always do my enemas and will aim for one-a-day to start the day which will be like reaching an incredible milestone. The menu won't revert, of course fresh food is perfectly normal and I have all I could ever ask for.

I'm alive and I want to make good of it. Join me? Let's get this story out there and start to make difference where it really matters.

Working with Keith and Alice has been truly inspirational. Their devotion and tenacity in healing Keith has been amazing. A former nurse of 25 years, and having a vaccine damaged child and feeling very let down by orthodox medicine, I happened across the VEGA principle. This changed mine and my family's health so much for the better and I have been a VEGA practitioner for over 18 years. I believe passionately in this technology and I have never come across a couple so driven to use VEGA to its full potential. I am SO privileged to have been a part of this amazing journey and to personally witness such an astonishing recovery from such a devastating prognosis. The medical profession has its place but it needs to wake up and embrace other more natural solutions beyond such harmful chemicals. There is so much more out there.

Caroline Warren

My haematologist and I have been together since 2013 and in 2017 he asked what I did at home to heal so I kept my word and volunteered a hospital appointment I didn't need a year later so we could update him. He was clearly happy to see me, we bounced off each other and we went through the motions. I told him what I did to get in this state as he scribbled notes. The nurse in the room joined in, clearly grasping the point of flushing toxins from the body. Alice and I sat mesmerised as she and the good doctor debated the merits of this element of my protocol like it mattered to them! This was a small thing but a very special moment in our journey.

"Excellent", he repeated after examining me and my blood work and assessing my outlook. *"Excellent! Keep up the good work."*

Good advice to wrap up our relationship. I shall, kind sir, I shall. He later wrote to my GP:

I reviewed this gentleman in clinic. ***It is a year since I last saw him. He was looking very well and had no symptoms. He has now as you may know dropped dairy, processed food, sugars and alcohol and has gone purely organic. He has also taken to drinking ozone water and treating himself with magnetic pulsing therapy. Examination revealed no pathology. His blood count was entirely normal. No intervention is therefore required.*** *I will review him in a year's time or sooner if there are concerns.*

Dr Xxxxx Xxxxx, 12 February 2018

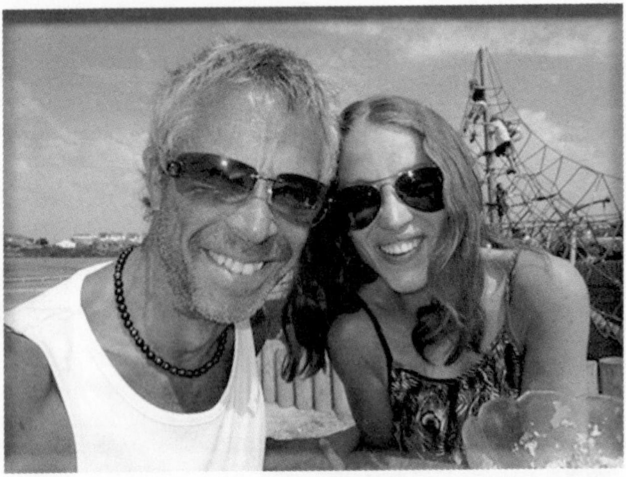

Where there's love there's life. 2018 thriving.

Must read more

It's in the blood where it's always been, sometimes hidden sometimes seen.
He comes our foe when the blood ain't clean.
Keith Mann

Books I'd read if I hadn't just:

Vaccine A -The Covert Government Experiment that's Killing our Soldiers and Why GI's are Only the First Victims - Gary Matsumoto
Living Proof - Michael Gearin-Tosh
The Cancer Conspiracy - Dr Robert E. Netterberg & Robert T. Taylor
World Without Cancer - Edward Griffin
A New Earth - Eckhart Tolle
Healing The Gerson Way – Charlotte Gerson & Beata Bishop
The Gerson Therapy - Charlotte Gerson
Fats That Heal Fats That Kill - Udo Eramus
Behind Closed Doors - Diana Holmes
Knockout - Suzanne Sommers
The Politics of Cancer, Revisited - Samuel Epstein
Cancer Free - Bill Henderson & Carlos M. Garcia
The Great Thyroid Scandal and How to Survive it - Dr Barry Durrant-Peatfield
Dr Mary's Monkey - Edward T. Haslem
Naked Empress - Hans Ruesch
Mum's Not Having Chemo - Laura Bond
Cancer - Why We Are Still Dying To Know The Truth - Phillip Day
The Vaccination Superstition - J W Hodge MD
Radical Remission - Kelly A Turner
The Cancer Cure That Worked - Barry Lynes
The Cancer Industry - Ralph Moss
Questioning Chemotherapy - Ralph Moss
The China Study - T. Colin Campbell & Thomas M Campbell
Where Did The Towers Go - Judy Wood B.S, M.S, PhD
Dispelling Wetiko - Paul Levy
The Trial and Persecution of Gaston Naessens - Christopher Bird
Dr Max Gerson: Healing The Hopeless - Howard Straus
You Can Eliminate Your Cancer. Healing Through the Gerson Therapy - Yushiro Watanabe M.D
The Cancer Microbe - Alan Cantwell
The Conquest of Cancer - Virginia Livingston-Wheeler
The Virus and the Vaccine - Debbie Bookchin & Jim Shumacker
A Cancer Therapy - Results of Fifty Cases – Dr Max Gerson
What Vets Don't Tell You About Vaccines - Catherine O'Driscoll
Vaccine Guide for Dogs & Cats - Catherine J.M. Diodati, MA
Thimerosal - Let the Science Speak – Robert F Kennedy JR
The Vaccine Papers - Janine Roberts
How to Immunize Your Dog Without Vaccines - Aleksandra Mikic, DHHP, DVHH, DPh

Dissolving Illusions - Suzanne Humphries MD, Roman Bystrianyk
Callous Disregard - Andrew J. Wakefield
Vaccination Policy and the UK Government: The Untold Truth - Christina England & Lucija Tomljenovic PhD

And watched:
The Truth About Cancer
The Truth About Vaccines
Vaccines Revealed
Vaxxed

All the links cited in this book are stored @ www.iamkeithmann.com

Thanks also to www.lymphomasurvival.com
www.gersonmedia.com/natural-healing-radio-show
www.cancertutor.com
www.vaccine-injury.info/curing-autism.cfm
www.vaxxedthemovie.com
www.parentsandcarersagainstinjustice.weebly.com
The Gerson Support Group, in particular
Kathleen Blake & George Lane:
www.facebook.com/groups/Gersonsupport
Nobivac 4 - Our Experiences:
www.facebook.com/groups/322967551247441
www.bobbeck.com
www.drsircus.com
www.sharinghealth.com
Holistic Help for Dogs with Mast Cell Cancer:
www.facebook.com/groups/6053799421/

The vaccines. At a glance

The Scotch Covenantors, Ann Askew, John Wyecliffe, and the apostles of old were told that their persecutors were "only the administrators of the law," but they defied the law, and the proudest privileges and blessings we possess have been won for us by the law-breakers of this country. It is not a question merely of the health but of the very lives of the children which are at stake in this matter; and I believe that the present century shall not close until we have placed our foot upon the dragon's neck, and plunged the sword of liberty through its heart. (Cheers.) They tell us we are trying to rouse the country with a "crazy cry"-- the cry of liberty of conscience-- and, we are not ashamed of that cry. It is that "crazy cry" which snapped the shackles of despotism in the past. That "crazy cry" is spreading at the present time throughout the length and breadth of the country. We are told that the intelligent portion of the population is against us; it's false. That "crazy cry" is ascending higher and higher, into a raging and tremendous storm; that liberty which has been won by the blood of our forefathers for the theological conscience, is the liberty we demand for the scientific conscience. (Loud cheers.) Already it is thundering at the door of the House of Commons, and it shall be heard. Yes, we are going forward with the "crazy cry" of liberty of conscience upon our unfurled banner, and we never intend to rest until we get it. (Loud and prolonged cheering).

The Case Against the Compulsory Vaccination Act.

January 25, 1896.

Address by Dr Hadwen, J.P., M.D., L.R.C.P., M.R.C.S., L.S.A., Etc

(Gold Medallist in Medicine and in Surgery)

At the Goddard's Rooms, Gloucester.

The soul is the same in all living creatures, although the body of each is different.
Hippocrates

- Vaccines are unavoidably dangerous especially when delivered in multi-dose hits. They harbour cellular debris from dead animals and birds and unwanted viruses that cannot be removed; many contain mercury and/or aluminium and other cancer causing agents.
- None have been properly tested against unvaccinated controls in double blind 'sugar pill' trials either for safety or efficacy when taken alone or when multiplied with other unproven vaccines. True placebo trials are now rare.
- All untested medical products are assumed to be unsafe, unnecessary and ineffective until proven otherwise.
- Vaccines impose an unnatural route of infection, they cause target disease, novel disease and allergies.
- Mass vaccinating has transformed natural viral infection into chronic illness.

MMR	**The Autistic MMR**, the CDC's Dr William Thompson's extensive and devastating whistleblower files and testimony prove a high risk of autism with this vaccine, large scale scientific fraud at the highest level and a cover up. [306] **Measles** according to NHS UK *"can be unpleasant, but will usually pass in about 7 to 10 days without causing any further problems".* [307] MMR contains WI-38, derived from lung tissue of an aborted female foetus. Propagated in chick embryo cell culture and in MRC-5 cells from an aborted white male foetus. Contains bovine serum and human albumin. Atypical Measles Syndrome is caused by the measles vaccine. **Mumps** *"symptoms of mumps include headaches, joint pain and a high temperature. It's most recognisable by the painful swellings at the side of the face under the ears (the parotid glands), giving a person with mumps a distinctive 'hamster face' appearance. The infection should pass within one or two weeks".* [308] **Rubella** (German measles) *"is a viral infection that's now rare in the UK. It's usually a mild condition that gets better without treatment in 7 to 10 days".* [309]
DTP	**Boostrix-IPV: (DTaP(polio)**, adsorbed on aluminium hydroxide and aluminium phosphate propagated in Vero monkey kidney cells. Boostrix-IPV *"was co-administered with MMR/V vaccines in 2 clinical studies with 406 children aged 3-6 years. In*

306 http://vaxxedthemovie.com/

307 https://www.nhs.uk/conditions/measles/

308 https://www.nhs.uk/conditions/mumps/symptoms/

309 https://www.nhs.uk/conditions/rubella/

	these studies, upper respiratory tract infection and rash were commonly reported. Fever, irritability, fatigue, loss of appetite and gastrointestinal disorders (including diarrhoea and vomiting) were very common.... the degree and duration of protection afforded by the vaccine are undetermined". The DTP vaccine has a long standing reputation for causing serious neurological damage in young children. **Diphtheria** is rare and another disease of slum living and poor nutrition. **Tetanus** bacteria *"are commonly found in soil and the manure of animals such as horses and cows. If the bacteria enter the body through a wound, they can quickly multiply and release a toxin that affects the nerves, causing symptoms such as muscle stiffness and spasms.* [310] *Most people who develop symptoms of tetanus eventually recover".* 233 cases of tetanus were reported to the CDC for the entire USA between 2001 and 2008 with a handful fatal and just 4 recorded infections in the UK last year. Tetanus can take over a week to show symptoms, leaving time to act once wounded and the sooner an infection is treated the better. Vaccine contains formaldehyde + thimerosal + aluminium phosphate + aborted human foetal lung cell tissue from a 14 week old male + a 12 week old female foetus (WI-38). **Pertussis/whooping cough** vaccine doesn't protect. Causes serious neurological illness. Wide spread vaccine uptake mirrors an increase in disease prevalence. It has been known for decades that the B. pertussis bacteria have evolved both whole cell and acellular pertussis vaccines.
Polio	The cancer causing vaccine for humans. Used for infecting hundreds of millions of innocent victims with the oncogenic simian virus known as SV40. • According to the Lancet in 2016: *"Vaccine-derived polio constitutes an increasing proportion of overall polio infections".* [311] • The iron lung we have been programmed to fear has evolved to be today's ventilator, a simple piece of life saving medical equipment to aid breathing in severe cases. As the patient recovers the aid can be removed. • *"While India has been polio-free for a year, there has been a huge increase in non-polio acute flaccid paralysis (NPAFP). In 2011, there were an extra 47,500 new cases of NPAFP. Clinically indistinguishable from polio paralysis but twice as deadly, the incidence of NPAFP was directly proportional to doses of oral polio received".* [312] • *"Up to 95% of all polio infections are completely*

310 https://www.nhs.uk/conditions/tetanus/

311 https://www.thelancet.com/journals/laninf/article/PIIS1473-3099%2816%2900147-X/fulltext

312 https://www.ncbi.nlm.nih.gov/pubmed/2259187

	asymptomatic. Approximately 5% of polio infections consist of a minor, non-specific illness consisting of an upper respiratory tract infection (sore throat and fever) and gastrointestinal disturbances (nausea, vomiting, abdominal pain, and diarrhoea). This influenza-like illness, clinically indistinguishable from the myriad of other viral illnesses, is characterized by complete recovery in less than a week with resultant life time immunity. Less than 1% of all polio infections result in paralysis. Most importantly, the vast majority of individuals who contract paralytic poliomyelitis recover with complete - or near complete - return of muscle function." [313] Outbreaks of polio caused by cVDPVs (vaccine-derived polioviruses) have been reported across the world.
Varicella Chickenpox	*"Chickenpox is a common illness that mainly affects children and causes an itchy, spotty rash. Most children will catch the pox at some point. It can also occur in adults who didn't have it when they were a child. It's usually mild and clears up in a week or so".* [314] And provides life-long immunity! Suppressing this virus has created a more unpleasant shingles experience in the older generation no longer boosted by circulating virus exposure. Grown in embryonic lung cells (HEL) and human diploid cells (WI-38). *"Vaccine recipients should attempt to avoid, to the extent possible, close association with high-risk individuals susceptible to varicella for up to 6 weeks following vaccination."* [315]
Flu	Flu vaccine doesn't protect. Grown in contaminated poultry proteins. Contains thiomersal, squalene, polysorbate 80 (which takes the vaccine contents across the blood brain barrier), cancer causing formaldehyde and the mutagenic carcinogen octoxynol 10. Risk of narcolepsy.
Shingles	Doesn't protect. Causes shingles, chicken pox, disease of the central nervous system, and brain-swelling/encephalomyelitis.
Hepatitis B	Vaccine is injected into one day old babies (in the US, it's 8 weeks of age in the UK) with a syringe of what is an IV drug user/sexually transmitted disease and an unproven cocktail of chemicals, live animal organisms, foreign DNA, formaldehyde, aluminium and polysorbate 80.
HPV	There is no evidence this has prevented a single cancer. *"It and all the new vaccines are contaminated with genetically engineered DNA. Gardasil was the worst thing we had ever seen in terms of the symptoms that were showing up. Gardasil has amazing list of reactions that stand out... and they include some very serious things. Coma... death... unconsciousness... suicide...*

[313] https://www.newswithviews.com/Tenpenny/sherri3.htm

[314] http://www.nhsdirect.wales.nhs.uk/encyclopaedia/c/article/chickenpox/

[315] https://www.fda.gov/downloads/BiologicsBloodVaccines/Vaccines/ApprovedProducts/UCM123793.pdf

	Aluminium is strongly associated with depression. I think the vaccine makes them so incredibly depressed they can't cope." Stephanie Seneff, PhD Senior Research Scientist, Massachusetts Institute of Technology.
BCG/ Tuberculosis	*"Most people who have TB infection will never develop TB disease. In these people, the TB bacteria remain inactive for a lifetime without causing disease. But in... those who have weak immune systems the bacteria may become active and cause TB disease".*[316] All the vaccines stand out in their own way. The BCG used in newborn babies since 1927 is the same one used in cows and the same one injected into wild animals, such as badgers and possums. And yet if we ask the vaxers what of their product we find an abundance of issues. • *Although over 2 billion people have been immunized with BCG, and it is currently an officially recommended vaccine in more than 180 countries... the efficacy of BCG as a vaccine against tuberculosis remains controversial.* [317] • *There are significant gaps in our knowledge regarding the impact that the vaccination of either badgers or cattle.* • *Does not induce full protective immunity in all individuals* • *Has, so far, not been used extensively to control chronic bacterial infections such as TB in wildlife.* • *The duration of immunity from BadgerBCG remains unknown.* • *Field data suggest that BCG vaccination provides a similar spectrum of protection in badgers as well as cattle and other species whereby some individuals are fully protected, some are partially protected by having reduced disease, and the remainder are afforded no protection at all, but it is not possible to attribute precise figures to these categories.* • *Has not been evaluated for carcinogenic, mutagenic potentials or impairment of fertility.* • *Animal reproduction studies have not been conducted.* • *The need to bring effective and cost-effective vaccines to market that can be used to tackle the problem of bovine TB in England and Wales remains an urgent one.* [318] There is a product for treating BCG but there is no vaccine to protect against it!

316 https://www.gov.uk/

317 https://www.fda.gov/downloads/BiologicsBloodVaccines/Vaccines/ApprovedProducts/UCM202934.pdf

318 http://veterinaryrecord.bmj.com/content/175/4/90

	The first experiment on badgers started in January 2002 on twelve badgers who were snatched from an Irish island and held in four separated groups in the BROC facility in Ireland. All were killed four months later having been sacrificed on behalf of the pro-vax activists, the drug pharma and the cow farmer, and what were the findings? More badgers needed. In the second experiment one of the captured badgers was pregnant and gave birth to two cubs two months after receiving the second dose of BCG vaccine. The good news is that the second experiment yielded results. Yeah! - go animal researchers! According to the wildlife-vivisecting scientists, the vaccine *"did not appear to affect... foetal development."* Phew! This sounds reassuring and I do like a happy ending but this is neither. What this is is half a story. *"Although the cubs did not survive longer than approximately one month, the fact that live cubs were born to a vaccinated badger supports the view that BCG vaccination does not affect fecundity."* [319] I hazard a guess before looking up the meaning of words but this little baby had me stumped. Fecundity, I found, is the 'ability to produce an abundance of offspring; fertility'. See the sleight of hand? In a single vaccine experiment a side effect was not death of foetus and so to these people this makes for a good vaccine. Talk about cup half full! Fecundity makes this experimental vaccine a place of comfort for some to park up; a happy place where the vaccine almost produces babies! But just how well are the babies doing?
Meningitis	Vaccine protection is only short-lived and even then does not target the most common forms of the disease. *The majority of the safety experience with Meningitec [the most commonly used vaccine used from 1999] comes from a single study conducted in the United States... in which Meningitec was compared with [another vaccine]. Infants in this study received Meningitec or [other vaccine] on a 2, 4, 6 month schedule, along with routine immunisation with either DTP/Hib... or DTPa... The infants may also have received other routine childhood vaccines".* [320]
	DOGS
Rabies	Not generally a UK issue but every bit a welfare issue. Contains aluminium and mercury. *"The most common disturbances following rabies vaccination are aggressiveness, suspicion,*

[319] randd.defra.gov.uk/Document.aspx?Document=SE3216_3326_FRP.doc

[320] http://experimentalvaccines.org/wp-content/uploads/2014/12/Meningitec.pdf

	unfriendly behaviour, hysteria, destructiveness (of blankets, towels), fear of being alone and howling or barking at imaginary objects." * Sounds like autism! And what of the mercury being poo'd out everywhere, or does it stay in the dogs? * Dr Pitcairn's Complete Guide to Natural Health for Dogs and Cats.
Distemper	Puppies. Rare. Canine cell line origin.[321] Vaccines such as this are seriously hazardous to dogs. Cause of encephalitis.
Hepatitis	Puppies. Rare. MDCK canine cell line vaccine, contains foetal bovine serum. Cause of encephalitis.
Parvo	Puppies. Canine cell line. Doesn't protect. Studies on dogs vaccinated with CPV-2 parvovirus show that the virus can remain in the bloodstream and be shed via faeces for as long as four weeks after vaccination. *"The canine parvovirus was isolated from a rectal swab taken from a clinical case of parvovirus infection that occurred in an eight week old beagle puppy in a breeding kennel. The virus was inoculated to a culture of FEFs [feline embryo fibroblast] and passaged a further time in these cells before transfer to cultures of the canine A72 cell line [from 8 year old female Golden Retriever cancer tumour]. The virus was subsequently attenuated through 41 passages in this cell line, in the course of which 4 cloning steps were made... then inoculated back into FEF cultures and the harvest of the 2nd passage in FEFs was layed down as a "MASTER SEED" LOT".* [322] To finish the recipe it gets mixed with a heap of other serious risk factors to be passaged into our puppies.
Kennel cough/ Bordetella	A mild human-like cold of close confinement. Vaccine doesn't work.
Leptospirosis	A rare disease. Vaccines offer poor protection against only some strains and contain mercury. Lethal with high risk of injury and death.
	CATS
Feline calicivirus vaccine	Not protective.
Feline herpes/cat flu	Minimal protection. With medication, good nutrition and tender loving care, most cats will make a successful recovery from infection.
Feline Panleucopenia (FPL)	No protection. *"Our study revealed serious problems associated with primary vaccination against FPL. A significant proportion of kittens failed to develop active immunity following the recommended vaccination scheme."*[323]

321 Canine cell line extracted from Cocker Spaniel in 1958.

322 https://www.google.com/patents/CA1278513C?cl=en

323 https://www.ncbi.nlm.nih.gov/pmc/articles/PMC3475090/

Feline Leukaemia (FeLV)	The cancer causing vaccine for cats. A cat that exists 100% indoors with no other cats is very unlikely to ever get FeLV. Cats over 4 months are much less susceptible to infection.
FIV vaccine	Is not protective and enhances viral replication.
Infectious Peritonitis (FIP) vaccine	Not protective. Many different strains of the virus can infect cats, but most don't cause serious disease, the vaccine causes worse disease symptoms.
Bordetella	Not protective. Affects a small number of cats held in colonies. Infected cats may cough, have a runny nose or runny eyes, sneeze, and occasionally have a fever. Vaccine causes similar symptoms and worse. Vaccine may reduce some symptoms. The signs of disease are very similar to those caused by herpes virus and calici virus.
Rabies	No risk to cats in UK. Same vaccine dogs get with mercury and aluminium included.
Ringworm	Not protective, may suppress symptoms, does induce sarcomas. Contains mercury.
	HORSES
Tetanus	Horses get less but it only takes one. Our friend Cassie was a strong fit horse. She had the flu + tetanus vaccine in May 2017 3 months later she developed colic requiring extensive surgery. By the October she was dead.
Influenza	See flu vaccines
Encephalo... ..myelitis	*"Fertilised chicken eggs are susceptible to a wide variety of viruses.* ***All the egg based vaccines are contaminated****... influenza measles mumps yellow fever and smallpox vaccines. As well as the vaccine for horses against encephalomyelitis virus."* Dr Andrew Lewis head of DNA Virus laboratory in the Division of Viral Products. To the Vaccine and Related Biological Products Committee. Transcript of meeting 19 Nov 1988 (Page 19: The Vaccine Papers, Janine Robert)

The answer to the VACCINATION calculation is of course 666.

-

East Sussex Healthcare NHS
NHS Trust

Direct Dial
Haematology Secretaries:
Appointments:
Appointments:

NHS Number:

Clinic Date: 12/02/2018

Dr.

Dear Dr.

Mr Keith Mann DOB: 20/05/1966
East Sussex,

Diagnosis: **Low grade non-Hodgkin's lymphoma.**
6 x Rituximab and Bendamustine 2015.

I reviewed this gentleman in the clinic. It is a year since I last saw him. He was looking very well and had no symptoms. He has now as you may know dropped dairy, processed food, sugars and alcohol and has gone purely organic. He has also taken to drinking ozone water and treating himself with magnetic pulsing therapy.

Examination today revealed no pathology.

His blood count was entirely normal, haemoglobin 165 g/L, white count 6.64 $\times 10^9$/L with a normal differential and platelets 325 $\times 10^9$/L. Chemistry was normal, his LDH normal at 253 U/L.

No intervention is therefore required. I will review him in a year's time or sooner if there are concerns.

Kind Regards,

Yours sincerely

Checked and authorised

Dr FRCP, FRCPath
Consultant Haematologist

Private & Confidential
cc Mr Keith Mann

East Sussex

East Sussex Healthcare NHS
NHS Trust

Direct Dial
Haematology Secretaries:
Fax:

Appointments:
Appointments:

NHS Number:

Clinic Date: 08/08/2016

Dear Dr.

Mr Keith Mann DOB: 20/05/1966
East Sussex,

Diagnosis: **Low grade non-Hodgkin's lymphoma**.

Treatment: Completed six cycles of Rituximab and Bendamustine.

Full blood count: Hb 146 g/l, white cell count 7 $\times 10^9$/l, platelets 254 $\times 10^9$/l, ESR 5 mm/Hr , LDH 841 U/L.

I met this gentleman in Dr Haematology Clinic today. He is doing well in himself and has no B- type symptoms. From our records his weight has dropped by approximately 1.5 Kg. However Mr Mann tells me he feels his weight is stable.

On examination today there are numerous small volume lymph nodes bilaterally. Previously he had lymph nodes recorded on the left side of the neck. They are palpable in the anterior and posterior chain on the right side. He also has axillary lymph nodes bilaterally of approximately 1 cm. His abdomen is soft and non-tender without evidence of splenomegaly.

In the context of the increased number of lymph nodes and the slightly raised LDH I would like to repeat Mr Mann's imaging so that we can re-assess his disease status. Mr Mann is very keen to not have interventions unless he is feeling unwell and has concerns about radiation exposure.

Mr Mann would consider having non-irradiation scans such as MRI. This is not a usual assessment but I will discuss this with Radiology.

I have explained to Mr Mann that I think there is a risk/benefit advantage in having scans so that we can properly assess disease. If we wait to treat him only when he feels unwell as this may make initiating chemotherapy more difficult. However, I appreciate his standpoint and his wish to undergo as few interventions as possible unless he feels unwell and that treatment is entirely necessary.

I would like to see him back in four weeks' time hopefully with a scan to monitor his progress.

Yours sincerely

Checked and authorised

Dr FRCPath PhD
SpR Haematology

cc Mr Keith Mann

East Sussex

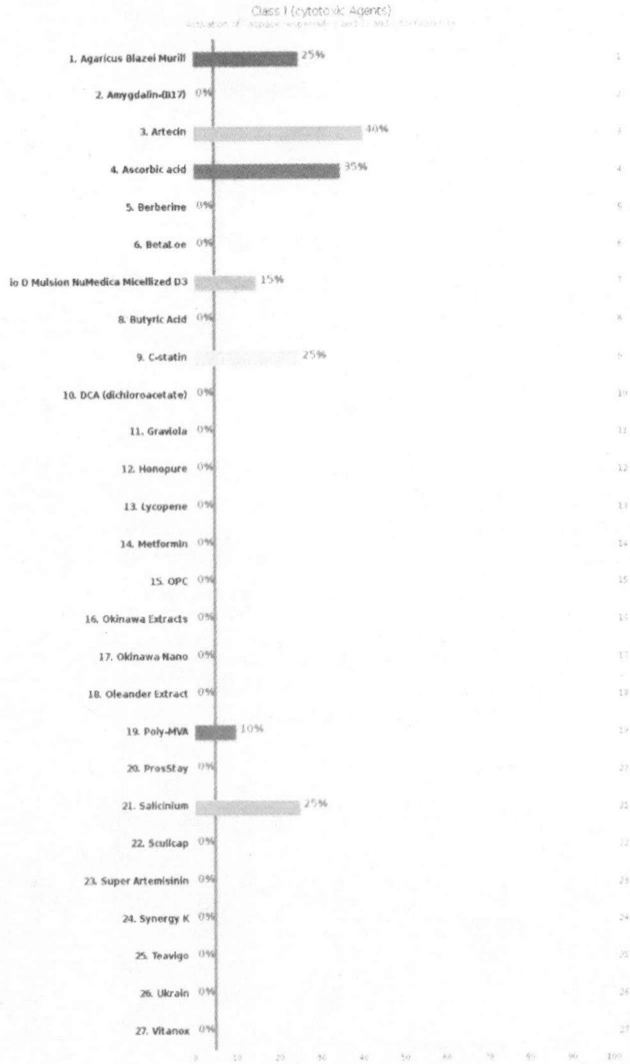

Mr Keith Mann
Industrial Area of Florina, GR 53100 – Florina, Greece
Tel.: +30 23850 41950, 41951, 41960, 41961, Fax.: +30 23850 41931
Website: www.rgcc-genlab.com E-mail: papasotiriou.ioannis@rgcc-genlab.com

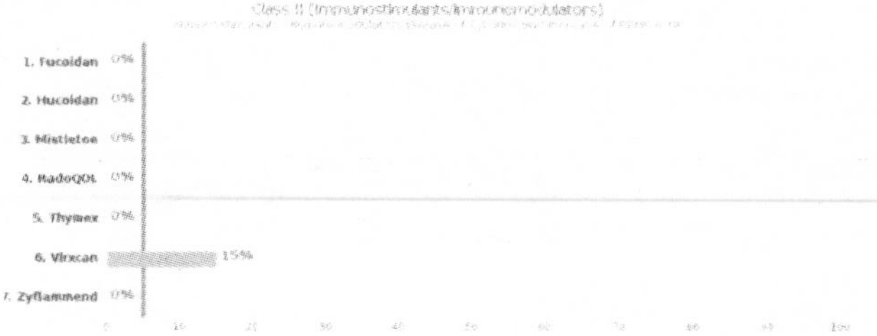

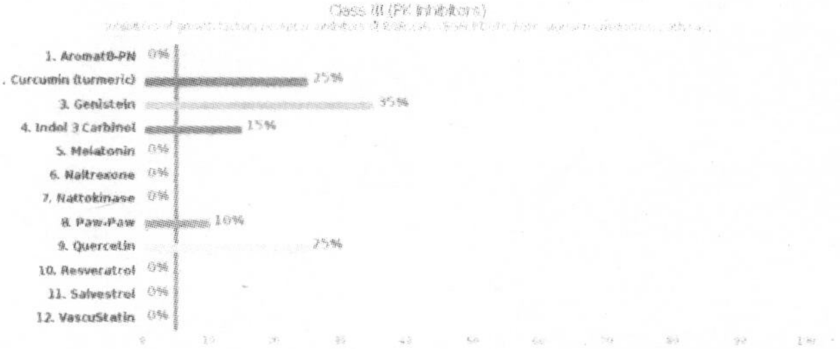

<u>CONCLUSION:</u> It seems that this specific population of malignant cell have greater sensitivity in Agaricus Blazei Murill, in Artecin, in Ascorbic acid, in Bio D Mulsion NuMedica Micellized D3, in C-statin, in Poly-MVA, in Salicinium, in Virxcan, in Curcumin (turmeric), in Genistein, in Indol 3 Carbinol, in Paw-Paw, in Quercetin and less in Amygdalin-(B17), in Berberine, in BetaLoe, in Butyric Acid, in DCA (dichloroacetate), in Graviola, in Honopure, in Lycopene, in Metformin, in OPC, in Okinawa Extracts, in Okinawa Nano, in Oleander Extract, in ProsStay, in Scullcap, in Super Artemisinin, in Synergy K, in Teavigo, in Ukrain, in Vitanox, in Fucoidan, in Hucoidan, in Mistletoe, in RadoQOL, in Thymex, in Zyflammend, in Aromat8-PN, in Melatonin, in Naltrexone, in Nattokinase, in Resveratrol, in Salvestrol, in VascuStatin .

Sincerely,

Ioannis Papasotiriou MD., PhD
Head of molecular medicine dpt. of
R.G.C.C.-RESEARCH GENETIC CANCER CENTRE LTD

DISCLAIMER

This study is known as an Ex-Vivo type study (testing the actual tumor stem cells of an individual outside their body). This test will tell us what natural substances will induce apoptosis via the cytochrome c (esp. caspase 3 & 9 pathways) after the tumor stem cells and a single product have been in contact, in a well plate for 48 hours. We have found this test to be very accurate over the past 10+ years and thousands of test. However, it cannot take into account the many combinations of natural substances or the physiological dynamics of each individual that are required for life We are also aware that natural substances can have a wide variety of additional benefits that may assist healthy individuals, as well as those with cancer. Therefore, even if a product shows not to induce apoptosis, on this test, it most likely will have many other benefits especially when used in combination with other therapies your health care provider may use. This is when you must rely on the skill, knowledge and training of your health care provider and their years of clinical experience (successes and failures) with the many various combinations which they have found to work in a clinical setting. The body is a wonderful, magnificent, dynamic organism and very complex.

Mr Keith Mann
Industrial Area of Florina, GR 53100 – Florina, Greece
Tel.: +30 23850 41950, 41951, 41960, 41961, Fax.: +30 23850 41931
Website: www.rgcc-genlab.com E-mail: papasotiriou.ioannis@rgcc-genlab.com

Elemental Analysis Hair

Genova Diagnostics Europe

Patient: KEITH MANN
DOB: May 20, 1966
Sex: M
MRN:

Order Number:

Route Number:

Genova Diagnostics Europe
Referring Laboratory
Parkgate House
356 West Barnes Lane
New Malden, Surrey KT3 6NB
Great Britain and Northern Ireland

Toxic Elements

Element	Reference Range	Reference Range in µg/g
Aluminum	0.9	<= 17.3
Antimony	0.032	<= 0.016
Arsenic	0.075	<= 0.080
Barium	0.27	<= 1.70
Bismuth	<dl	<= 0.178
Cadmium	0.006	<= 0.022
Gadolinium	<dl	<= 0.0005
Lead	0.159	<= 0.700
Mercury	0.07	<= 1.32
Nickel	0.09	<= 0.55
Rhodium	<dl	<= 0.0005
Rubidium	<dl	<= 0.040
Thallium	0.0005	<= 0.0004
Tin	0.117	<= 0.149
Uranium	0.0066	<= 0.0057

Nutrient Elements

Element	Reference Range	Reference Range in µg/g
Calcium	605	192-1,588
Chromium	0.03	0.01-1.58
Cobalt	0.002	0.001-0.129
Copper	13	8-136
Iron	6.2	5.2-24.4
Magnesium	16	11-122
Manganese	0.07	0.04-1.93
Molybdenum	0.03	0.01-1.24
Phosphorous	138	104-206
Selenium	0.67	0.58-1.13
Sodium	5	14-426
Strontium	1.15	0.01-4.40
Sulfur	44,468	41,781-60,894
Vanadium	0.007	0.003-0.108
Zinc	138	119-245

Element	Reference Range	
Lithium	<dl	<= 0.302
Potassium	3	<= 174

Ratios

	Inside Range	Outside Range	Reference Range
Ca/Mg		38	5-29
Ca/P	4		1-9

© Genova Diagnostics · CLIA Lic. #34D0655571 · Medicare Lic. #34-8475

HARG2 RMS 60 Rev 5

Pre-diagnosis hair mineral test.

KEITH MANN - DOB: 20-May-1966 < Previous Result
Specimen No: - Specimen Type: Lymph node
Request Date: 17/07/2013 16:13:00 - Reported Date: 01/08/2013 13:44:11

Reasons for Request:
Form undated, specimen received 17.07.13. URGENT multiple
neck lymph node black centre
Specimen Suffix:1
Tissue Code: Lymph node

Showing Result 3 of 11 Back to Index < Newer Result Older Result >

Test	Result	Units	Reference Range
TEST GROUP UNKNOWN			
			-

Labelled lymph node right neck. Part of a lymph node measuring
10mm x 8mm x up to 6mm. On section some slightly darker areas are
seen centrally. 3 transverse total, ntr.
HISTOLOGY
Sections show replacement of the lymph node architecture by
numbers of follicular structures which lack tingible body
macrophages and lymphocyte mantles.
Immunohistochemistry shows the follicular structures to be
positive for CD20 and CD79 but with B-cells spilling out into the
interfollicular tissue. The follicles are positive for CD10 and
BCL6 and also BCL2. CD23 and CD21 stain follicular networks.
Significant numbers of CD3 and CD5 positive T-cells are seen.
CD68 stains very few macrophages. Kappa and Lambda staining
suggests Lambda light chain restriction. Cyclin D1 is negative.
Ki67 shows a relatively low proliferative index with no evidence
of polarisation within the follicular structures.
Overall the appearances are those of a low grade follicular
lymphoma.
In addition, some black pigment is present within the lymph node.
The cause of this pigment is not certain but it might represent
black tattoo pigment and it would be worthwhile checking whether
the patient has any tattoos in this area. An alternative
possibility, depending on the level of the lymph node, might be
carbon pigment spread from the lungs.
Material from this case is being referred to King's Hospital for
an expert opinion and a supplementary report will be issued when
more information is available.
Assessment agreed with Dr S Mathe.
SUPPLEMENTARY REPORT
Material from this case has been referred to King's College
Hospital and has been reported as follows:
"The lymph node architecture is effaced by confluent neoplastic
follicles predominantly composed of centrocytes and occasional
centroblasts. There is extracapsuler spread is seen. There is also
black pigment seen suggesting Tattoo.
Immunohistochemistry is positive for CD20, CD79a, bcl2, CD10 and
bcl6, with staining of the extra follicular lymphocytes by CD10
and bcl6. CD23 is also expressed (CD23 expression is seen in a
subset of follicular lymphomas). CD5 and CD3 stain the reactive
T-cell population and cyclin D1 is not expressed. CD21 highlight
the slightly expanded follicular dendritic cells meshwork.
The ki67 proliferation index is low (20%).
The features are those of low grade follicular lymphoma (WHO or
grade 1-2).
There is no evidence of transformation seen.
DIAGNOSIS
Outside slides-Right neck lymph node (excision): Low grade
follicular lymphoma (WHO or grade 1-2). "
Reporting Pathologist(s):
Ramesar, Dr K.

Key:

¬ In Lab	= Awaiting Validation	~ Interim	Final	Out of Range *

Showing Result 3 of Back < Older

INDEX

E

F

K

M

N

O

P

Q

R

S